"Psychology, psychiatry, and have been captured by an (agenda."

Before dismissing this claim as right-wing conservative backlash, it must be noted that it comes from two lifelong liberal activists whose careers have been defined by radical positions and actions, many of which were enacted through their leadership roles within the American Psychological Association itself. To back it up, Rogers H. Wright and Nicholas A. Cummings have assembled a truly impressive collection of leading scholars, practitioners, and researchers in this unprecedented insider's critique of the present and future of mental health care.

Operating under the premise that special interest groups have used faulty—even false—science to promote political agendas, contributing authors critically examine contemporary issues such as homophobia, the psychology of victimhood, cultural sensitivity, ADHD, managed care, and intelligence research. Controversial chapters challenge the APA's recent politically motivated stances on gay marriage, pedophilia, abortion, and boxing, exposing a disturbing trend in which ideology trumps science at the highest levels of a supposedly empirically based professional organization. The argument here is not against high-minded goals such as cultural or sociopolitical diversity, but rather warns of the dangers of actively discouraging valid scientific inquiry when it could lead to results that might not be politically correct.

Destructive Trends in Mental Health presents compelling arguments for a re-evaluation of the practices and policies of professional organizations in the mental health fields, the needs of the public they ultimately serve, and how practitioners deliver care to their patients. Wright and Cummings demonstrate that unless steps are taken to reverse these destructive trends, the mental health professions will suffer fatal blows to their credibility and, in the long term, their economic viability. An eye-opening read from cover to cover, the information contained in this volume will undoubtedly challenge your views of the APA and the field of professional psychology, but also more generally your faith in health care systems and the purity of scientific inquiry.

Destructive Trends
in Mental Health

Advance praise for

Destructive Trends in Mental Health

Buttressed and burnished by a glittering Who's Who in scientific and professional psychology, Wright and Cummings persuasively and forcefully dramatize how the mental health professions will enhance patient benefits by removing from the therapeutic process such destructive barriers as political correctness and intrusive ideologies.

Robert Perloff, Ph.D.
Distinguished Service Professor, Katz Graduate School of Business, University of Pittsburgh, and Former President, American Psychological Association

Organized psychology has been captured by a small group that is dumbing down psychology while pursuing its own agenda. This book shows how this oligarchy threatens to destroy the science and profession of psychology, and wreak harm on an unsuspecting public that trusts and depends on psychology. It deserves very wide readership.

Arnold A. Lazarus, Ph.D., ABPP
Distinguished Professor Emeritus, Rutgers University

This book brings into sharp focus the intrusion of social and economic policies that are distorting what should appropriately be the emphasis in mental health: best practices for the benefit of those served.

Martin Kalb, J.D., LLM
Of Counsel, Greenberg Taurig

Want to avoid foolishness, stupidity and harm? Read this book; highly recommended.

Michael Hoyt, Ph.D.
Chief of Adult Psychiatry, Kaiser Permanente, author of *Some Stories Are Better Than Others, Interviews with Brief Therapy Experts*, and *The Present Is a Gift*

Destructive Trends in Mental Health could not be more timely, confronting issues that bedevil U.S. healthcare, namely, the physician glut that has arisen, transforming medicine and mental health from science-based, health-seeking, Hippocratic endeavors to pharma-mandated, dollar-seeking enterprises, saying whatever to embellish diagnosis and treatment.

Fred Baughman, M.D.
Nationally recognized Neurologist and Pediatric Neurologist, and author of *The ADHD Fraud—How Psychiatry Makes "Patients" Out of Normal Children*

The authors provide cogent examples of how in mental health circles today misguided idealism and social sophistry guarantee that good science and practice will not go unpunished.

Jack G. Wiggins, Ph.D., Psy.D.
Former President, American Psychological Association

No matter how intelligent, the public needs to be educated by organized psychology and psychiatry to make a distinction between sound practice and psychobabble. This book illustrates in painful detail not only how psychiatrists and professional psychologists have failed to educate, but how often, to enhance stature and income, they have embraced psychobabble and practiced it.

Robyn M. Dawes, Ph.D., Charles J. Queenan Jr.
Professor, Department of Social and Decision Sciences, Carnegie-Mellon University

This book brings together outstanding and respected mental health scholars to challenge the permeation of mis- and disinformation being foisted on the public, the medical profession, and the mental health communities. With such noted scholars challenging these trends, the public has greater insight into what has heretofore been blindly accepted.

David Stein, Ph.D.
Professor of Psychology, Longwood University, and author of *Unraveling the ADD/ADHD Fiasco: Successful Parenting without Drugs*

Destructive Trends in Mental Health

THE WELL-INTENTIONED PATH TO HARM

Edited by

Rogers H. Wright and
Nicholas A. Cummings

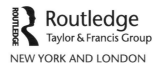

Routledge
Taylor & Francis Group

NEW YORK AND LONDON

Published in 2005 by
Routledge
Taylor & Francis Group
711 Third Avenue,
New York, NY, 10017, USA

Published in Great Britain by
Routledge
Taylor & Francis Group
2 Park Square
Milton Park, Abingdon
Oxfordshire OX14 4RN

First issued in paperback 2015

Routledge is an imprint of the Taylor and Francis Group, an informa business

© 2005 by Taylor & Francis Group

International Standard Book Number-13: 978-1-138-96745-8 (pbk)
International Standard Book Number-13: 978-0-415-95086-2 (hbk)

The co-editors are appreciative of the permission to reprint all or portions of the following journal articles:

O'Donohue, W. (2002). Cultural sensitivity: A critical examination. *New Ideas in Psychology, 20,* 15–48. Permission granted by Elsevier.
O'Donohue, W. and Caselles, C.E. (1993). Homophobia: Conceptual, definitional, and value issues. *Journal of Psychopathology and Behavioral Assessment, 15*(5), 177–1195. Permission granted by the Journal.
O'Donohue, W. and Dyslin, C. (1996). Abortion, boxing and Zionism: Politics and the APA. *New Ideas in Psychology, 14*(1), 1–10. Permission granted by Elsevier.
Redding, R.E. (2001). Sociopolitical diversity in psychology: The case for pluralism. *American Psychologist, 56*(3), 205–215. Permission granted by the American Psychological Association.
Zur, O. (1994). Rethinking "Don't blame the victim": The psychology of victimhood. *Journal of Couples Therapy, 4*(3/4), 15–36. Permission granted by Haworth Press.

Library of Congress Cataloging-in-Publication Data

Destructive trends in mental health: the well-intentioned path to harm/ Rogers H. Wright and Nicholas A. Cummings, editors.
    p. cm.
Includes bibliographical references and index.
ISBN 0-415-95086-4 (hardback)
    1. Mental health services. 2. Psychiatry. 3. Psychology. 4. American Psychological Association. I. Wright, Roger H. II. Cummings, Nicholas A. III. Title.

RA790.5D47 2005
616.89—dc22

2004019946

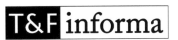

Visit the Taylor & Francis Web site at
http://www.taylorandfrancis.com

Taylor & Francis Group
is the Academic Division of T&F Informa plc.

First of all, do no harm

Hippocrates
The Physician's Oath
Circa 400 B.C.

Contents

Preface

Why would two lifelong activists, I an octogenarian and my colleague nearly so, edit this controversial book when our lives have been characterized by progressive social and political advocacy? Why, when we could be resting on our laurels at the twilight of our careers, do something that is certain to ignite accusations that we are rightwing extremists? Why, after decades of fighting to establish the rightful role of professionalism in psychology, do we now question the validity and integrity of some of the prevalent practices in our profession? The answer is simple: psychology and mental health have veered away from scientific integrity and open inquiry, as well as from compassionate practice in which the welfare of the patient is paramount.

Despite sentiment among our mental health colleagues that there should be a forum for a host of legitimate psychological topics that are avoided because they would bring an avalanche of criticism, no one is willing to step forward. These taboo topics typically unleash a silencing array of unwarranted charges ranging from political incorrectness, insensitivity, and lack of compassion to (in the extreme) bigotry. We are troubled that disciplines such as psychology, psychiatry, and social work, which pride themselves on diversity, scientific inquiry, intellectual openness, and compassion for those who need help, have created an atmosphere in which honest, albeit controversial, points of view are squelched.

We decry the extremism on the right, but we do not address it in this volume because that is not the problem within organized mental health today. Psychology, psychiatry, and social work have been captured by an ultraliberal agenda, much of which we agree with as citizens. However, we are alarmed with the damaging effect it is having on our science, our practice, and our credibility.

In 1973, American Psychological Association (APA) President Leona Tyler enunciated the principle under which we would advocate in the name of psychology and when we would do so as concerned citizens. This principle became APA policy. In speaking as psychologists, our advocacy should be based on scientific data and demonstrable professional experience. Absent such validation, psychologists are free to speak as any concerned citizen, either as individuals or collectively through dedicated advocacy organizations. This separation is necessary if society is to ascribe credibility to advocacy when psychologists are speaking authoritatively as psychologists. Violation of this principle erodes the credibility of the science and profession to represent fact and evidence, and we become another opinionated voice shouting to be heard in a vast arena.

Since enunciation of this principle, advocacy for scientific and professional concerns has been usurped by agenda-driven ideologues who show little regard for either scientific validation or professional efficacy. Although I am in agreement with many of APA's stances, I am opposed to the process that has diminished its credibility. It is no longer perceived as an authority that presents scientific evidence and professional facts. The APA has chosen ideology over science, and thus has diminished its influence on the decision makers in our society.

Let no one presume that ideology does not influence science. Within psychology today there are topics that are deemed politically incorrect, and they are neither published nor funded. Journal editors control what is accepted for publication through those chosen to conduct peer reviews. Although it can be argued that journals have the right to determine their areas of primary interest, this can be used to stifle controversy or political incorrectness even when these are important topics for scientific inquiry. Censorship exists, and if the *Psychiatric News* and the *Monitor on Psychology* published all the news of interest to psychiatrists and psychologists, there would be no market for the *Psychiatric Times* and *The National Psychologist,* both published outside the two APAs. One wag recently observed that although the *Monitor on Psychology* detests managed care, it loves managed news.

Within the profession of psychology there is currently debate over treatment techniques and interventions that have not been scientifically validated. Admittedly, there are two sides to this question. Practitioners are aware that transposing therapies from the laboratory to practice is fraught with problems, inasmuch as the multiple diagnoses found in most patients do not respond in the same way that single-case experimental subjects do. Furthermore, a simple protocol—for example, on smoking cessation—will have a much different outcome depending on whether the patient is an alcoholic, a schizophrenic, or a sociopath, to name only three. Who is having a psychological problem is at times even more important than the psychological problem being addressed by a standard, one-size-fits-all protocol. This fact is known to all competent practitioners. On the other hand, and rightly so, the science is alarmed by ever-proliferating therapies that are not only without validation but are irresponsible, and often later shown to be harmful.

Unfortunately, questioning the efficacy of certain popular therapies is equated by many practitioners with a lack of compassion toward those who are ostensibly benefiting from such dubious treatments. A prime example is the decade-long controversy over repressed memories of incest, and whether these were implanted by well-meaning therapists. A task force appointed by the APA to look into the controversy became politically paralyzed, and the matter was finally settled by the courts. Society spent a number of years sentencing fathers to prison based on false memories, followed by years of releasing them with the court's apology as accusers became aware of the implanted memories. Practitioners lost their licenses, and many were subsequently sued by those they had accused. Meanwhile, the APA remains politically polarized over the issue.

Both my co-editor and I lived through the McCarthy era and the Hollywood witchhunts and, as abominable as these were, there was not the insidious sense of intellectual intimidation that currently exists under political correctness. In the previous era you knew who your oppressors were (e.g., the John Birch Society, anti-Semites, segregationists, and, more benign, the evangelist in the tent down the street who wanted to save my soul). Now misguided political correctness tethers our intellects. Those viewed as conservative are looked down upon as lacking intelligence. Reminiscent of the Puritan religious shunning in a bygone era, we are witnessing a type of secular shunning by those who see themselves as the self-appointed guardians of truth and the saviors of the planet. Dr. Wright and I did not realize how pervasive this shunning and intimidation could be until we began talking with potential contributors, many of whom declined to be included, fearing loss of tenure or stature, and citing previous ridicule and even vicious attacks, described by several chapter contributors. One colleague agreed to contribute as long as her name was removed as a chapter contributor.

This shunning is almost automatic, and often totally thoughtless. At the 2002 APA convention in Chicago, the Association for the

Advancement of Psychology held a black tie fundraising dinner for three psychologist candidates for Congress: Ted Strickland (D-OH) and Brian Baird (D-WA), incumbents who were subsequently reelected, and Tim Murphy (R-PA) who was subsequently elected for the first time. Murphy received a much different reception from the attendees than the two Democrats, even though he made the most engaging of the three speeches. At the table where I was sitting a prominent APA political type remarked that there were no Republicans at our table: "Otherwise I would not be sitting here." When it came time for Tim Murphy to rotate to our table, she immediately and indignantly got up and left. This was not only rude, but politically stupid inasmuch as we were wooing friends in the Congress on behalf of psychology, yet no one at the table but I thought her behavior outrageous. One of those who expressed admiration that she had the courage of her convictions also exited soon after. This was a triumph of ideology over dignity, grace, and political savvy.

After soon-to-be-Congressman Murphy left our table, a conversation ensued that left me with the fear my tablemates might be historical illiterates. To the categorical imperative echoed by several, "There has never been a Republican I could like," I asked about Abraham Lincoln, Wayne Morse, and John McCain. "Well, they aren't real Republicans because they did not stand in the way of progress," was the defensive reply. The disbelief at my pointing out that a Republican president emancipated the slaves and the Democrats blocked desegregation in the 1960s by filibuster confirmed my deepest concern that even among psychologists ideology rewrites history. My statement that the Vietnam War was launched by a Democratic president (Kennedy) when he sent the first military "advisers" to Saigon, that another Democratic president (Johnson) escalated the war, and that the war was ended by a Republican president (Nixon) resulted in hostile defensive silence.

Political diversity is so absent in mental health circles that most psychologists and social workers live in a bubble. So seldom does anyone express ideological disagreement with colleagues that they believe all intelligent people think as they do. They are aware that conservatives exist but regard the term intelligent conservative as an oxymoron. In fact, depending on how left the vantage point is, moderates are seen as conservative and conservatives are lumped in with rightwing extremists. Together they comprise the vast rightwing conspiracy that impedes all progress. The existence of intelligent, scholarly, and reasoned conservatives such as Thomas Sowell or Richard Rodriguez would be a fiction.

This bubble is so encapsulating that psychologists were shocked when the House of Representatives and the Senate of the United States censured the APA for publishing in one of its journals a meta-analysis and interview study of college students who had been molested as children. The publication challenged the notion that these experiences had been deleterious, setting off a firestorm led by radio talk show host "Dr. Laura" Schlessinger, which culminated in the APA being the only professional society in the history of America to be censured by the Congress. To be sure, Dr. Laura cleverly used her talk show pulpit and was joined by powerful conservatives in the Congress, particularly Tom Delay, then majority Whip and now majority Leader in the House. However, no amount of conservative clout could have engineered a unanimous condemnation of the APA were there not already a backdrop of distrust for psychology. Most psychologists are not aware of these events, and those who are do not realize the extent of the humiliation. They blame Dr. Laura and her powerful allies in the Congress, but the finger pointing fails to note that the condemnation was unanimous in both the House and Senate. It further fails to note that not one of psychology's traditional friends voted against the resolution, and even the two psychologist members of the House abstained rather than vote nay. The humiliation was complete.

Psychologists are largely unaware of how inept the profession's testimony before the Congress was. It came down heavily on the side of academic freedom and uncensored scientific research, and only secondarily against pedophilia. Such is the disconnect between psychology and society at large. Americans' support of the notion of academic freedom without the yoke of scientific inquiry does not override their concerns with pedophilia and the need to protect children. This disconnect is curious in a profession that sees itself as expert in human behavior. We not only purport to understand society, but also to treat its problems and its members who need help. Had the APA testimony unequivocally condemned pedophilia first, and then secondarily defended scientific freedom, the vote might not have been completely one-sided. In private, several members of Congress confided that the APA testimony was so ambiguous that voting against condemning the APA would have given the appearance of endorsing pedophilia.

Another example of psychology's disconnect with society at large was the publication by four social psychologists of a painstaking analysis of authoritarianism (Jost, Glaser, Kruglanski, & Sulloway, 2003), in which certain strong statements by President Bush branded him in the authors' conclusions as an authoritarian personality. It is interesting that the statements quoted (e.g., "I know what I believe and I believe I am right") are temperate compared to some of the speeches of Prime Minister Winston Churchill and President Franklin D. Roosevelt during World War II, President John F. Kennedy during the Cuban missile crisis, and President Harry Truman almost anytime. Yet these personalities were not deemed authoritarian. Strong leaders at times of crisis make statements that are commensurate with the need to energize the nation.

In rebuttal, Greenberg and Jonas (2003) point out that the criteria of conservatism set forth by Jost et al.—for example, a desire to return to an idealized past, intolerance of ambiguity, lack of openness to experience, uncertainty avoidance, personal needs for order, structure, and closure, fear of death, and system threat (p. 383)—can apply not just to Ronald Reagan and George W. Bush but equally to Adolph Hitler, Benito Mussolini, and Joseph Stalin, who all wanted to return to "an idealized past." A University of California at Berkeley press release did, in fact, label all of these figures as authoritarian and conservative. On these dubious dimensions Stalin, Castro, and Mao, all radical Marxists, qualify as conservative.

Any "psychological scale" that equates U.S. presidents with ruthless genocidal dictators who murdered millions must be woefully deficient in its ability to differentiate personality. Ostensibly Jost et al. are intelligent and well-meaning, but they demonstrate the triumph of ideology over science and professionalism. Predictably, and unfortunately, psychology once again became a media laughingstock, a reputation it could ill afford following the pedophilia debacle. Perhaps the kindest thing said was the remark of one commentator that it was all unimportant because no one any longer pays attention to the strange conclusions of psychologists. Clearly, we have lost much of our ability to speak with credibility and authority.

Psychology has an impressive record of promoting racial, ethnic, and cultural diversity in its membership and organizational structure. We have become an admirable microcosm of America in this regard. However, sociopolitical diversity is sorely lacking. It is obvious that we need a greater diversity of ideas and a counterbalance to the prevailing ideologies within mental health circles today. If psychology is to soar like an eagle, it needs both a left wing and a right wing. We must broaden the debate by reducing the ridicule and intimidation of ideas contrary to the thinking of the establishment in the field of psychology. We must return to the principles on which psychology—and, indeed, the entire field of medicine—was founded: above all, to do no harm and to act for the public good. This entails acting with prudence and foresight so that we can once again assume a leadership role in matters where our expertise is invaluable.

The intent of this book is to acquaint the reader with the often well-meaning, but frequently self-interested destructive trends that have permeated the mental health professions, threatening harm to the patients who seek their help, and betraying the society they are sworn to serve. Three general topics have been selected, with the first addressing political correctness, misguided sensitivity, and overemphasis on diversity. In chapter 1 Cummings and O'Donohue trace how psychology has surrendered its science and profession to political correctness, and in chapter 2 O'Donohue gives a critical analysis of the limitations in the current concept of cultural sensitivity. Victimhood and how it deprives patients of best practices is the theme of Zur's chapter 3, and O'Donohue and Caselles in chapter 4 examine the misuses and intimidations of the word homophobia.

The second section looks at mental healthcare economics, a totally neglected area in psychology, psychiatry, and social work. In his chapter 5 Cummings demonstrates how the economic pinch of too many practitioners has led to artificial and harmful methods of expanding a diminishing revenue; Glasser in chapter 6 augments this by pointing to the financial incentives to sacrifice psychotherapy and counseling, the traditional mainstays of mental health, to inappropriate and even harmful medication. Wright in chapter 7 discusses how attention deficit/hyperactivity disorder has been expanded beyond all neurological proof, and he rounds out the section in chapter 8 revealing that the laws intended to protect the public by requiring professional continuing education have turned into a profitable industry that has forgotten its original mission.

The last section is the longest, addressing the many-faceted subject of how politics influences both science and practice. Gottfredson in chapter 9 has compelling evidence of how the fear of being labeled racist has all but eliminated research on intelligence, ultimately hurting those we intend to help. Lilienfeld, (chapter 10) a widely recognized authority on pseudoscience in psychology, along with his colleagues, challenges some of the most popular, and perhaps more lucrative, of the many dubious diagnoses. In chapter 11 psychology columnist John Rosemond, writing in his usual journalistic style, meets head-on how politics is determining misdiagnoses in our children. Getting specific on how politics has determined many stances and declarations by the American Psychological Association is the subject of O'Donohue's and

Dyslin's chapter 12, and Zur in chapter 13 addresses the politics that has undermined psychology's Code of Ethics, especially in its intimidation that has led to risk management rather than practice in the patient's best interest. Community psychology, founded in the 1960s, was intended to research and advocate social justice, but Lillis and his colleagues in chapter 14 demonstrate how it has been captured by a one-sided agenda. Finally Redding (chapter 15), both a lawyer and a psychologist, carefully demonstrates the remarkable lack of sociopolitical diversity in a profession that champions ethnic and racial diversity.

The chapters in this volume are controversial, and although the editors may not agree with everything proffered by the contributors, their ideas deserve the forum that is often denied them. The common thread in all fifteen chapters is to reveal how well-intended but destructive forces have invaded the very foundation of mental health, threatening its credibility, distorting its science, and exposing its patients to possible harm. The lack of sociopolitical diversity among the mental health professions, with its accompanying atmosphere of intellectual intimidation, has made the publication of this book compelling.

Nicholas A. Cummings

REFERENCES

Greenberg, J. & Jonas, E. (2003). Psychological motives and political orientation—The left, the right, and the rigid: Comments on Jost et al. (2003). *Psychological Bulletin, 129*(3), 376–382.

Jost, J.T., Glaser, J., Kruglanski, A.W., & Sulloway, F.J. (2003). Political conservatism as motivated social cognition. *Psychological Bulletin, 129*(3), 329–375.

Acknowledgments

Our profound appreciation to Dr. George Zimmar, Publishing Director, Routledge, Taylor & Francis, for his patience and skillful guidance in bringing this book to publication. We also gratefully acknowledge the assistance of Joanne Freeman, whose editorial expertise was essential to the editing and shaping of this volume.

In addition, we and the chapter contributors owe a debt of gratitude to Dr. Janet L. Cummings, president of The Nicholas and Dorothy Cummings Foundation, for making possible the extensive distribution of advance copies of this volume to key leaders in healthcare, the legislature, and the media.

Nicholas A. Cummings and Rogers H. Wright

INTRODUCTION

Rogers H. Wright

In the late 1950s, *The Demolished Man,* a whimsical novel written by a psychologist, postulated a future, highly stratified culture in which psychologists, who could read people's minds, were given the society's fourth highest rank. In return for this exalted status they were expected to take an oath limiting the use of their extraordinary power and knowledge to dispensing justice with fairness and equity. The author wryly noted that such dedication was not strenuously observed, indicating a general attitude toward compliance with oaths, claims, and codes of ethics that may have considerable current relevance among mental health service providers.

The novel captured the interest of a society that at the time was obsessed with parapsychology and mind-reading. Psychologists seriously conducted "experiments" in these activities, into which the federal government poured substantial research grant funds. The parapsychology fad has faded, but two aspects of that era persist: (1) the federal government and private institutions continue to waste millions of dollars on hobby psychological and politically correct research while neglecting to fund more basic, meaningful research; and (2) society continues to believe that mental health practitioners possess some kind of omniscience when it comes to human affairs. Unfortunately, this point of view is not only unchallenged but is shared by some mental health providers.

There has been a fundamental shift in the way we perceive mental health problems. Until the last third of the twentieth century, psychosis and insanity were viewed with shame and embarrassment. These diagnoses were underreported and swept under the rug, much the way many parts of the world attempt to deal with the current AIDS epidemic. Following World War II, psychologists, psychiatrists, social workers, and mental health consumers coalesced around the goal of diminishing the stigma associated with mental health problems. Seemingly overnight there developed an enormous interest in psychotherapy, and the nation's training facilities responded by turning out ever-increasing numbers of mental health providers.

These professionals became very articulate in addressing the stigma of mental illness. One of the strategies they employed was to substitute less sensitive appellations for terms: that is, mental health for mental illness, emotional condition for mental disease, problems in living for neurosis/psychosis, diminished capacity for feeble-mindedness or insanity. No one then would have predicted that the time would come when individuals would not be held responsible for their problematic/destructive behavior because they were "victims." In an attempt to eliminate the stigma, we may have thrown out the baby with the bathwater.

In the latter part of the twentieth century, these same interest groups worked with considerable success to persuade public policy makers, Congress, state legislatures, and public and private insurers to broaden the availability of mental health services as part of health coverage. The advent of insurance reimbursement for psychotherapy swelled the ranks of psychologists, psychiatrists, social workers, and counselors.

The co-editors of this volume have been privileged to serve and participate in the remarkable growth and availability of mental health services over the past five decades as providers, educators, researchers, and public policy activists. Our myriad experiences have provided what we believe is a unique perspective from which to view changes in the mental health field. Although the quality and availability of many mental health services has increased, there has also been a proliferation of philosophies, practices, and procedures that, at best, are self-serving and, at worst, destructive to the integrity of psychology and contrary to the concept of helping patients become mentally healthy and independent.

These changes stem from a variety of considerations. However, our focus is on three major factors, echoed in the three sections of this volume: (1) the broad social pattern of the culture, reflected in an obsession with political correctness, sensitivity, and diversity; (2) the way mental health service providers view themselves and their products, reflected in psychology's service and economic practices; and (3) an emphasis on ideology, reflected in the influence of politics on science and practice.

The ongoing interaction between psychology and culture blurs cause and effect. What is clear, however, is that value systems, acceptance, permissiveness, and nonjudgmental attitudes—essential to all forms of psychotherapy and counseling—are now valued behaviors in our culture. This despite the fact that such behaviors may have little or no direct relevance to education, business, the military, parenting, or other nonpsychotherapeutic endeavors. Indeed, in broad cultural applications these behaviors have been demonstrably ineffective and frequently shown to have significant and lasting deleterious results. A component of this migration of psychological practice to our culture has been the convoluted use of the concept of disease and/or victimization to excuse individuals and groups from responsibility for their behavior.

Profound changes, largely unappreciated at the time, began with the mid-1960s passage of Medicare and Medicaid. In effect, responsibility for one's health passed from the individual to a third party. Health care became a "right" and contributed to the escalating belief that "needs" translate into "rights." Aided and abetted by the mental health disciplines, this concept generalized into a philosophy of life for much of our culture. When our "rights" were denied, we became "victims."

Such victimhood, which allows escape from personal responsibility and elicits redress by others, has often reached the point of absurdity, fostered by those anxious to help the "aggrieved," including trial lawyers and some mental health providers. Thus, spilling hot coffee is not due to personal carelessness but reflects its being served at an incorrect temperature. A weight problem is no longer overeating but the result of food addiction exploited by fast-food interests. Lung cancer following a lifelong consumption of cigarettes is the fault of a conspiracy among the tobacco companies to addict large numbers of the public, the warning label on the cigarette package notwithstanding.

An entire industry exclusively dedicated to helping "victims" assert their "rights" has developed around the nation's Workers' Compensation Program. Victims' claims that the workplace is "too stressful, abusive" or otherwise inimical to their mental well-being all too frequently involve both compensation for the "injury" and long-term paid disability. In California, investigation of excessive workers' compensation losses revealed "compensation mills," with fraudulent claims being processed by psychology students who had never seen the claimants. This resulted in laws demanding that all mental health claims be written by the provider signing the report.

Accompanying the renunciation of individual responsibility for decisions and life choices are profound changes in child-rearing practices in this country. With the wholesale migration of women from the home into the workplace, large numbers of our children are being raised by uncredentialed, unsupervised, and frequently incompetent "child care" personnel. It is very difficult to assess what long-range impact the absence of the natural mother will have, but emerging evidence suggests that if it impairs the child's bonding, there are significantly negative psychological consequences.

The way in which our culture views the childhood years also has profound consequences. Formerly considered a preparation for adulthood, childhood is now regarded as endless playtime. Parents are so intimidated by the threat that structure and discipline may irreparably harm their children that they make only the most modest demands. Children are praised elaborately for doing little or nothing, in the misguided hope that this builds self-esteem. What gets lost in all this is that interpersonal comfort, self-acceptance, and self-esteem derive from mastery and accomplishment. Would it not be more helpful to teach our children personal responsibility and that choices have consequences rather than encourage irresponsibility and feel-good permissiveness?

In the field of education, the shrinking of individual and parental responsibility is glaringly apparent. The California Board of Education has consistently resisted implementation of competency exams for high school graduation, hoping to avoid its failure to educate, underscored by statistics indicating that a majority of current high school graduates in Los Angeles County repeatedly failed such an exam (Los Angeles Board of Education, 2002). Wholesale failures in education are attributed to an uncaring school system, socioeconomic factors, and the perennial lack of money. Never mentioned are the lack of standards and discipline, student irresponsibility, uninvolved parents, fear of parental and student complaints or retaliation and, most destructive of all, social promotion. Unfortunately, organized mental health has done little to address the decline in education, and when it has, it has weighed in with more of the same rationalizations and so-called solutions tediously offered by the teachers' unions.

Public attitudes and beliefs dictate public policy actions that may have major and long-lasting consequences. The wide application of nonjudgmental attitudes to violent and criminal behavior, coupled with the myth that counseling is a viable solution to chronic violence and habitual criminality, is a demonstrated failure. The idea that the behavior of a chronologically mature adult acting like a perpetual adolescent by manifesting "road rage" can be materially influenced by "anger management" misunderstands the basic problem.

Counseling, psychotherapy, and personal coaching have much to be modest about when it comes to the amelioration of criminality and other antisocial behaviors. Often therapy is merely an alternative to our crowded prison system. Sound statistics are difficult to come by, but the most optimistic estimates presage a less than forty percent "cure rate" for criminal behavior and substance abuse, a low success rate accomplished at an enormous expenditure of tax dollars (U.S. Department of Labor, 2001; White & Wright, 1999). Yet despite the scant return on investment, there is substantial interest within the body politic to "decriminalize" substance abuse by replacing incarceration with counseling or psychotherapy.

Another major area of social change has been our flirtation, to the point of obsession, with political correctness (see chapter 1). This has profound implications for the way we skew reality, interpersonal relationships, and internal and external responsibilities. Thought police are everywhere, and panels of experts arbitrarily dictate what words are to be eliminated from usage because they might hurt someone's feelings. In this fashion such words as "elite" and "yacht" are excluded from school textbooks on the premise that doing so will spare the feelings of underprivileged students. Words long identified with categorizations of intellectual performance have been changed to terms of such innocuousness that it becomes impossible for professionals, let alone the public, to tell what a person's performance level is on an intelligence test

Unfortunately, psychology has allied itself with a misguided viewpoint that has prevented education from addressing a compelling need: the differential rates of intellectual prowess. Research on intelligence is now regarded as potentially racist, and studies of intellectual functioning among cultural subgroups have all but disappeared in the psychological literature. Such research that continues to be conducted encounters substantial difficulty in being published or cited. Perhaps one of the most egregious examples is the pseudoscientific personal attacks on the internationally known psychologist, Dr. Arthur Jensen of the University of California, Berkeley (see chapter 9), whose research on intelligence goes against the grain of current political correctness.

Self-appointed advocates have sprung up for ever-proliferating groups of victims. Such widespread and lucrative activity also accrues significant social and political power to the organizations involved. The educator, politician, government official, journalist, or professional who incurs the wrath of such groups is frequently accused of being racist, judgmental, biased, or guilty of discriminatory practice. Often one need not say a thing. My co-editor, on the verge of agreeing with the positions of a prominent female psychologist, was publicly attacked before he could open his mouth: "I don't know what you are going to say; but we could never agree because I am a lesbian and you are a straight white male."

Accusations of bias, racism, and bigotry are intended to have a chilling effect on those who question any aspect of political correctness. Political correctness, and its attendant issues of affirmative action and diversity, also have had considerable impact on the training of mental health professionals and the delivery of scientifically based mental health services.

Despite the absence of hard evidence as to its value, the concept of diversity that found immediate and widespread favor in academia now has broad currency in the American vernacular. Diversity has been ardently embraced by most university training programs for mental health professionals and by professional societies. Education, training, research, and service delivery are frequently shaped more by diversity for the sake of diversity than by hard data, the reality and needs of the marketplace, and/or the populations to be served.

Not all identifiable subgroups within our culture are given favorable treatment in the interest of diversity. The groups favored for purposes of diversity are women, African Americans, and Hispanics. At the same time, Asian Americans and American Jews are often discriminated against in the selection process. If the point of diversity is its contribution to learning and professional function, should not diversity mirror our society as a whole by including right-wing conservatives, religious extremists, Marxist ideologues, and students whose annual family income is aggregated at $30,000 intervals? (See chapter 15.)

Traditionally, therapists have suppressed their own personalities and value systems in the interest of the therapeutic enterprise. This was calculated to maximize the freedom of the patient to express personal values, concerns, fantasies, feelings, problems, and even solutions within the confines of the therapeutic session. With the advent of affirmative action/diversity programs in both training and service delivery, a new mythology was propagated and repeatedly asserted: namely, that the psychotherapy process is less efficacious if the consumer and the therapist are not of the same subgroup. The ostensible rationale can be summed up as "you got to be one to treat one" (Wright, 1983) and is based on the highly questionable premise that shared backgrounds between therapist and patient facilitate the therapeutic process, broaden the therapist's understanding of the patient's problems, and promote growth and healthier lifestyles because the therapist constitutes a subgroup role model. This approach is potentially fraught with major problems for the patient. Not only do therapist and patient share the same "blind spots," but the aim of psychotherapy is to facilitate patients' understanding and accepting of themselves, not to make them clones of the therapist.

The shared-experience philosophy has spawned a long list of subgroup therapists, including ethnic minority, feminist, gay, and lesbian. All too frequently, assertions about the efficacy of patient/therapist subgroup identity or "specialization" of the therapist are blatantly self-serving, reflecting a glut of providers attempting to carve out a "fiefdom" in a very tight mental healthcare market. Another problem posed by these approaches is "classification": that is, to which of many possible subgroups does the prospective consumer belong?

Proponents of patient/therapist subgroup identity have repeatedly attempted to amend ethical codes of professional associations to prohibit therapists from treating consumers of differing cultural backgrounds. Although these efforts have largely failed, they have had substantial informal impact and have succeeded (again absent substantial credible evidence of the efficacy or necessity for such training) in persuading professional and governing groups to require more cultural and "sensitivity" training in the education of therapists (see chapter 2).

Equally without credible evidence, many proponents are attempting to turn psychotherapy into advocacy for their subgroups and psychotherapists into advocates for positions and goals of the given subgroup. Psychologist–advocates write about the need to explore the cultural heritage of the patient (Sue, 1998; Sue & Zane, 1997), and some proponents go so far as to assert "… that individuals from different cultural backgrounds cannot understand each other" (La Roche & Maxie, 2003, p. 181). Given a nearly hundred-year history of therapists/patients of different backgrounds working together successfully, such assertions border on the nonsensical. La Roche wisely noted later, "Unfortunately, the empirical research on the effectiveness of addressing cultural differences in psychotherapy is limited" (La Roche & Maxie, 2003, p. 181).

Nevertheless, La Roche has identified no less than ten areas of "cultural differences" that the author feels merit exploration, a position which fails to take into account that virtually all mental health service currently takes place in a climate where third-party payers are increasingly demanding justification for each and every therapeutic session. Perhaps a better and less costly vehicle for cultural exploration would be classes taught by experts equipped to teach appreciation of a given cultural heritage. Many experienced therapists would be troubled about a situation in which the provider, rather than the patient, determines the nature of the therapeutic work. Our position is that the best therapist is likely to be one who nonjudgmentally treats a broad spectrum of patients and is not compelled to visibly demonstrate identification with any philosophy, movement, or ideology. This, coupled with experience and effectiveness, helps ensure that psychotherapy will focus on patient needs, not the therapist's agenda.

In the current climate, it is inevitable that conflict arises among the proponents of the various subgroups in the marketplace. For example, gay groups within the APA have repeatedly tried to persuade the association to adopt ethical standards that prohibit therapists from offering psychotherapeutic services designed to ameliorate "gayness," on the basis that such efforts are unsuccessful and harmful to the consumer. Psychologists who do not agree with this premise are termed homophobic (see chapter 4). Such efforts are especially troubling because they abrogate the patient's right to choose the therapist and determine therapeutic goals. They also deny the reality of data demonstrating that psychotherapy can be effective in changing sexual preferences in patients who have a desire to do so.

Mental health providers must also recognize when they take themselves too seriously. The extent to which various patients can benefit is often limited by lack of motivation, adverse circumstances, unfortunate and irreparable choices in life, chronic illness, and even lack of accessibility to mental health services. Fifty years ago psychotherapy was heady with promise: "Give us enough therapists and we can cure every individual mental illness." The advent of community psychology and psychiatry (see chapter 14) trumped this arrogance with the attitude "Give us the personnel and we can cure society."

These are extreme examples, but psychotherapists who experience the gratitude of patients day in and day out may develop an exaggerated sense of importance. Success in the psychotherapy realm does not necessarily qualify us as experts in the broad arena of human affairs. Many of our colleagues have the propensity to extrapolate nonjudgmental therapeutic techniques into a philosophy of human behavior, concluding with the ideal of a valueless, relativistic, nonjudgmental society (see chapter 2). Indeed there are such things in life as good and bad, productive and unproductive, worthwhile and worthless. Whereas the application of a unique and dogmatic value system can be problematic, the failure to make any judgment as to value, appropriateness, or merit sentences us to a life that lacks direction. Children do misbehave. Criminals break the law. Violence is rampant.

The search for etiological factors does not preclude our making a judgment about these activities; rather, it leads to seeking change. Not every behavioral aberration is reflective of some environmental deficiency. Sometimes people are just too lazy to make an effort to change. In such a context, the rationalization "Let's not be judgmental," or "Don't judge me; I'm a victim," has no value in solving the problem.

Many factors interact in the broad arena of health economics. In the 1990s, as managed behavioral care sought to control soaring costs by the often arbitrary curtailment of services, providers found themselves with decreased patient loads and ever-increasing amounts of unremunerated time. Some of the new applications they sought for their skills were beneficial; others were questionable. Suddenly there were such therapies as grief counseling, anger management, and treatment for an expanded conceptualization of post-traumatic stress syndrome. These services, even when offered pro bono, had the advantage of enhancing provider visibility in the community.

Such services as grief counseling and trauma counseling lack solid evidence of lasting merit. In fact, evidence emerging from therapists treating workers and survivors of the 9/11 tragedy suggests that the immediate "counseling" prevents some individuals from assimilating the experience. At best, the long-term effects of these unproven psychological interventions need to be more carefully studied; in the short term, consideration needs be given to the possibility that they may contribute to normalizing histrionic behavior (see chapter 10). Another consideration is their impact on impairing the ability (especially among children and adolescents) to address life's stresses.

Meanwhile, the scope of other mental health problems has been broadened and new problems defined. Posttraumatic stress disorder, originally identifying a response to extreme combat, was extended to include civilian populations. Behavior disorders, associated with various substances such as red dyes, sugar, and food additives, began receiving widespread attention in the media and in alternative medicine. The recollection of deeply repressed memories of sexual exploitation reached a peak and then crashed in the courts as practitioners lost their licenses for having inadvertently induced such memories through hypnosis or frequent and suggestive questioning in psychotherapy (see chapters 5 and 10). Attention deficit disorder and attention deficit hyperactivity disorder were reformulated to apply to as many as thirty to forty percent of all children manifesting any behavioral problems (see chapters 6 and 11).

Not to be left out of this economic bonanza, psychiatry suddenly discovered that forty percent of all patients visiting the doctor were depressed enough to warrant antidepressant medication. Now five percent of all prescriptions issued to children are for antidepressants. The *New York Times* of August 8, 2003 reported several studies that showed SSRI antidepressants to be only "moderately effective," and the increased suicide risk among adolescents receiving Paxil has been reported both in British and American journals and by the FDA. The *Times* article also reported on studies demonstrating that the treatment of adolescent depression by antidepressants yields no better results than a placebo. Other studies corroborate the extensiveness and ineffectiveness of behavioral drugs on children and adolescents (Johnson, 2004; Fredenheim, 2004). Meanwhile television infomercials repeatedly advise adults who are distracted, tense, or unable to finish tasks that they may be sufferers of ADD/ADHD. These new or broadened mental health services have expanded the mental health economy, but to the benefit of whom? (See chapter 6.)

The American Psychiatric Association has played a significant role in this market expansion by modifying the criteria underlying its diagnostic manual. Adding the words "disorder" or "syndrome" has markedly increased the number of conditions requiring mental health treatment. This is significant because psychiatry's official diagnostic manual is the basis for reimbursement of mental health services. Are these disorders and syndromes helpful in treating the problem? Not particularly. Are they helpful in filling out insurance claim forms? Absolutely! Do they help hide the fact that we know only the symptom and not the cause? Most assuredly!

Mental health personnel have demonstrated endless creativity in expanding personal income, not the least of which is exploiting state licensing laws mandating continuing education (see chapter 8). Professional associations turned to political action to achieve these mandates, then captured the lucrative approvals process, making certain that courses without their imprimatur would not qualify in renewing professional credentials. No matter that CE offerings often tend to be of poor quality, dubious value, poorly taught, frequently misinformative, and contributors to the rising costs of all professional services.

American trial lawyers, never to be outdone at the cash register, discovered the lucrative market of championing abused persons and populations. They received help from mental health practitioners who impressed the courts with the depth of the psychological trauma and the need for years of corrective psychotherapy following real or imagined abuse. Lawyers also saw psychologists' vulnerability to laws requiring the "duty to warn" and well-meaning but ill-conceived codes of conduct that subjected mental health professionals to vague prohibitions such as "dual relationships" (see chapter 13). Lawsuits against mental health providers became commonplace, with many providers eager to testify against their colleagues. This litigation has resulted in defensive practice, needless hospitalization, frequent refusal to treat high-risk patients, and escalating costs.

Psychology is in need of a makeover. That there is much to be concerned about is underscored by the 2003 report of the President's New Freedom Commission on Mental Health, which concluded that mental health in America is often inadequate and requires fundamental transformation. This volume addresses some of the more destructive fads, mythologies, expectations, practices, and procedures. It strives to present information that will assist consumers in thinking more productively about mental health issues, both personally and in the broadest sense, and encourage mental health providers to view ourselves as others might see us.

The contributors to this book are nationally visible figures in the mental health field with an impressive list of citations, honors, and publications. One served as APA president, another as president of the American Psychological Foundation, and still another as executive director of the Association for the Advancement of Psychology. Two have served as presidents of state psychological associations, and two are recipients of the American Psychological Foundation's Gold Medal for Lifetime Achievement in Practice, psychology's highest award. They hold prestigious academic positions in universities or are leaders in business and professional organizations. Each has attained sufficient stature in the field to be able to present straightforward information and viewpoints unencumbered by concerns for political correctness or disapproval. Dr. Cummings and I are grateful for their courage, time, and commitment in sharing their views and expertise.

REFERENCES

Fredenheim, M. (2004, May 17). Behavior drugs lead in sales for children. *New York Times*, pp. B1, B3-4.

Johnson, L.A. (2004, May 17*).* Spending soars for kids' behavior drugs. Trenton, NJ: Associated Press.

La Roche, M.J. & Maxie, A. (2003). Ten considerations in addressing cultural differences in psychotherapy. *Professional Psychology: Research and Practice, 34,* 180–186.

Los Angeles Board of Education. (2002). *Progress Report on the County's Schools.* Los Angeles: Author.

President's New Freedom Commission on Mental Health. (2003). *An Interim Report to the President of the United States.* Washington, DC: The White House.

Sue, S. & Zane, N. (1997). The role of culture and cultural techniques in psychotherapy. *American Psychologist, 43,* 37–45.

Sue, S. (1998). In Search of Cultural Competency in Psychotherapy and Counseling. *American Psychologist, 53,* 440–448.

U.S. Department of Labor. (2001). *Facts and Figures about Alcohol, Drugs, and Criminality in the Workplace.* Washington, DC: Author.

White, R.R. & Wright, D.G. (1999). *Addiction Intervention: Strategies to Motivate Treatment-Seeking Behavior.* Binghampton, NY: Haworth.

Wright, R.H. (1983). You can't treat one if you ain't one. *Psychotherapy In Private Practice, 1*(2), 35–43.

Wright, R.H. & Cummings, N.A. (Eds.) (2001). *The Practice of Psychology: The Battle for Professionalism.* Phoenix, AZ: Zeig, Tucker & Theisen.

Section A

Political Correctness, Sensitivity, and Diversity

1

PSYCHOLOGY'S SURRENDER TO POLITICAL CORRECTNESS

Nicholas A. Cummings and William T. O'Donohue

"I used to think I was poor," cogently wrote the cartoonist Jules Feiffer (2003). "Then they told me I wasn't poor, I was needy. They told me it was self-defeating to think of myself as needy, I was deprived. Then they told me underprivileged was overused, I was disadvantaged. I still don't have a dime. But I have a great vocabulary."

The prescient Aldous Huxley (1935) in his novel *Brave New World* characterized future society as exhibiting two characteristics that were thought fanciful and improbable half a century before his prediction was to take place. First, most of the populace would be taking a drug called "soma" to alleviate even the slightest anxieties and mood swings that accompany life's daily vicissitudes. This would not be imposed by a totalitarian government exercising mind control; rather, people would clamor for it. As unlikely as this seemed in the 1930s, many authorities are now sounding the alarm that our current society is overmedicating itself rather than addressing and solving everyday problems, thus rendering itself and future generations less and less able to face the normal exigencies of living (Glasser, 2003; Healy, 2004; Kirsch & Antonuccio, 2004). In response to extensive, unrelenting TV advertising, an increasing number of patients are demanding medications from their primary care physicians, preferably medications that have in their names the letters xyz (Prozac, Zoloft, Luvox, Paxil, with Zyprexa being a *nom magnifique*). Particularly disturbing is the trend to prescribe psychotropic medications to adolescents, children, and even preschoolers, possibly endangering the delicate maturational balance that is still in progress (Cummings & Wiggins, 2001; Minde, 1998; Zito et al., 2004).

It is not the purpose of this chapter to address the advent of Huxley's soma but to look at the second of his predictions: the subtle changes in language he termed "double-speak," the renaming of nouns to reflect or impose changes in attitudes and behaviors. In an equally prescient novel whose title *1984* actually pinpointed the date the phenomenon would be extant, George Orwell (1961) named it "newspeak" and described how its beginning as revisions in language would soon become a censor of thought and behavior. No totalitarian state would be necessary to dictate this censorship; it would be the self-creation of a misguided society. With its roots in the social upheaval of the 1960s, often referred to as the counterculture era, the assaults on language and attitudes have increased steadily over the next several decades to culminate in the rubric "political correctness."

This seemingly harmless renaming of nouns has resulted in a surprisingly pervasive conglomerate of attitudes that are imposed on the populace by a noncodified set of pressures, stigmas, name-calling, and other disapprovals that constitute a cultural fascism. Job promotions, college grades, admission to graduate school, popularity, election to public office, and even success itself may depend on being politically correct. It is the intent of this chapter to trace how political correctness, the fulfillment of Orwellian society, insinuated itself into psychology and psychiatry, distorting the science and corrupting the profession. Make no mistake: the distortions in the mental health field have paralleled the sad social state, wherein an impeached president can dodge a question concerning his possible misconduct by answering under oath, "It all depends on what the meaning of 'is' is" (Clinton, 1999). Double-speak is not a harmless set of changes in nouns; it is a pervasive shift in attitudes that can profoundly corrupt not only our legal system, but other institutions as well. This has already occurred in mental health with psychology's surrender of its professionalism and its science to political correctness.

GENERAL PRINCIPLES OF POLITICAL CORRECTNESS

Although the focus of this chapter is primarily psychology, the commentary applies to psychiatry and social work, as well. It is important to look at some general characteristics of political correctness, which will be helpful in understanding their extrapolation to the mental health field.

Pervasive Use of Chicken Little's "The Sky Is Falling"

Once noun changes have been accepted into the language, political correctness thrives on scaring people into changing their behaviors. For example, it is not enough to rename "world climate change" to "global warming"; it is then incumbent upon everyone to prevent the extinction of the planet by drastically changing lifestyles, even to regressing to more primitive modes of existence. Most scientists believe the earth is warming, but they are sharply divided on whether this is the result of eons of cyclical climate changes or of greenhouse gases. Having failed to convince the scientific community of its position, radical environmentalists are now trying to create a new crisis: because of the earth's warming, half of the species on the planet will become extinct in the next fifty years.

This and other fallacies are discussed and refuted by the dedicated but contrarian Danish environmentalist Bjorn Lomborg (2000), who, after an extensive compilation of the evidence, concludes that the earth is getting healthier. There is less pollution, more forest, and more food per person. Although he believes there is global warming, he feels it would be more effective to adapt and continue to manage it rather than attempt to turn back the civilization's clock.

Imperviousness to Critical Self-examination

Politically correct thinking has spawned some monumental and near universally accepted inaccuracies that had ostensibly intelligent and educated authorities sounding the alarm that doomsday was coming. If the intent was to raise awareness—newspeak for scaring the dickens out of people into altering their attitudes and behaviors—they succeeded, at least until the myth was discredited. Among many examples is Paul Ehrlich's (1968) *The Population Bomb,* which predicted the world would run out of food and other resources before the twenty-first century, and Rachel Carson's *Silent Spring,* which in 1962 predicted the total disappearance of birds within twenty years because of pesticide use. These were widely accepted fears in their time and were given much publicity, but neither turned out to be a credible prediction. However, each accomplished its purpose: it advanced the cause of political correctness, set the stage for the broad acceptance of even greater myths, and then was quietly buried in the graveyard of politically correct absurdities. Political correctness, coated with Teflon® by its proponents, is then moved to invent yet another crisis.

So successful are burials of past inaccurate alarms that few people living in the early part of the twenty-first century remember that thirty years ago society was bombarded with predictions that the use of fossil fuels was rapidly bringing about another ice age. The cooling of the planet was so rapid, we were told, that meteorologists could not keep up with the climate changes. The government was urged to stockpile provisions because in twenty to thirty years the earth would be too cold to grow food. Schemes were proposed to slow down the impending ice age, with one of the most preposterous being to melt the polar icecaps by covering them with black soot. The reader is referred to an extensive landmark publication in *Newsweek* (April 28, 1975, "The Cooling Earth"), which chronicled what was widely accepted as the inevitable consequence of air pollution. In the ensuing thirty years, however, instead of planet cooling and the inability to grow food, there has been a 180-degree turn, and it is now politically correct to predict that the burning of the same fossil fuels will bring about global warming and the extinction of millions of plant and animal species.

False alarms of lesser magnitude abound, among them the now-discredited overestimation by severalfold of the number of homeless in America (Whittle, 1992; Revel, 1991). For years the fabricated figures spouted by self-appointed champions of the homeless were accepted and repeated as fact by either a lazy or politically correct media until finally some conscientious journalist actually checked (U.S. Bureau of the Census, 1991). The feminist movement disseminated false information, again accepted by a politically correct press, which stated that hundreds, if not thousands, of young women were dying annually from anorexia because they were trying to be thin to please unreasonably demanding males. Finally, the National Institute of Mental Health (NIMH), when pressed to check, suggested that in a ten-year period there may have been no more than seventeen such deaths (Sommers, 1994).

One alarm that certainly should have been sounded was the early contamination of our blood supply by HIV, but a life-saving solution was too long delayed because it clashed with misplaced gay rights. In *The Band Played On*, Randy Shilts (1987) chillingly described how a politically correct public health system literally endangered lives rather than risk being accused of homophobia.

Political correctness is unable to self-correct its own internal contradictions. It promotes wind power, and on the other hand it tries to ban windmills because they have killed thousands of birds, including at least one eagle. Plastic grocery bags introduce more chemicals into the environment, but paper bags come from cut forests. Electrical power is clean, but it is mostly generated by coal, which pollutes the air. Similarly, mandated MTBE added to gasoline results in cleaner air, but it contaminates the groundwater and the law should be repealed. Herbal medicine is alternative medicine and thus is politically correct, but the harvesting of wild plants to obtain the herbs is endangering many exotic species and must be stopped. These are serious considerations, but sometimes it gets downright entertaining, as when animal rights and gay rights clash. In San Diego the People for the Ethical Treatment of Animals (PETA) picketed a motorcycle meeting of gay bikers because the latter, also known as "leather queens" and "dykes on bikes," have a fetish for leather, ostensibly resulting in thousands of needlessly killed animals. The bikers responded that PETA is homophobic.

Promotion of a Feel-Good Attitude Even without a Solution

Politically correct terminology can make people feel good in the absence of any real solution. It may be relatively harmless that the "used car" has given way to the "pre-owned vehicle," a term that may lull the buyer into the false assumption that the pre-owned vehicle has none of the mechanical defects of a used car. More important examples are those that make people feel good without tackling serious problems. Thus, Chicago, Detroit, and Philadelphia no longer have black ghettos, and Los Angeles has lost its barrio; all have inner cities instead. The blight is still there and the inner city inhabitant is no better off, but others may feel good that ostensibly something has been accomplished. We no longer have jungles, only rain forests that continue to be destroyed at an alarming rate. Having wetlands instead of swamps has not reduced their endangerment, and the fact that backward countries are now underdeveloped does not make them less backward. Ah, but the new more politically correct language makes us feel better without the need to do anything tangible.

POLITICAL CORRECTNESS INVADES MENTAL HEALTH

The introduction of double-speak into mental health began innocently enough during the post-World War II era, and with the noblest of intentions. The purpose in renaming was to remove the stigma that discouraged or even prevented many needy patients from seeking psychological help. As Wright has noted in the introduction to this volume, mental health was substituted for mental illness, emotional condition for mental disease, problems in living instead of neurosis/psychosis, intellectually challenged instead of mentally retarded, and diminished capacity rather than insanity. During this noble phase of renaming, no one would have predicted that the day would come when it would become politically correct to absolve all aberrant behavior because it was "hard-wired"; that is, an individual has no choices in life, and no one should be held responsible for problematic or destructive behavior.

In the effort to eliminate the stigma, we had exceeded the bounds of science and common sense. A contradiction ensued: aberrant behavior was normalized and tolerated, but because no one was responsible for its consequences, this "normalized" behavior could be used as a defense in court. The new terms led to a broad concept of victimology, where everyone is a victim but no one is crazy (see chapter 13). Before this could be fully accomplished, however, two hurdles had to be surmounted. First, the diagnostic nomenclature had to be reconstituted and expanded so that all of this normalized behavior would continue to be reimbursable through health insurance under its new, nonillness terminology. Also, there needed to be instituted some kind of societal acceptance of a system that lacked scientific credibility for its assertions.

The breakthrough came in 1954 when Judge David L. Bazelon, Chief Justice of the Circuit Court of Appeals for the District of Columbia, expanded the insanity defense in criminal law. In the landmark *Durham vs. United States* decision, Judge Bazelon referred several times to the "science of psychiatry" and firmly established a science where there was none, and where intrinsically there still is none (Bazelon, 1987). During the 1960s the concept of responsibility was progressively eroded, and psychologists and psychiatrists were called as experts to render "scientific" testimony that more often than not was contradictory and sometimes crossed into the theater of the absurd. Thus, we had the Twinkie defense in the murder of San Francisco Supervisor Harvey Milk, in which experts on diminished capacity resulting from too much sugar intake prevailed and set the stage for even less likely expertise to follow (see chapter 5). Those with appropriate professional degrees and credentials (psychologist or psychiatrist) were hereafter recognized as experts in the *science* of psychiatry, and thus empowered to utter some of the most unscientific statements ever recorded in the courtroom.

As the nation emerged from the expanded legal defense concepts that proliferated in the 1960s, the 1970s began in earnest the reformulation of psychiatric diagnosis. *The Diagnostic and Statistical Manual* of the American Psychiatric Association yielded suddenly and completely to political pressure when in 1973 it removed homosexuality as a treatable aberrant condition. A political firestorm had been created by gay activists within psychiatry, with intense opposition to normalizing homosexuality coming from a few outspoken psychiatrists who were demonized and even threatened, rather than scientifically refuted. Psychiatry's House of Delegates sidestepped the conflict by putting the matter to a vote of the membership, marking the first time in the history of healthcare that a diagnosis or lack of diagnosis was decided by popular vote rather than by scientific evidence.

The point here is not what was done, but how it was done. The coauthor of this chapter (Cummings) not only agrees with the outcome, but also during 1974 introduced in the Council of Representatives of the American Psychological Association (APA) the successful resolution that homosexuality is not a psychiatric condition. The year after that he introduced a successful followup resolution that stated there is no occupation for which being homosexual should be a barrier to employment. These resolutions carried with them the proscription that appropriate and needed research would be conducted to substantiate these decisions. Cummings watched with dismay as there was no effort on the part of the APA to promote or even encourage such required research. The two APAs had established forever that medical and psychological diagnoses are subject to political fiat. Diagnosis today in psychology and psychiatry is cluttered with politically correct verbiage, which seemingly has taken precedence over sound professional experience and scientific validation.

POLITICAL CORRECTNESS AS AN ALTERNATIVE TO SOLUTIONS

The field of psychology is severely fractionated into almost sixty formal divisions and fifty state associations, which compete for seats on the organization's governing body, the Council of Representatives. These divisions range from the subfields within psychology, such as experimental psychology, clinical psychology, counseling psychology, military psychology, and psychopharmacology, to the more ideological groups, such as the Society for Consumer Psychology, humanistic psychology, Society for the Psychology of Women, Society for the Psychological Study of Lesbian, Gay and Bisexual Issues, ethnic minority issues, peace psychology, and international psychology. Originally intended as units organized around special interests and concerns within psychology, they have become power bases and self-interest groups that fiercely vie against one another for the limited number of seats on the Council of Representatives in order to influence the course and commitments of the APA.

As pervasive as this fractionation is, it pales when compared to the chasm that divides scientific psychology from professional (practice) psychology. The animosities are deep and go back almost three-quarters of a century when the clinical psychologists, feeling ignored by the academically dominated APA, bolted and formed a separate organization. They subsequently returned and set out to change the APA from within (Wright & Cummings, 2000). Scientists have since formed their own American Psychological Society, which continues its only partially effective existence. The APA remains the overarching battleground for the accelerating clash between science and practice. The latest hostilities involve scientists' insistence on evidence-based therapies (EBTs), whereas practitioners reject such protocols as having no credible applicability in the real world. Neither is advancing its cause, yet neither will give ground.

With each side dug in, American psychology is facing a kind of stagnated trench warfare in which not very much gets done. Complete paralysis would surely have been the case were it not for a third force, the politically correct group that can tilt the battle one way or another and thus has become the deciding power. It was inevitable that both the academic and scientific sides would pander to this power, moving the organization farther into runaway political correctness. The official name for this politically correct group is public interest psychology. Although most psychologists are generally sympathetic to its tenets, the psychologists who primary identify with the name represent the fanatics who have moved the APA perilously closer to extreme stances.

While this internecine warfare rages, the practice of psychology has become beleaguered. Fixated on its internal battles, psychology was totally unprepared for the industrialization of healthcare, particularly the behavioral healthcare that burgeoned in the latter two decades of the last century. It continues to be unable or unwilling to change to meet the new challenges, and practitioners' incomes are declining. Solutions are proffered and rejected by a fractionated constituency, and depression and paralysis would ensue were it not for the feel-good nonsolution of passing resolution after resolution on diversity, sensitivity, homophobia, purging of the language, and a plethora of other politically correct concepts that divert attention from the failure to solve the crises facing the science and profession.

This is not to diminish the importance of social action, but when it serves as a diversion or masks a failure to solve a problem, it can be destructive. Psychology could become the most diverse and politically correct doctoral profession in healthcare and at the same time be its lowest paid and most economically depressed. The failure of the psychological field to solve its problems is a chronic phenomenon. Mental health is replete with feel-good nonsolutions that have corrupted its professional practice and crippled its science so it no longer can curb its excessive political correctness. Meanwhile, the most basic problems remain.

When someone gets into trouble because of aberrant behavior that we have normalized, we blame it on "diminished capacity" and excuse the conduct. This makes everyone a victim, and no one mentally ill. This attitude impedes us from helping the patient toward resiliency, self-sufficiency, and autonomy, which should be the goals of psychotherapy. Turning "emotional problems" into "issues" does not lessen the magnitude of these problems. Being "emotionally challenged" rather than "neurotic" does not make one less abnormal. Research on intelligence has virtually come to a halt because those conducting such studies are branded as racists. As a consequence, we are stymied in solving such pressing problems as poor results in our inner city schools (see chapter 9). Everything in nature is distributed along a bell curve, except intelligence, at least according to political correctness. However, referring to someone as "intellectually challenged" rather than "mentally retarded" does not raise IQ.

Psychology Has No Definition of Competence in Practice

The Boulder Conference in 1948 determined that the science of psychology had not sufficiently progressed to warrant a profession of psychology, and that practicing psychologists should be trained primarily as scientists and only secondarily as practitioners. This was termed the scientist–professional model. Although it was too early at that time to develop a definition of professional competence, in the ensuing half century dozens of conferences have been convened and there has been no consensus on a definition of competence. Manifestly, if psychologists do not know what constitutes a competent psychologist, the public has even less of a clue. It should not be a surprise that practitioners range from very competent to incompetent, with some bordering on quackery. As an example, when a group of psychologists in Sedona, Arizona, began practicing mineral therapy that involved having patients enhance therapeutic insights by holding minerals during the session, they defended their behavior before the licensing board by saying that they were practicing within their community's standards. Sedona is identifiably a new-age community, however, it is still incumbent on the profession to eliminate quackery and educate the public on what constitutes sound practice. The APA Code of Ethics, upon which state licensing boards base their investigations, states merely that it is unethical for a psychologist to practice beyond his or her competence, which is tantamount to saying nothing.

The Training of Practitioners Has No Nationally Accepted Core Curriculum

The consensus at the Boulder Conference that the enunciation of a universal core curriculum for the training of professional psychologists should be left to the future has been replaced after dozens of conferences with the dictum, "Let a thousand flowers bloom" (apparently with no apologies to Chairman Mao, who coined the phrase before being denounced by his own people). In short, there is no universal core curriculum, and it is left to individual institutions to set a core curriculum commensurate with their educational goals (see Benjamin, 2001; Cummings, 2003). So while we wait for a thousand flowers to bloom, the garden is inundated with weeds. The various psychotherapies are in conflict with one another, and some interventions are considered outrageous and/or dangerous. Psychological experts line up in court hearings to testify and contradict one another, leaving the public bewildered and skeptical of psychology.

Yet although a consensus on a core curriculum is lacking, the APA does not hesitate to mandate courses on diversity, sensitivity, multiculturalism, and other subjects that bring kudos from an often self-serving, politically correct group, absent an iota of evidence that such politically correct interventions are effective. These same proponents would make treatment of patients from ethnic or sexual minorities by therapists of different groups unethical unless such therapists have taken a course in sensitivity, typically taught by one of the politically correct elite. We have in the 112 years since the APA's founding failed to identify the learning basic to professional psychology, but we can still feel good because we have made significant progress in social issues.

POLITICAL CORRECTNESS DICTATES TREATMENT

Psychological practice is replete with examples in which political correctness has altered the treatment process, sometimes for the better but often for the worse, as the following few examples illustrate.

Victimology Replaces Resiliency

People make choices in life that are followed by consequences. However, in today's psychological climate, everyone is considered a hapless victim and not responsible for the consequences of his or her own actions. Thus, the widow of a lifelong smoker, who was urged by his physician for the past twenty years to quit, can sue the tobacco company for addicting her husband. And it does not stop there. No sooner had articles been published in the 2004 medical journals stating that women are harmed more than men by smoking than the daughter of a smoker filed a lawsuit claiming the tobacco company had not acknowledged in its package warning label that women were more prone to lung cancer than men. Thus, the company was responsible for her mother's death.

Similarly, obesity is "caused" by McDonald's and Dunkin' Donuts because they sell fattening food, and TV (not parents) is responsible for the growing sedentary problem among children. And now the Social Security Administration has pronounced that obesity is a disease, paving the way for a plethora of stomach stapling. Although tremendous pressure exists to do something about the epidemic of obesity, once again we have removed all personal liability and the impetus to behave responsibly. Stomach bypass will become the implant litigation of the future, and the long-term effects will be severe. Negating personal responsibility goes on and on, influencing psychotherapy as well as the legal system (see chapter 3).

Psychology not only has uncritically accepted victimology, it enforces this concept by accusing practitioners who do not subscribe to its tenets of "blaming the victim." Forgotten is the work of Seligman (1975, 1994) and others who demonstrated that "learned helplessness," such as that promoted inadvertently by victimology, can prevent or retard the individual from emerging from adversity, trauma, loss, or disability. Patients who feel helpless are relieved of responsibility and might welcome a sympathetic psychotherapist who tells them they are victims, thus creating a dependency and perhaps ensuring the steady income of the practitioner. In the meantime, the patient becomes further entrenched in helplessness. This outcome is not the basis upon which therapy is founded, which is to restore the individual to optimum functioning and well-being as soon as possible and with the least intrusive intervention.

Crisis Counseling Can Impair Recovery

During the past two decades there has been a growing trend to rush psychological counselors to the scene of a disaster, be it San Francisco's 1989 earthquake, the Columbine High School massacre, or the World Trade Center terrorist attack. This tactic has mushroomed until a common incident such as the automobile accident death of a high school student requires the stepping in of counselors to console the entire school population, many of whom barely knew the deceased. In fact, use of counselors in even mundane misfortunes has become pro forma, and institutions fear that failure to provide them may be the basis for a lawsuit.

Recently, however, a growing body of research (McNally, 2003; see also Lebow, 2003) says that such early interventions are of marginal help at best and can be deleterious at worst; at the very least, they encourage histrionics and may prolong the crisis and impair healing. Following a crisis, it is better to make psychotherapeutic services readily available through regular channels for those in whom the emotional reaction persists, rather than blanket a whole population as in need of immediate intervention. But it has become politically correct to rush counselors to any scene of tragedy, whether major or minor. Again, extensive crisis counseling can ensure employment for counselors, but is it good or necessary for the public?

Americans Ostensibly Live under Stress

All kinds of questionable studies allege that Americans live under constant stress, resulting in all sorts of malfunctioning. Most of these studies involve those who are, in fact, stressed-out, rather than the population at large. So generally accepted is this notion within psychology that one APA president (Max Siegel) officially declared that everyone can benefit from psychotherapy. In spite of evidence that unnecessary psychotherapy can foster dependency and other untoward effects, the more the public believes this concept, the more likely psychologists will experience full employment.

Recent research casts serious doubts on the notion that most individuals are stressed beyond what is healthy. In reviewing the evidence, it can be concluded that psychology has considerably underestimated the human capacity for resilience (see, for example, Bonanno, 2004), and that fostering such beliefs can negatively alter brain chemistry to hurt rather than heal (Ray, 2004). Even the hoped-for surge of stressed-out patients has backfired; patients who believe they are stressed or depressed turn to the expediency of psychotropic drugs rather than psychotherapy, thus enriching drug manufacturers and poorly trained physicians and psychiatrists, not psychology. While the demand for medication increases, the demand for psychotherapy decreases, spurring psychologists to fight even harder to obtain prescription authority as a way of saving the profession.

Best Practices Do Not Exist in Organized Psychology

The concept of "best practices," or the need to separate the wheat from the chaff in healthcare, exists in nearly every branch of medicine, even though it may vary in terms of success or failure. This concept can be dated back two millennia to Hippocrates, who said that the obligation of every physician is to first do no harm, and then provide the patient with the best practice available. A system to determine best practice does not exist in organized psychology, and separating good practice from questionable practice is left to the scientific process of research, replication, debate, and, more often than not, inconclusiveness. "Tried-and-true" methods are, by necessity, the scientific way, but the practice of psychology does not have such luxury because in the interim it can do harm.

The first attempt by the APA to address a pressing practice issue came in response to the surge a few years ago of the so-called recovery of repressed incest memories that sent many innocent fathers to prison. Researchers in recovered memory (such as Loftus, 1993) found evidence that such "memories" could be created in the susceptible individual, especially under conditions of hypnosis or the repeated prodding of an overly zealous practitioner.

The debate became so compelling that the APA appointed a taskforce to make recommendations on the matter because society was in dire need of a scientific and professional resolution to a psychotherapeutic procedure that was getting out of hand. The taskforce met for several years and was bogged down by political correctness. Those who proposed caution and attention to the pertinent research were accused of being antifeminist, indifferent to the plight of incest survivors, or supportive of male paternalism that was the root cause of incest. The matter was settled not by psychology but by the courts, which determined that the propensity for the recovery of false memories was overwhelming. The judicial system spent the next decade releasing fathers from prison and punishing the overly zealous practitioners who had inadvertently implanted the false memories.

The debate still rages within psychology, while society has settled the matter in its own way and without definitive professional or scientific input from psychology. Even the most ardent proponents of recovered incest memories no longer press their patients to seek legal redress because of the chilling effect on such practice not by the profession but by the courts.

Within the concept of letting a thousand flowers bloom, psychology has rendered itself incapable of addressing the issue of best practices. In the interim, questionable and sometimes harmful practices are settled by the courts: from rebirthing, in which children have suffocated, to eye movement desensitization response (EMDR), which awaits the long process of scientific scrutiny (Lebow, 2003). In rebirthing there was immediate harm; in practices like Werner Erhardt's EST (now thankfully defunct) and EMDR the worst might be that many patients wasted a lot of money and were deprived of real treatment in the meantime. Even the latter is no small matter and makes the striving for best practices by the profession of psychology a compelling one. While organized psychology does nothing, behavioral managed care companies have addressed the issue of best practices. This is a step in the right direction, but without the expert participation of the profession, best practices might become just another way for managed care to limit services. As the courts by default have defined certain best practices in their own way, managed care may do the same.

Because political correctness is often the force that breaks the science versus practice deadlock, decisions may be dictated by ideology rather than either scientific facts or practice experience. Let us look at two examples.

Capitulation to Nader's Raiders

In the mid-1970s, Ralph Nader mounted an attack on standardized psychological tests during a time when testing in the schools and at work was under scrutiny. This so intimidated the APA board of directors that it invited Mr. Nader to Washington, where he was wined and dined. Most, if not all, of Nader's assertions could have been refuted, but psychology had already accepted him as an icon and had pretty much sympathized with the politically correct notion that psychological testing can be deleterious to minorities and others. In short, the board was hoping to appease him and reach an amicable resolution.

During the course of his dialogue with the APA board, it was discovered that the basis of the attack came from the work of two Nader's Raiders who were undergraduates, with no graduate courses in psychology and absolutely no training in test construction or in measurement. Their report was mostly rhetorical, inflammatory, and with little substance. The two editors of this volume were members of the board at the time and wanted to expose this attack as scurrilous, making public its amateurish and grossly unscientific/unprofessional basis. The intimidated board balked, and instead wrote a polite letter to Nader, who then went on to bigger game. In the meantime, the report attacking psychological testing stood in its most unsubstantiated form, and was later widely quoted in lawsuits against school districts, as well as in other matters. The board referred the matter to its Board of Social and Ethical Responsibility in Psychology, which was the most politically correct group within APA. There the request that the Nader report be refuted brought contempt, accusations, and name calling against its proponent (Cummings), without a semblance of scientific or professional counterargument. This is just one incident in which psychology surrendered to political correctness.

Is Treating Homosexuality Unethical?

Although the APA is reluctant or unable to evaluate questionable practices and has thus avoided addressing the issue of best practices, this did not prevent its Council of Representatives in 2002 from stampeding into a motion to declare the treatment of homosexuality unethical. This was done with the intent of perpetuating homosexuality, even when the homosexual patient willingly and even eagerly seeks treatment. The argument was that because homosexuality is not an illness, its treatment is unnecessary and unethical. Curiously, and rightly so, there was no counterargument against psychological interventions conducted by gay therapists to help patients be gay, such as those over many decades by leading psychologist and personal friend Donald Clark (the author of the best-selling *Living Gay)* and many others. Vigorously pushed by the gay lobby, it was eventually seen by a sufficient number of Council members as runaway political correctness and was defeated by the narrowest of margins. In a series of courageous letters to the various components of APA, former president Robert Perloff referred to the willingness of many psychologists to trample patients' rights to treatment in the interest of political correctness. He pointed out that making such treatment unethical would deprive a patient of a treatment of choice because the threat of sanctions would eliminate any psychologist who engaged in such treatment. Although the resolution was narrowly defeated, this has not stopped its proponents from deriding colleagues who provide such treatment to patients seeking it.

DEADLOCK, STAGNATION, AND THE CONTINUED DECLINE OF PRACTICE

In the deadlock between the science and profession of psychology, it is difficult to imagine a situation where both sides could be so right and, at the same time, so wrong. The blanket opposition to evidence-based treatments is indefensible, inasmuch as all healthcare strives for scientific verification. Yet it is difficult to translate pristine laboratory findings based on pure cases for experimental purposes into real-life patients who characteristically have co-morbidities. Psychologists whose training has centered on "manualized" techniques have been shown to be poor therapists, stilted and unimaginative at best. Conversely, psychologists trained with insufficient scientific foundation are subject to espousing faddist therapies and even promoting harmful ones. Treatments subjected to research are those that are easily quantified, not those most needed. Manuals, by default, may prematurely become the standards of practice in courts of law, leaving therapists practicing outside of manuals helpless to defend their interventions. In the meantime, financially beleaguered malpractice insurance carriers may limit coverage to EBTs, effectively curbing effective therapy that is not "manualized." Finally, the managed care companies that in the courts and legislatures have lost the ability to override the recommendations of the doctor may seize on the movement to limit reimbursement to EBTs only, thus creating a new way of withholding care.

What is needed is the field testing of EBTs in large delivery systems. Few scientific psychologists have the inclination to conduct this kind of research, and practitioners do not know how to do it. Yet the template exists. During the years it was psychologically driven, American Biodyne subjected validated treatments to field research in a system with 14.5 million covered patients and 10,000 psychotherapists. Formulating treatment that was both effective and efficient was a race without a finish line, as protocols and training were subjected to the field, then back to the laboratory, and back to the field again in a never-ending cycle of fine-tuning. The result was that in the ten years the system was in place in a large population spanning 39 states, there was not a single malpractice suit or patient complaint that had to be adjudicated. The methodology does exist. The APA needs to appoint a commission to promote this solution, a commission that will not be sidetracked by the diversionary issues of political correctness.

POLITICAL CORRECTNESS DEFINES WHAT IS PERMISSIBLE

Political correctness attempts to define permissible and impermissible behavior, particularly pertaining to beliefs and speech. There are four major problems with this practice:

1. Proscriptions and prescriptions associated with political correctness are generated by fiat rather than by reasoned argument.
2. PC frequently rests on the notion that a speech or belief is "offensive" to someone, often because of an individual's membership in a group that allegedly is experiencing discrimination or other unfair treatment. However, such phenomenological reports of offensiveness (or "uncomfortableness") are difficult to verify independently, and, more important, may result from the person's hypersensitivity (perhaps even carefully cultivated), rather than a substantive offense.
3. By focusing exclusively on "offensiveness," political correctness misses more overriding considerations such as legal rights to free speech.
4. The remedies and punishments for real or apparent transgressions of the PC rules tend to be overly severe (e.g., loss of job, ruined reputation, large monetary awards) and often are tendered based on problematic investigatory and administrative processes (Avina, Bowers, & Donahue, 2004).

To be critical of political correctness is not to condone unfair treatment towards certain individuals or to deny that prejudices and problematic practices exist. Rather, it involves concern with the way political correctness defines the problems and the remedies for these situations. We believe, for example, that some groups are discriminated against and that this prejudice needs to be understood so it can be eradicated. But we also believe that the social problems facing many individuals are complex and may involve factors that are not condoned by the PC worldview (e.g., reverse prejudice or other problematic behaviors of the "victim" group). We do not discuss the epistemic problems with PC claims and practices or the associated social injustice inasmuch as this has been discussed elsewhere (e.g., Kors & Silvergate, 1998). Rather, the next two sections discuss two other major issues: the psychology of political correctness, and the negative influence political correctness can have on scientific psychology.

THE PSYCHOLOGY OF POLITICAL CORRECTNESS

It is unfortunate that psychologists (perhaps because they have been swept up in the movement) have not empirically studied the psychology of political correctness. Thus, currently we have little data to go on. In short, it is politically incorrect to question political correctness. Here we attempt to provide a response to the question, "What psychological functions does political correctness fulfill for the individual?" and the related question, "What is the attraction of political correctness to certain personalities?" What follows are some hypotheses that we have constructed in an effort to understand this behavioral phenomenon and spur its study.

Political Correctness Harbors Hostility

Political correctness allows significant hostility to be expressed in ways that have become socially sanctioned and even valued. This is essentially the view expressed by the German philosopher Friedrich Nietzsche when he said that "to claim victimization is the most hostile, aggressive act." Individuals may feel hostile toward the values of their parents or the perceived establishment, or toward some groups such as males. Their involvement with political correctness allows them to attack these entities.

Daphne Patai (1998), for example, has argued that much of what she calls "the sexual harassment industry" is oriented toward punishing any evidence of heterosexuality rather than really protecting women from a violation of their rights. She sees this as evidence of what she interestingly calls "heterophobia." The question then becomes, to what extent is a PC approach to sexual harassment a mechanism to express hostility toward heterosexuals, particularly male heterosexuals, rather than simply a way of addressing the problem of women being harassed? Similar questions can be addressed toward other favorite targets of the PC movement.

Political Correctness Reflects Narcissism

Political correctness, with its unarguable dogmatic presentation (with any counterargument being construed as evidence of a moral failing on the part of the dissenter rather than a reasonable expression of a differing view) is evidence of a type of narcissism. To use Thomas Sowell's (1995) felicitous phrase, it is an expression of "the vision of the anointed." It can involve a process in which one can conspicuously display one's exquisite sensitivity ("I'm offended by your failure to include any X in your subject sample or in your committee") or one's sensitivity to the wonderful sensitivity of others ("I feel your pain"). This psychological mechanism involves a strange game of sensitivity one-up-(person)ship in which the victor gains the moral high ground.

Political Correctness Masks Histrionics

Political correctness may be associated with histrionic tendencies. Problems in the PC worldview often become tremendous crises that contain dramatic exaggerations: for example, the prominent feminist Catherine McKinnon's (1987) claim that "All men are rapists." Instead of a sober description of a problem that can lead to effective problem solving, the problem and its solutions (Take Back the Night marches) are handled in dramatic, attention-grabbing style.

Political Correctness Functions as Instant Morality

Political correctness is an easy way to appear moral (concerned, active) on certain important issues relevant to justice and morality, without, in fact, exerting much effort or making any sacrifices. The more traditional moral view involves sacrifices such as tithing, good works such as volunteering in soup kitchens, and even "tough love" to help those leading harmful lifestyles learn responsibility and more ethical conduct (Olasky, 1995). Instead, political correctness offers simplistic remedies such as the correct semantic labeling of minority groups ("African Americans," not "Blacks") and affirmative action, which forces younger generations to have different employment opportunities than those that were available to individuals currently holding jobs. For some reason, political correctness proponents feel very moral when they force others—younger, poorer individuals in the current job pool— to bear all the costs of the "solution" to the employment problem.

Political Correctness Wields Power

Political correctness is a way for certain individuals to gain control and power in situations that are difficult or that may raise self-doubts about worth and efficacy. Thus, simply due to their demographic characteristics, individuals become "experts" whose input must be gathered and factored into decision making, without any consideration about whether they actually are experts on the issues at hand. Ann Coulter (2002) in her book *Slander* describes how in the politically correct arena individuals are intimidated into acting or speaking in certain ways because the PC are ready to trot out very damning, slandering labels that can cause significant injury to those who dare to differ.

Political Correctness Serves as Distraction

Political correctness may be a way of conveniently distracting attention from certain aspects of one's self or one's group. Having others defend themselves in response to serious accusations can keep the attention of others away from problems that political correctness does not want to address.

Political Correctness Involves Intimidation

Acceptance and tolerance of political correctness involve a combination of guilt and lack of assertiveness. Individuals can be intimidated and lack the courage or assertiveness to respond adequately to this coercion. This is the case with society's attack on and general devaluing of masculinity and behaviors generally associated with being male. So true is this that strong active resistance to these threats and intimidation is seen as more problematic than the slander and intimidation associated with the PC attack in the first place.

Political Correctness Lacks Alternatives

Political correctness may stem from the fact that some individuals do not understand how to implement other less harmful and more effective ways of addressing existing problems. Critical thinking and liberal education have largely failed (Bloom, 1988), and the many individuals who adopt their values and political beliefs from media such as television and Hollywood tend to dole out the politically correct doctrine.

It would be interesting to investigate to what extent these hypotheses can be corroborated or falsified. We are not claiming that these propositions are true. Our argument is that most issues are more complex than they appear at first and do not lend themselves to a quick politically correct fix, however psychologically attractive the "solution" appears to certain individuals. Psychologists should empirically investigate this psychological complexity. We admit that our hypotheses are oriented to finding out what is psychologically wrong with those endorsing political correctness and are mindful that some may find this approach misguided. We certainly countenance the possibility that some individuals endorse politically correct views for relatively innocuous psychological reasons. However, others do not.

POLITICAL CORRECTNESS AND PSYCHOLOGICAL SCIENCE

O'Donohue (1989) in an *American Psychologist* article, notes how general background beliefs affect the practice of science. This view was based on the argument of the prominent science philosopher Karl Popper: that science springs from our folk beliefs about the world. O'Donohue's view was also shaped by the prominent analytic philosopher W.V.O. Quine, who argued that our entire web of belief (his phrase) is always involved both semantically and epistemically in any claim or any test of any claim (see O'Donohue, 1989 for an elaboration of the logic associated with these claims). Here we briefly describe the pernicious effects of political correctness on the practice of psychological science.

First, note that the popular *bête noir* of the politically correct with respect to science is the Roman Catholic Church. Their claims include assertions that the Church is hostile to science and interferes with research, which results in jeopardizing the jobs of psychological scientists, especially in Catholic universities. Furthermore, it is alleged that the Catholic Church brooks no dissent on certain moral issues, ostracizing scientists who dare to believe differently. There's also the assertion that the Church makes certain questions off limits for research, such as the moral status of homosexuality. These allegations are also used to justify tenure, picturing faculty as hapless pawns without such protection.

These claims constitute a red herring. Careful examination reveals that the Catholic Church has not interfered with the independence of science and the freedom of academia for well over a half-century, and the consistent playing of the Galileo card after four centuries suggests lack of a better scapegoat. To be sure, there are a number of evangelical colleges and universities that require a creedal oath from its faculty; as a result these institutions are not known for their unfettered research accomplishments. Furthermore, these evangelical campuses attract faculty that are in sympathy with the religious dogmas, and internal challenges to their academic freedom (or lack of it) simply do not occur. In academia today faculty members and researchers do not fear losing jobs or tenure because their views clash with the Church. And because modern psychology is little more than a century old, it has never experienced negative influence from the Catholic Church. Clearly, something else is going on.

If one merely substitutes the "politically correct" for "the Church" in the previous paragraphs, as we have done below, then these statements are true. It is interesting, albeit alarming, that this real threat to the free practice of science is unrecognized while the red herring is widely blamed.

- Political correctness is hostile to science. At times the PC view holds that science itself is biased because of some alleged fault (e.g., its association with big business), or because it is Eurocentric or based on a male viewpoint. Thus, the PC can dismiss any scientific finding that they consider to be problematic and instead dogmatically assert claims more in line with their ideology or agenda. Thus, political correctness and the postmodernism that currently pervades academic psychology go hand in hand.
- Political correctness is associated with hostility toward certain research questions: for example, false allegations of sexual abuse, genetic basis of intelligence, or the role of out-of-wedlock births in poverty. Scientists pursuing these questions often face hostility and a variety of negative consequences (e.g., note reactions in academia to Herrnstein and Murray's *The Bell Curve* (1994), as well as to the Gottfredson article that constitutes a chapter in this volume). This can have a chilling effect on science as the PC movement creates real dangers in posing certain questions.
- Political correctness can view certain questions as settled moral issues rather than empirical questions requiring investigation. Thus, those dissenting from the PC view are viewed as morally problematic or as simply holding an incorrect empirical belief. As we discussed previously, the status of homosexuality is a settled moral question to those in the PC movement. The National Endowment of the Arts would see those objecting to *Piss Christ* as infringing on the freedom of expression of certain artists but would simply see something like *Piss Gay* as offensive and morally wrong.

- Political correctness is entrenched in many of the institutions of science, including universities (see Kors and Silvergate, 1998) as well as government agencies that influence research; thus, PC can dictate priorities and policies affecting science. Two cases in point are determining funding priorities (AIDS vs. breast cancer) and the contemporary practice of evaluating grants by federally determined categories of minority inclusion.

SOLUTIONS

A first step in solving a problem involves recognizing the problem. Thus, we think it is crucial that psychologists recognize and respond to all threats to free scientific inquiry, sound practice, and free political speech rather than be satisfied with a false sense of courage as they quixotically bluster against windmills (e.g., the contemporary Catholic Church, the Republican Party, and the skeptics of come-and-go Chicken Little warnings that the sky is falling). This will require them to review how their own political and ideological biases affect their behavior and possibly harm others. We think it is critically important that psychologists embrace and enforce free speech rights. Free speech has legitimate limits—such as hate speech—which psychologists should rigorously condemn. But at the same time no Orwellian moves should be countenanced in which "uncomfortableness" or other such proxies are substituted for actual hate speech.

Another solution is to embrace and enforce an ethic surrounding the allegations associated with the PC movement. It has become too easy to accuse. Persons who are members of a federally determined protected class are rarely held accountable for their allegations (e.g., witness that an individual prominently involved in false rape allegations against White police officers was able to become a presidential candidate for the Democratic party). This laxity has allowed many to accuse first, and then try to muster facts later, if at all. Some politically correct proponents make accusations against entire groups (all males are rapists) or against some individuals (X is a racist). These accusations are serious matters and have tremendous potential to do lasting harm. If there is evidence that all males are rapists, it is a reasonable and just claim. If this evidence does not exist, then it is a false and harmful allegation. The ethic of accusation should involve something similar to an indictment process. The accuser should be able to immediately muster some fairly convincing evidence that such claims are warranted. If such evidence is clearly missing, the accused should not have the burden of further clearing his or her name; rather, the accuser should experience appropriate consequences.

REFERENCES

Avina, C., Bowers, A., & O'Donohue. W. (2004). Sexual harassment. In W. O'Donohue & E. Levensky (Eds.), *Handbook of Forensic Psychology.* New York: Academic Press.

Bazelon, D.L. (1987). *Questioning Authority: Justice and Criminal Law.* New York: Knopf.

Benjamin, L.T. (2001). American psychology's struggle with its curriculum: Should a thousand flowers bloom? *American Psychologist, 56,* 67–73.

Bloom, A. (1988). *The Closing of the American Mind.* Chicago: University of Chicago Press.

Bonanno, G.A. (2004). Loss, trauma and human resilience. *American Psychologist, 59*(1), 20–28.

Carson, R. (1962). *Silent Spring.* New York: Houghton Mifflin.

Clinton, W.J. (1999). President's testimony before the grand jury investigating the Monica Lewinsky matter.

Coulter, A. (2002). *Slander.* New York: Crown Forum.

Cummings, N.A. (2003). Just one more time: Competencies as a refrain. *Register Report, 29* (Spring), 4–5.

Cummings, N.A. & Wiggins, J.G. (2001). A collaborative primary care/behavioral health model for the use of psychotropic medication with children and adolescents. *Issues in Interdisciplinary Care, 3*(2), 121–128.

Ehrlich, P.R. (1968). *The Population Bomb.* New York: Sierra Club–Ballantine.

Feiffer, J. (2003). Thoughts on the business of life. *Forbes, 171*(7), March 21, p. 126.

Glasser, W. (2003). *Psychiatry Can Be Hazardous to Your Mental Health.* New York: Harper-Collins.

Healy, M.C. (2004). Testimony before the Federal Drug Administration, Feb. 2. www.FDA.gov or sscpnet@listserve.it.northwestern.edu.

Herrnstein, R. J., & Murray, C. (1994). *The Bell Curve.* New York: Free Press.

Huxley, A. (1935). *Brave New World.* New York: Random House.

Kirsch, I. & Antonuccio, D. (2004). Testimony before the Federal Drug Administration, Feb. 2. www.FDA.gov or sscpnet@listserve.it.northwestern.edu.

Kors, A.C. & Silvergate, H.A. (1998). *The Shadow University: The Betrayal of Liberty on America's Campuses.* New York: Free Press.

Lebow, J. (2003). War of the worlds: Researchers and practitioners collide on EMDR and CISD. *Psychotherapy Networker,* September/October, 79–83.

Loftus, E.F. (1993). The reality of repressed memories. *American Psychologist, 68*(5), 518–537.

Lomborg, B. (2000). *The Skeptical Environmentalist.* London: Cambridge University Press.

McKinnon, C.A. (1987). *Feminism Unmodified: Discourses on Life and Law.* Cambridge: Harvard University Press.

McNally, R. (2003). As extensively quoted in S. Begley, Is trauma debriefing worse than letting victims heal naturally? *Wall Street Journal,* September 12, B1.

Minde, K. (1998). The use of psychotropic medication in preschoolers: Some recent developments. *Canadian Journal of Psychiatry, 43,* 571–575.

Newsweek (1975). The cooling earth. (April 28, pp. 11–53). New York: Author.

O'Donohue, W.T. (1989). The (even) bolder model: The clinical psychologist as metaphysician-scientist-practitioner. *American Psychologist, 44*(12), 1460–1468.

Olasky, M. (1995). *The Tragedy of American Compassion.* New York: Regnery.

Orwell, G. (1961). *1984.* New York: New American Library.

Patai, D. (1998). *Heterophobia: Sexual Harassment and the Future of Feminism*. New York: Rowman and Littlefield.

Ray, O. (2004). How the mind hurts and heals the body. *American Psychologist, 59*(1), 29–40.

Revel, J.F. (1991). *The Flight from the Truth: The Reign of Deceit in the Age of Information*. New York: Random House.

Seligman, M.E.P. (1975). *Helplessness: On Depression, Development and Death*. San Francisco: W.H. Freeman.

Seligman, M.E.P. (1994). *What You Can Change and What You Can't*. New York: Knopf.

Shilts, R. (1987). *And the Band Played on: Politics, People and the AIDS Epidemic*. New York: St. Martin's.

Sommers, C.H. (1994). *Who Stole Feminism? How Women Have Betrayed Women*. New York: Simon & Schuster.

Sowell, T. (1995). *The Vision of the Anointed*. New York: Basic.

U.S. Bureau of the Census (1991). *Current Population Reports*, Series P60–185. Washington, DC: U.S. Government Printing Office.

Whittle, R.J., Jr. (1992). *Rude Awakenings: What the Homeless Crisis Tells Us*. San Francisco: ICS Press.

Wright, R.H. & Cummings, N.A. (2000). *The Practice of Psychology: The Battle for Professionalism*. Phoenix, AZ: Zeig, Tucker & Theisen.

Zito, J.M., Safer, D.J., dosReis, S., Gardner, J.F., Boles, M., & Lynch, F. (2004). Trends in prescribing psychotropic medications to preschoolers. *Journal of the American Medical Association, 283*, 1025–1030.

2

CULTURAL SENSITIVITY: A CRITICAL EXAMINATION

William T. O'Donohue

This chapter critically evaluates the increasingly important issue of cultural sensitivity, including problems parsing and validly attributing cultural status, the lack of clarity about what constitutes cultural sensitivity, the implications for ethically mandated behaviour, as well as the unintended negative effects that can result.

BACKGROUND SKETCH

For much of its first century, psychology was little concerned with "culture." To be sure, even in psychology's early years there were some reservations about differences from nation to nation: for example, concerns about American rats acting American (or at least interpreted as doing so), British rats acting British, and German and Russian rats acting German and Russian, respectively. Later, culture came to play a more systematic and formal role in the subdiscipline of cross-cultural psychology (e.g., Berman, 1989). One of the major questions this subfield addressed was the generalizability of regularities across international groups, although it mainly investigated the extent to which North American results could be generalized to other countries.

In the last two decades, however, the construct of cultural sensitivity has played an increasingly central role in mainstream psychology. As the demographics of the United States continue to shift to include greater proportions of people representing ethnic minority populations, what has come to be known as "cultural sensitivity" is stressed, and even ethically prescribed, for many of the major activities of the psychologist. These activities include formulating problems, devising adequate explanatory theories, constructing measurement instruments, analyzing and interpreting data, disseminating research findings, training students, designing effective therapies, forming goals in therapy, delivering services, and eliminating barriers to services (Bernal & Castro, 1994; Betancourt & Lopez, 1993; Closser & Blow, 1993; Dumas et al.1999; Korchin, 1980; Matthews, 1997; Rogler, 1999; Sasao & Sue, 1993; Sue & Zane, 1987). As a case in point, research grants are now judged by the National Institutes of Health on their gender and minority inclusiveness (i.e., cultural categories); if these are determined to be insufficient the grant will not be funded.

Although the need for cultural sensitivity is repeatedly cited in the mainstream literature, exactly what constitutes cultural sensitivity is generally left unspecified. A concern is that mainstream psychology may be paying lip service to cultural sensitivity as acceptable, necessary, and ethical without defining how this concept can be used to enhance the field. We need to look beyond a superficial acceptance of cultural sensitivity and conduct a critical examination of its role in contemporary psychology. We agree with researchers such as Betancourt and Lopez (1993) who assert that the study of culture, ethnicity, and race can be approached by testing "theoretically derived hypotheses" and by directly measuring specified cultural elements. We believe that the study of culture and its cognates constitutes open empirical questions.

WHAT IS CULTURE?

What is the substance of a culture? Farley (1994) offers one definition (apparently "transcultural") of culture as "a complex and global variable that represents the beliefs, language, rules, values, and knowledge held in common by members of a society" (cited in Matthews, 1997, p. 35). Currently, there is no consensus on a definition of culture, and therefore no consensus as to how one goes about conducting culturally sensitive research or how one provides culturally sensitive therapy.

One interesting reflexive issue is whether the notion of culture is itself relative to culture: that is, do various groups differ on what constitutes what we late twentieth century, North American, relatively affluent, highly educated professionals see as culture? It would be somewhat ironic if the construct itself were not inclusive of the variability found across groups on this dimension. It would be particularly ironic if this construct were heavily influenced by a particular set of cultural concerns, say those of upper middle class, highly educated, ameliorative-minded individuals. We have not conducted the proper empirical studies to see how many of the people thought to be helped by the construct of cultural sensitivity actually view it in the same way that scholars and professionals do.

In order to examine the role of culture in psychology, one must both define culture and decide how to parse individuals into these cultural categories. As Dumas et al. (1999) stated, researchers must be aware of the "salient within-group cleavages" (p. 179). Because there is no consensus on what these groups might be, they are left to vary with each study.

Culture Defined by Race and Ethnicity

Two of the most utilized cognates of culture have been race and ethnicity. Ethnicity is a popular distinguishing characteristic used to determine group membership. This construct, however, raises a host of issues. One complicating factor is that the definition of ethnicity is not agreed upon, and at times is used interchangeably with terms such as race and culture. According to Betancourt and Lopez (1993), race, in general, is defined in terms of physical characteristics. Zuckerman (1990), however, argues that "racial groups are more alike than they are different" (p. 1300). Even if physical characteristics are held in common, they do not typically result in the formation of what commonly would be considered a culture. Ethnicity, according to Betancourt and Lopez, is usually used in reference to groups that are characterized in terms of a common nationality, culture, or language. For example, ethnic status defined by Eaton (1980) is "an easily identifiable characteristic that implies a common cultural history with others possessing the same characteristic. The most common ethnic 'identifiers' are race, religion, country of origin, language, and/or cultural background" (cited in Okazaki & Sue, 1998, 160). The amount of commonality necessary is determined by each researcher. As a result, commonality can involve a theoretically driven, thoughtful decision process or be a simple category of convenience.

It is interesting that group categorizations made by the researcher/ therapist may differ from the subject/client's perceived group membership. Sasao (1992) provides an example of the possibility for this type of incongruity in a southern California study of high school students in which "approximately 20 percent of the Chinese students indicated their primary cultural identification was Mexican" (cited in Sasao & Sue, 1993, p. 343). In this study, the "self-perceived ethnicity" of these children was Chinese, but the "cultural identification" was Mexican because of the Mexican-American community in which they lived and the interracial climate at school.

Problems with Group Membership

Regardless of the method chosen to determine identity with a group there are complications. If one assigns group membership, there is a risk of loss of precision resulting from a potential discrepancy between assigned group membership and self-defined group membership. If one allows the subject to self-identify using predetermined group choices, it is possible that because of the nonexhaustive nature of the groups, the subject's self-identified group is not an option. If one allows the subject to self-identify in an open-ended format, there is a trade-off of consistency and standardized definitions for idiosyncratic identifications.

One must also consider the question of category stability versus fluidity. Are categories/groups stable across time, development, and settings (i.e., school, recreation, home)? Sasao and Sue (1993) call for recognition of the "fluid nature" of ethnic–cultural groups inasmuch as group membership may change with maturity, acculturation, or settings. They point out that the majority of identity or acculturation measures "have been developed to measure the concepts at *one particular point in time*" (p. 7).

If one therefore identifies a subject (or the subject self-identifies) as belonging to a particular group at one point in time, or in one particular setting, there is no guarantee that the group membership will not change at another point in time or in a different context. A subject, could, for example, self-identify as Korean at one point in time and then self-identify as American later. The cultural categories themselves could depend on the temporal parameters, as well. Currently, for example, we use the term American Indian/Native American to refer to a particular group of indigenous people. However, these terms did not exist before the European immigrants arrived in the Americas.

The distinction did not even exist at that time. Thus, culture is a somewhat ephemeral quality.

Closser and Blow (1993, p. 199) list the limitations of research concerning populations such as groupings of race. These include the internal heterogeneity of groups, the lack of mutual exclusion within groups, and the lack of exhaustive groups. In particular, the "race differences" (Korchin, 1980, p. 263) approach to psychology has been criticized for ignoring within-group heterogeneity (Korchin, 1980; Olmedo, 1979; Sue, 1983), thus risking the formation of "exaggerated stereotyped images," one important potential iatrogenic effect of group difference findings (Campbell, 1967, cited in Sue, 1983, p. 585). Some researchers working with ethnic minority groups have therefore called for an approach that examines phenomena within groups (Korchin, 1980; Olmedo, 1979).

In a within-group approach, for example, a researcher could choose to look within the American Indian group rather than at the American Indian group compared to the White European group. Researchers working in northern Nevada (who are familiar with group membership as defined by the groups themselves) might find the distinction between the Paiute and Washoe tribes more useful than looking at an implied homogeneous American Indian group. They might further parse the groups and look at particular bands or clans (such as the Pyramid Lake band). Researchers in the southwest United States, however, might find the distinction between band and tribe as used in the North to be inapplicable. Instead, they might use the tribe distinction (e.g., Navajo) and break down the tribes into clans defined in terms of family affiliation (e.g., Beaver clan).

The lack of mutual exclusion within groups complicates the categorization process. How does one, for example, categorize a subject who identifies with or is identified as belonging to multiple groups/cultures under consideration? In the example given above, people in the Reno/Sparks Indian Colony include people from different tribes (e.g., Paiute and Washoe). An individual then could belong to the Reno/Sparks Indian Colony and the Washoe tribe, just as a child of a Latino mother and an African-American father would have a dual group membership. Sasao and Sue (1993) raise the following questions: "Is it appropriate or possible to define a multicultural or mixed-race community for research? Or, does it warrant a separate community-based research for this often neglected group of individuals" (p. 711).

The lack of exhaustive groups is another issue with culture/ethnic group research. Group classification is inconsistent and may depend more on the interests of the researchers or therapists than on other considerations (i.e., a gay therapist may use the homosexual/heterosexual distinction more often than the Latino researcher who sees the world in ethnic terms). There is no end to the number of categories/groups that can be formed.

Closser and Blow's (1993) limitations—internal heterogeneity, lack of mutual exclusion, and lack of exhaustive groups—can be illustrated by an attempt to parse the graduate student group. If we are partitioning graduate students, we must decide who will constitute our cultural groups: graduate students as a whole (here culture is defined on an occupational dimension); clinical psychology graduate students (a finer grain occupational distinction); female clinical graduate students (an added gender dimension); female clinical, Protestant graduate students (an added religious dimension); Pacific Islander, female, clinical, Protestant, graduate students (an added geographical dimension); black, Pacific Islander, female, clinical, Protestant, graduate students (an added skin color dimension); and so on.

Deciding how to parse culture and define group membership is sufficiently difficult with clearly defined variables such as graduate program or gender. However, the process becomes even more complex when nonexclusive, nonexhaustive, and poorly defined categories such as race and ethnicity are used. Some philosophers have suggested that in order to have categories of existence, one must have some principle of individuation (e.g., Quine, 1960). That is, one must be able to reliably and validly recognize individual exemplifications of abstract entities. However, it is not clear that this criterion is met regarding cultures; neither is it clear that culture, as used in contemporary psychology, breaks down into nonarbitrary natural divisions. As Dumas et al. (1999) point out, the following question remains unanswered: "When is a group sufficiently distinct to constitute a 'cultural group' (rather than a set of individuals)?" (p. 180).

Benefits and Costs of Using Ethnic Groups as Variables

Using ethnic groups as variables provides researchers with a convenient way to talk about phenomena and groups of people, and generates data on a more diverse population. However, there are costs associated with using ethnic groups as variables.

Stereotypes Researchers and therapists are encouraged to take culture into consideration, yet they are warned not to fall into the trap of stereotyping. Martinez (1994) argues that the concept of cultural sensitivity "has evolved into a caricatured concept that has led to stereotypic overgeneralizations of entire ethnic populations" (p. 12). It has been claimed that between-group comparisons perpetuate "exaggerated stereotyped images" of group difference findings (Campbell, 1967, as cited in Sue, 1983, p. 122) and may contribute to racist conceptions of human behavior (Betancourt & Lopez, 1993). There is an inherent tension that exists between categorizing and avoiding stereotypes. We can categorize people with the goal of increased homogeneity for variance control purposes, but when we look to utilize this commonality, we risk stereotyping.

Overlooking a More Useful Variable When focusing on ethnicity as a main variable, there is the possibility that one is overlooking a more important or useful variable. Montalvo's 1988 "stereotypic ethnic vacuums" are described by Martinez (1994) as resulting from the practice of taking cultural variables into account to the point of overemphasis. "The stereotypic ethnic vacuum refers to the implication that, by identifying a cultural reason for the existence of a behavior, the behavior is understood as being inherent to the culture and therefore dismissed or minimized. This sometimes preempts intervention or prevents change" (p. 76).

Proximal versus Distal Variables A related issue involves the choice of a distal variable over a more proximal variable. Investigators specializing in cultural research advocate the use of more proximal sociocultural variables (as opposed to the distal variables of ethnicity) in the study of ethnic group behavior (Betancourt & Lopez, 1993; Okazaki & Sue, 1998). The findings of Betancourt and Lopez's (1993) study with schizophrenics, for example, suggested that ethnicity was a more distal variable and religious affiliation a more proximal variable (i.e., Catholicism accounted for a greater proportion of the variance.) They consider racial group to be inadequate as a general explanatory factor of between-group phenomena and encourage researchers to focus more on cultural elements and the relevant variable, "not on racial groupings alone" (p. 631). Korchin (1980, p. 263) advises the consideration of "the pervasive importance of class, education, and other social-status variables" when examining racial group differences. On a more basic level, other examples of potential causal variables include climate/temperature (tropical, cold, etc.) and exercise habits.

Betancourt and Lopez (1993) summarize the implications: "It is important to note that the 'cultural differences' thought to underlie the observed group differences are frequently not directly measured or assessed. It is assumed that because these two groups are from two distinct cultural or ethnic groups, they differ from one another on key cultural dimensions. This may or may not be the case" (p. 634). Researchers, for example, might use the groups "Latinas" and "Persian women" in an attempt to obtain commonality and distinction, but what is actually achieved is unknown. At a minimum, the more proximal differences need to be directly measured to observe if the hypothesized differences actually exist.

Manipulation Unavailability The unavailability of ethnic manipulation as an option is a methodological cost of using the ethnic group as an independent variable. Therefore, we cannot examine directly the possible causal roles of ethnicity. Using the ethnic group as an independent variable limits the researcher to correlational studies. One must then keep in mind that third variables may actually be involved in the casual relationship.

Terminology Confusion There is a lack of consensus regarding ethnic group operational definitions, and terms are used inconsistently. As a result, the literature is vulnerable to confusion, miscommunication, and dissemination complications. In the area of cultural research, there has been a call for specificity in the reporting of studies to combat this problem. As Okazaki and Sue (1998) caution, we cannot know if researchers are studying and communicating about the same constructs unless each study explicitly states its assumptions regarding the use of such categorical variables.

THE APPLICATION OF CULTURAL SENSITIVITY TO CONTEMPORARY PSYCHOLOGY

The Dual Roles of the Psychologist

One way to view the foundational and regulative role of cultural sensitivity is in terms of the roles this notion and its cognates play in conjectures of what will best further the growth of psychological knowledge, as reflected in the APA's Ethical Principles of Psychologists and Code of Conduct (1992). The preamble may set the stage for what we claim is the ameliorative agenda associated with this construct when it states that the goal of psychologists is to "broaden knowledge of behavior and, where appropriate, to apply it pragmatically to improve the condition of both the individual and society" (p. 1599).

The role of the psychologist, therefore, is not only to understand behavior and social relations but to enhance these concepts. This dual role of psychologist as scientist and a socially responsible member of society has been debated in the literature. On one end of the continuum, there are those who claim that the science of psychology is purely objective and value free, and that the task of the psychologist is to look at the "brute facts" and "allow[ing] the facts to speak for themselves" (Hansen, 1958, cited in Howard, 1985, p. 257). The more prevalent view, however, is that the scientific method itself is a cultural product, and that all human behavior (including that of psychologists) occurs in cultural contexts (Dumas et al., 1999; Ridley, 1985; Tharp, 1991; Yee, Fairchild, Weizmann, & Wyatt, 1993).

Applied psychologists work to make things better (as do many experimental psychologists, albeit less directly) and for some their concerns move from individuals to more molar entities such as groups. Psychologists have generally parsed groups along the lines that are generally found to predominate in general political discourse. When psychologists in the United States focus on culture and cultural sensitivity, they tend to study groups protected by federal mandate. This tendency, we conjecture, reflects their ameliorative agenda in that these groups face more severe economic and social problems than others. Unfortunately, however, legitimate concern with these significant social problems does not mean that these constructs will be scientifically useful. The fact that a problem can be defined using a construct does not mean that this construct will eventually be shown to play an essential role in scientific regularities associated with the problem, that useful applications of the construct will necessarily follow, or that it will not be used to harm particular groups.

A History of Harm

Caution is needed to navigate the slippery slope from usefulness/ helpfulness to harmfulness when dealing with issues of culture. The general ethical claim, for example, that discrimination is wrong and ought to be combated could be viewed as existing in tension with the goal of cultural sensitivity. For example, in Martin Luther King's "I Have a Dream" speech, delivered on the steps of the Lincoln Memorial on August 28, 1963, he stated, "I have a dream that my four children will one day live in a nation where they will not be judged by the color of their skin but by the content of their character" (Alvarez, 1988). How do we, as psychologists, then deal with the tension between attending to a person's culture (associated with "cultural sensitivity") and attending to "the content of their character?" It may be that seeing a person as a member of a group detracts from seeing the person's individual character. This raises the specter of whether an emphasis on cultural diversity may be inadvertently counterproductive because it has the unintended effect of actually increasing divisiveness by focusing on differences such as skin color.

These concerns are not just hypothetical. There have been clear precedents in which focus on group differences has had clearly undesirable aspects. The historical context of the study of culture and ethnic minority groups in psychology includes themes on what Sue, Ito and Bradshaw (1982) refer to as the inferiority model. Early research on ethnic groups suggested that certain groups were inferior to Whites both in social and intellectual domains because of hereditary factors but also at times because of the allegedly inferior environments constructed by these groups (Thomas & Sillen, 1972, cited in Sue, 1983). The deficit model followed the inferiority model. According to Sue (1983), "The deficit model's assumption was that prejudice and discrimination created stress and decreased opportunities for minority groups. As a result, many minority group persons were considered deficient, underprivileged, deprived, pathological, or deviant" (p. 587).

There are, nevertheless, pragmatic issues to consider. Closser and Blow (1993), for example, argue that neglecting to attend to the importance of culture may "contribute to existing barriers to treatment, including lack of relevance, language, and treatment access problems" (p. 199). With respect to mental health services, findings of underutilization of services and high attrition rates of ethnic minorities in therapy have been cited in the literature as reasons to take the role of culture in service delivery into consideration (Sue, Allen, & Conway, 1978, Sue, McKinney & Allen, 1976; Takeuchi, Sue, & Yeh, 1995). In a study of seventeen community mental health centers, Sue (1977) found that "regardless of utilization rates, all of the ethnic minority groups had significantly higher dropout rates than Whites" (cited in Sue & Zane, 1987, p, 37), and that "ethnicity was a significant predictor of premature termination even after other client demographic variables and treatment variables were controlled" (cited in Sue et al., 1991, p. 533).

Training culturally sensitive psychologists and increasing the number of ethnic minority psychologists (partly based on the notion that these psychologists will be more ethnically sensitive, at least to clients from their own group) have been emphasized in the literature as one approach to decrease underutilization rates, as well as offer diversity of thought in all roles of the psychologist (Iwamasa, 1996; Korchin, 1980; Martinez, 1994; Porter, 1994; Rogler, Malgady, Constantino, & Blumenthal, 1987; Sue, 1977; Sue & Zane, 1987). The APA ethics code (1992) and APA Guidelines for Providers of Psychological Services to Ethnic, Linguistic, and Culturally Diverse Populations (1993) have evolved, in part, as a response to this call from the literature, They attempt to hold psychologists accountable for these dual roles.

The Ethical Imperatives

Being culturally sensitive is not simply associated with conjecture on what practices will result in the best progress in psychology; it also has become ethically mandatory. This requirement, however, is problematic, given the confusion associated with cultural sensitivity. According to the APA ethics code (1992), a psychologist may be sanctioned for not behaving in a manner that could be considered "culturally sensitive." For example, ethical standard 2.04 (Use of Assessment in General and With Special Populations) of the code states:

> Psychologists attempt to identify situations in which particular interventions or assessment techniques or norms may not be applicable or may require adjustment in administration or interpretation because of factors such as individuals' gender, age, race, ethnicity, national origin, religion, sexual orientation, disability, language, or socioeconomic status (p. 1603).

The subspecialty of psychological testing was one of the first focus areas of cultural sensitivity in the field of psychology (Martinez, 1994). The reliability and validity of instruments and procedures developed for and normed on Caucasian samples and used with ethnic minorities were called into question. Researchers have asserted that consideration of the role of culture in psychology will facilitate the creation of instruments and interventions that will yield more accurate measurements by being more sensitive to a culturally heterogeneous population (Betancourt & Lopez, 1993; Matthews, 1997; Olmedo, 1981). The complication is that we do not know which relevant regularities should be taken into account. For example, what cultural variables need to be factored in for whom when constructing or using an intelligence test? As Okazaki and Sue (1998, p. 35) point out, it is even debatable whether some methods of assessment may be more likely to result in cultural or ethnic bias than others.

Principles within the APA ethics code also address concerns related to service delivery to ethnic minorities and the training of professionals. Principle A, Competence, reads:

> Psychologists are cognizant of the fact that the competencies required in serving, teaching, and/or studying groups of people vary with the distinctive characteristics of those groups.… They maintain knowledge of relevant scientific and professional information related to the services they render, and they recognize the need for ongoing education (p. 1599)

According to Principle C, psychologists have a "professional and scientific responsibility" to "uphold professional standards of conduct, clarify their professional roles and obligations, accept appropriate responsibility for their behavior, and adapt their methods to the needs of different populations" (p. 1599). Principle D, Respect for People's Rights and Dignity, maintains that:

> Psychologists are aware of cultural, individual, and role differences, including those due to age, gender, race, ethnicity, national origin, religion, sexual orientation, disability, language, and socioeconomic status. Psychologists try to eliminate the effect of their work of biases based on those factors, and they do not knowingly participate in or condone unfair discriminatory practices (pp. 1599–1600).

Thus, cultural sensitivity has achieved the status of an ethical imperative for psychologists. Unfortunately, the code fails to specify a rationale for this ethical decision (O'Donohue & Mangold, 1996). We suggest that currently this rationale is based on a number of empirical presumptions—for example, factual assertions that groups of people differ in significant ways on certain dimensions, as well as causal claims such as a specific cultural belief that causes a person to act in a certain way—that are generally unresolved, open, empirical questions. Because culture is not something that can be experimentally manipulated, it is difficult to make claims concerning the causal role of culture. Therefore, inasmuch as these questions are generally unanswered, the assumptions about the importance of culture and particular cultural elements are also currently unanswered.

Outlining the Dimensions of Cultural Sensitivity

Perhaps our early efforts have focused on culture but have not properly focused on "sensitivity." This raises the question of what exactly constitutes "sensitivity" toward a culture. We agree with Rogler's (1989, p. 296) assertion that "no single specific act or set of finite acts performed on research provides a complete answer to the question" of what culturally sensitive mental health research or the application of such research is. There are, nonetheless, superficial conceptions of cultural sensitivity that we do not accept as adequate.

We agree with those who claim that neither good intentions alone nor awareness of cultural differences is adequate to constitute cultural sensitivity (Dumas et al., 1999). We also contend that mainstream psychology's common approach to dealing with the ethical mandates of cultural sensitivity and funding agency requirements is unsatisfactory and even potentially harmful. We are referring to the tendency of psychologists to analyze their data by race/ethnic categories, what Scarr (1988) and Okazaki and Sue (1998) refer to as "afterthoughts." As Scarr explains, not incorporating these variables into the actual research design, not thoughtfully making an informed decision to use these variables, and not considering the potential most proximal uses of the data do not exonerate the psychologist from being culturally insensitive or from any of the blame resulting from outcomes of the research. It is not scientifically or socially responsible simply to include certain samples of populations in one's work and claim that one is being culturally sensitive.

In our search for a workable definition, we propose seven potential dimensions of cultural sensitivity.

First, it would seem that, at a minimum, being sensitive entails the ability to accurately identify the culture(s) to which a person belongs. This requires accurate taxonomies and assessment strategies.

Second, sensitivity involves accurately knowing factual regularities associated with a culture or cultures. For example, if it is the case that Culture X finds direct eye contact impolite, then a culturally sensitive person should know this. Well-defined research is necessary to uncover the nature and extent of these regularities.

Third, the notion of cultural sensitivity, at least for psychologists, seems to involve knowing when these regularities are potentially relevant for the task with which the psychologist is concerned. Specifically, cultural sensitivity seems to involve knowledge of how the relevant regularity can influence a goal. It is possible that even if a relevant cultural regularity exists, at times it would be properly judged as irrelevant and not have an impact on any implementation.

Fourth, sensitivity involves an ethical judgment that acting on or respecting this cultural regularity is not ethically impermissible. That is, there is also an important question of whether these cultural regularities should be taken uncritically. If not, what criteria (themselves "objective" or culturally biased) should be used to evaluate these regularities? If, for example, one subculture is judged as misogynist (e.g., practicing female infanticide) what constitutes "sensitivity" regarding this behavior? Such issues could just as easily refer to a Nazi culture that espouses obliterating particular ethnic minorities as it could to a celebration of diversity that respects all people.

Fifth, sensitivity involves knowing how to effectively implement any action in a culturally sensitive manner. In the many roles of the psychologist, this applies to testing, providing therapy, doing research, supervising graduate students, writing, and so on.

Sixth, if cultural sensitivity is regarded as a global construct, all of these issues are nested by all relevant cultures (e.g., ethnic, religious, sexual, etc.) and all possible permutations. For example, the relations between Latinos and Caucasians, Latinos and Asians, and Latinos and all other ethnic groups must enter into any sensitive judgment of the cultural identity of this group.

Seventh, cultural sensitivity involves an awareness that the psychologist's own culture, values, assumptions, and the like bring to the task at hand. It further involves the knowledge that these values and assumptions may bias every activity in which the psychologist participates. The research question chosen, design, methodology, interpretation of data, dissemination of data, content of therapy, and interactions with clients may all be affected (Dumas et al., 1999; Gil & Bob, 1999; Howard, 1985; Ridley, 1985; Rogler, 1999; Scarr, 1988; Sue, Arredondo, & Mc Davis, 1992; Yee et al., 1993). It is interesting to note that mainstream psychologists tend to equate cultural sensitivity with knowledge of cultures different from their own; however, in cultural research, awareness of one's own culture is stressed.

CONCLUSION

Given the complications, culture as a global general construct may not prove particularly useful to our activities as scientist–practitioners in psychology. It may also be premature to make ethical prescriptions based on this construct, given the state of our knowledge at this time.

We counsel a cautious stance. Before we rush to be accepted as culturally sensitive, we need to define the applicability of this concept to psychology and assess its potential contribution to the field. These benefits must then be weighed against the very real pitfall of allowing cultural considerations to weaken our ability to provide efficient therapy and effective research.

REFERENCES

Alvarez, A. (1988). Martin Luther King's "I Have a Dream": The speech event as metaphor. *Journal of Black Studies, 18*, 337–357.

American Psychological Association (1992). Ethical principles of psychologists and code of conduct. *American Psychologist, 47*, 1597–1611.

American Psychological Association. Office of Ethnic Minority Affairs (1993). Guidelines for providers of psychological services to ethnic, linguistic, and culturally diverse populations. *American Psychologist, 48*(1), 45–48.

Berman, J.J. (Ed.) (1989). Cross-cultural perspectives. *Nebraska Symposium on Motivation.* Lincoln: University of Nebraska Press.

Bernal, M.E. & Castro, F. (1994). Are clinical psychologists prepared for service and research with ethnic minorities? *American Psychologist, 49*(9), 797–805.

Betancourt, H. & Lopez, S.R. (1993). The study of culture, ethnicity, and race in American psychology. *American Psychologist, 48*, 629–637.

Closser, M. & Blow, F. (1993). Special populations: Women, ethnic minorities, and the elderly. *Psychiatric Clinics of North America, 16*, 199–208.

Dumas, J.E., Rollock, D., Prinz, R.J., Hops, H., & Blechman, E.A. (1999). Cultural sensitivity: Problems and solutions in applied and preventive intervention. *Applied & Preventive Psychology, 8*, 175–196.

Eaton, W.W. (1980). *The Sociology of Mental Illness.* New York: Praeger.

Farley, J. (1994). *Sociology,* rev. ed. Englewood, NJ: Prentice-Hall.

Gil, E.F. & Bob, S. (1999). Culturally competent research: An ethical perspective. *Clinical Psychology Review, 19*(1),45–55.

Howard, G.S. (1985). The role of values in the science of psychology. *American Psychologist, 40*(3), 255–265.

Iwamasa, G.Y. (1996). On being an ethnic minority cognitive behavioral therapist. *Cognitive and Behavioral Practice, 3*, 235–254.

Korchin, S. (1980). Clinical psychology and minority problems. *American Psychologist, 35*, 262–269.

Martinez, K. (1994). Cultural sensitivity in family therapy gone awry. *Hispanic Journal of Behavioral Sciences, 16*, 75–89.

Matthews, A. (1997). A guide to case conceptualization and treatment planning with minority group clients. *The Behavior Therapist, 20*, 35–39.

O'Donohue, W. & Mangold, R. (1996). A critical examination of the ethical principles of psychologists and code of conduct. In W. O'Donohue & R. Kitchener (Eds.), *Philosophy of Psychology.* London: Sage.

Okazaki, S. & Sue, S. (1998). Methodological issues in assessment research with ethnic minorities. In P. Balls Organista, K.M. Chun, and G. Marin (Eds.), *Readings in Ethnic Psychology,* (pp. 26–40). New York: Routledge.

Olmedo, E. (1979). Acculturation, a psychometric perspective. *American Psychologist, 34*, 1061–1070.

Olmedo, E. (1981). Testing linguistic minorities. *American Psychologist, 36*, 1078–1085.

Porter, N. (1994). Empowering supervisees to empower others: A culturally responsive supervision model. *Hispanic Journal of Behavioral Science, 16*, 43–56.

Quine, W.V.O. (1960). *Word and Object.* Cambridge, MA: MIT Press.

Ridley, C.R. (1985). Imperatives for ethnic and cultural relevance in psychology training programs. *Professional Psychology: Research and Practice, 16*(5), 611–622.

Rogler, L. (1989). The meaning of culturally sensitive research in mental health. *American Journal of Psychiatry, 146*, 296–303.

Rogler, L. (1999). Methodological sources of cultural insensitivity in mental health research. *American Psychology, 54*(6), 424–433.

Rogler, L., Malgady, R., Constantino, G., & Blumenthal, R. (1987). What do culturally sensitive mental health services mean? The case of Hispanics. *American Psychologist, 42*, 565–570.

Sasao, T. (1992). Correlates of substance use and problem behaviors in multiethnic high school settings. Unpublished manuscript, University of California, Los Angeles.

Sasao, T. & Sue, S. (1993). Toward a culturally anchored ecological framework of research in ethnic-cultural communities. *American Journal of Community Psychology, 21*, 705–727.

Scarr, S. (1988). Race and gender as psychological variables. *American Psychologist, 43*(1), 56–59.

Sue, D.W., Arredondo, P., & Mc Davis, R.J. (1992). Multicultural counseling competencies and standards: A call to the profession. *Journal of Multicultural Counseling and Development, 20*, 64–88.

Sue, S. (1977). Community mental health services to minority groups, some optimism, some pessimism. *American Psychologist, 32*, 616–624.

Sue, S. (1983). Ethnic minority issues in psychology, a reexamination. *American Psychologist, 38*, 583–592.

Sue, S. & Zane, N. (1987). The role of culture and cultural techniques in psychotherapy, a critique and reformulation. *American Psychologist, 42*, 37–45.

Sue, S., Allen, D., & Conway, L. (1978). The responsiveness and equality of mental health care to Chicanos and Native Americans. *American Journal of Community Psychology, 6*, 137–146.

Sue, S., Ito, J., & Bradshaw, C. (1982). Ethnic minority research: Trends and directions. In E.E. Jones & S.J. Korchin (Eds.), *Minority Mental Health.* New York: Praeger.

Sue, S., McKinney, H., & Allen, D. (1976). Predictors of the duration of therapy for clients in the community mental health system. *Community Mental Health Journal, 12*, 365–375.

Sue, S., Pujino, D., Hu, L., Takeuchi, D., & Zane, N. (1991). Community mental health services for ethnic minority groups: A test of cultural responsiveness hypothesis. *Journal of Consulting and Clinical Psychology, 59*, 533–540.

Takeuchi, D., Sue, S., & Yeh, M. (1995). Return rates and outcomes from ethnicity-specific mental health programs in Los Angeles. *American Journal of Public Health, 85*, 638–643.

Tharp, R.G. (1991). Cultural diversity and treatment of children. *Journal of Consulting and Clinical Psychology, 59*, 799–812.

Yee, A.H., Fairchild, H.H., Weizmann, F., & Wyatt, G.E. (1993). Addressing psychology's problems with race. *American Psychologist, 48*(11), 1132–1140.

Zuckerman, M. (1990). Some dubious premises in research and theory on racial differences. *American Psychologist, 45*(12), 1297–1303.

3

THE PSYCHOLOGY OF VICTIMHOOD

Ofer Zur

The psychology of victims and the dynamics of victimhood have been largely ignored by scholars and clinicians. Although the psychology of perpetrators and bystanders and the dynamics of posttraumatic stress disorder has been thoroughly examined (Ochberg & Willis, 1991; Viano, 1990; Walker, 1979), the psychology of victimhood as a personal and cultural phenomenon has not. In past years, the tendency was to blame victims; more recently, however, the tide has turned. It is now politically incorrect to explore the role of victims in violent systems. This is viewed as tantamount to blaming the victim.

In this chapter we shy away from blame and offer a typology of the victim, exploring the familial and cultural origins of victimhood, as well as the characteristics of victims and their relationships with the perpetrators. As we move from blame to a more complex understanding of violent systems and how our culture perpetuates these systems, we provide ourselves with better tools to predict and prevent further victimization.

Hierarchy, inequality, and violence have historically been part of human social structures. There have always been rulers and ruled, leaders and followers, the fortunate and the needy, and the powerful and the weak. Various cultures have treated disparities in status, power, fortune, and ability in different ways. Buddhists emphasize karma and destiny, whereas in the modern West the focus has been on freedom, choice, and the individual's control of destiny. In this Western world-view, inequalities and differences are often associated with injustice and victimization.

BLAME AND RESPONSIBILITY

Traditionally, two main approaches have dominated the way we look at victimization in the modern West. The first approach points the finger of blame at the victim (Brownmiller, 1975; Ryan, 1971; Sundberg, Barbaree, & Marshall, 1991; Walker, 1979). The victim may be a battered wife, a woman who was raped, a person of color, or someone who is economically disadvantaged. The second approach views men as solely responsible for violence, whether as soldiers on the battlefield, politicians in government, or husbands in domestic violence (Hughes, 1993; Keen, 1991; Zur & Glendinning, 1987). These two approaches to blame have not only failed to resolve the violence and suffering but actually tend to perpetuate and exacerbate them.

A complex relationship exists between the diverse and complementary roles that perpetrators and victims in general, and men and women in particular, assume in the dynamics of violence. Rather than blame, we seek to apply a systems analysis approach to increase our understanding of the dynamics and origins of victimhood and the varying types of victims. Our investigation concentrates on adult victims and on patterns of victimization established early in life, rather than on the effects of a single trauma. It focuses on intimate violence, not on random incidents among parties who have no past relationship.

Our intent is to help victims and victimizers end their abusive relationships. Blame is counterproductive. But it is also counterproductive to allow the politically correct attitude of nonblame to produce a climate that forbids exploration of the role of victims in systems of violence. Fear of blaming preserves and perpetuates systems of abuse and victimization.

Using the Blame Approach

Civil rights and feminist movements have shed light on the blatant injustice of holding the poor, rape or incest victims, minorities, or the handicapped responsible for their misfortunes (Ryan, 1971). The most obvious manifestations of this "blame the victim" approach are rape cases. Women victims are too often blamed for being provocative, seductive, suggestive, for proposing, teasing, or just plain "asking for it"

(Brownmiller, 1975; Keen, 1991; Russel, 1984). In this myth, men are seen as helplessly lusty, sexually frustrated beings, responding to the provocations of women.

A similarity exists in domestic violence cases in which women have been blamed for being masochistic, withholding, and, again, "asking for it" or "deserving it" (Sundberg, Barbaree, & Marshall, 1991; Walker, 1979, Yollow & Bogard, 1988). African Americans are viewed as lazy and incapable if they are unemployed (Ryan, 1971), girl victims of sexual abuse are accused of being seductive, and mothers of daughters who have been sexually abused are assumed to be sexually frigid, emotionally cold, and generally unsupportive of their husbands (Caplan & Hall-McCorquodale, 1985).

The second approach that concentrates blame for violence on men has been promoted by a brand of feminism that believes the patriarchal system existing in the West is responsible for the evils in the world. Men are regarded as the culprits in issues that range from wars and politics, domestic violence and sexual abuse, to toxic dumping by corporations, nuclear weapons, and the military–industrial complex. At the heart of this approach lies the split between men's aggressive and violent nature and women's inherent goodness. (For further discussion see Keen, 1991; Sykes, 1992; Zur, 1989; Zur & Glendinning, 1987).

The New Culture of Victimization

Former Washington, D.C. mayor Marion Barry, who was caught red-handed smoking crack, blamed it on that "bitch" who "set me up" and later insisted his prosecutors were racially motivated. Mrs. Rose Cipollone blamed the tobacco industry for the deadly lung cancer she developed after smoking for forty years. A man who jumped in front of a moving train in New York and had to have his legs amputated sued the engineer and the subway system for negligence.

Not only do people wish to claim the status of victim, the legal and political systems promote and legislate it as well. Marion Barry received only a slap on the wrist. The courts awarded Mrs. Cipollone $400,000 in damages to be paid by the cigarette manufacturer. And the man who deliberately and voluntarily jumped in front of a New York subway train collected $650,000 in damages.

Victimization is neither a recent nor an especially North American phenomenon. The American culture has nevertheless provided a unique and increasingly fertile ground for the cultivation of victimization. The American emphasis on freedom and choice implies that we are in charge of our destiny. Whether it is by working hard to get ahead, pulling oneself up by one's bootstraps, or by social and political activism, we believe not only that we can but that we must take total control of our individual and social destiny.

Unlike the Buddhist acceptance of evil, inequality, and hierarchy, Western culture—and particularly North American culture—has evolved notions about the individual's freedom to choose, the immoral nature of social inequality, and the inalienable right of each person to pursue happiness. Within this cultural psychology, and specific to psychotherapy, lies a belief in people's inherent ability to change themselves and their environment. Violence and victimhood, like evil and inequality, must be fought and eradicated. Accordingly, the occurrence of violence and suffering victims or the existence of equalities are interpreted not as acts of God or manifestations of karma but as failures that must be corrected. It is this focus on failure that leads to victimhood and blame.

Unlike Far Easterners, Middle Easterners, or Russians, Americans expect things to turn out well. The constitutional promise to all Americans that they have the right to the pursuit of happiness gives rise to the expectation that Americans are supposed to feel happy. Thus, not feeling happy indicates some sort of failure. The victim says, "It is definitely not my fault."

The culture of victimization is closely tied to what Amitai Etzioni (1987), a sociologist at Georgetown University, calls the "rights industry." This is a collective term for those who fight for the rights of groups such as women, abused children, minorities, the homeless, experimental animals, AIDS victims, or illegal immigrants.

The concepts of "rights" and "victims" are often closely related. Fighting for a "right" implies that a right was denied. Although this is not always the case, many claims for rights pose a moral claim on someone else, as in the battle between smokers and nonsmokers, and very often between men and women. Fighting for a right all too often means claiming victim status. Ironically, the rights movement often victimizes one group while liberating another. What seems to be a noble, justified, long-overdue act of protecting a victim can easily turn to blame and warfare. When this happens, conflict, injustice, and victimization are perpetuated, and the possibility of resolution and healing is destroyed.

Similar to the rights movements is the recovery movement. In the last decade, we have seen an explosion of twelve-step programs focusing on an endlessly growing list of addictions. Many of these programs help their members master recovery and discourage feelings of blame and victimhood. However, within the recovery movement, some programs like ACA (Adult Children of Alcoholics) and CODA (Co-Dependents Anonymous) can easily perpetuate members' sense of victimization instead of enhancing their sense of self-mastery and personal power (Kaminer, 1992; Tavris, 1993). Identifying oneself primarily and over long periods of time as an adult child of an alcoholic is to embrace the permanent identity of a wounded victim. Conscious acknowledgment of the original family dysfunction and its effect on the individual is frequently necessary for healing, however, it is only the first step. Remaining with ACA groups indefinitely not only keeps people in the mode of victim but also prevents them from moving to a place of empowerment and choice. Although programs such as Alcoholics Anonymous, Narcotics Anonymous, Gamblers Anonymous, and Overeaters Anonymous focus on specific addictions, the co-dependency movement ludicrously assumes that ninety-six percent of the population are victims of a disease they call co-dependency (Schaef, 1986).

We have become a nation of victims, leapfrogging over one another to compete publicly for the status of victim and defining everyone as some sort of survivor. Many people in recovery shamelessly compare their individual sagas of abuse in alcoholic families or sexual harassment on the job with the experiences of World War II Holocaust survivors who endured the atrocities of the concentration camps (Herman, 1992). Today it is fashionable to be a victim. Celebrities like Oprah Winfrey, Kitty Dukakis, Elizabeth Taylor, and Michael Reagan are leading this trend. Oprah's, Geraldo's, and Donahue's shows are saturated with victims from all walks of life, proudly confessing their victimization on national television (Hughes, 1993; Kaminer, 1992; Sykes, 1992; Tavris, 1993).

The blame–victim approach is not confined to recovery movements. It is also at the heart of attempts by the legal system to respond to injustice and violations by identifying and prosecuting the perpetrators and compensating the victims (Sykes, 1992; Hughes, 1993). The faulty part of this approach is the focus on simplistic, linear, short-term, and face-value justice. It is concerned with differentiating between polar opposites—right from wrong, guilty from innocent, conviction from acquittal—and it is insensitive to situations in which some responsibility should be shared by both defendant and plaintiff.

In claiming the status of victim and assigning all the blame to others, a person can achieve moral superiority while simultaneously disowning any responsibility for his or her behavior and its outcome. The victims "merely" seek justice and fairness. If they become violent, it is only as a last resort, in self-defense. The victim status is a powerful one. The victim is always morally right, neither responsible nor accountable, and forever entitled to sympathy.

At the heart of the blame approach is a system of warfare that centers on the outcome of moral or legal battles rather than on the resolution of conflict and the prevention of future violence. As such, it neither reduces pathology nor protects the victim. Sending an abusive husband to jail stops beatings and may give the wife a feeling of justice and revenge. However, it will not help the husband deal with his violent behavior, and it will not teach the wife about her more subtle role in the violent relationship. By confirming the wife's status as victim, the legal solution is likely to perpetuate further violence. The imprisoned husband may leave prison angrier and with more violent tendencies than he had before he was incarcerated, and the wife may simply find herself another abusive man. Whether their abusive husbands are charged, restrained, or jailed, women who were abused as children are likely to engage in abusive relationships unless some healing occurs (Viano, 1990). The hope for victims does not lie in the blame approach and the legal system. Hope is established when the victims acquire high self-esteem, learn to differentiate between love and violation, and can finally feel they are entitled to loving relationships.

Why, then, if mental health workers are devoted to healing and prevention, is the blame approach so pervasive? The answer lies in understanding that mental health workers not only mirror the general culture of victimization, they also abide by the unspoken, politically correct imperative that the role of the victim in violent systems is not to be explored.

Rethinking "Don't Blame the Victim"

In response to decades of racial oppression, the civil rights movement spearheaded the effort to stop blaming victims. In an understandable backlash, William Ryan (1971) wrote his book *Blaming the Victim*. In it he contends that blaming the victim is a method of maintaining the status quo of the group in power. Although valid within its historical context, the message "do not blame the victim" also resulted in silencing any exploration of victimhood during subsequent decades, inadvertently perpetuating further victimization.

Theories of victimology and research have concentrated mainly on domestic violence, on the effect of traumas on victims (including posttraumatic stress syndrome research), perpetrators, and bystanders, and on treatment. Very few writers have warned against the unrealistic and ultimately patronizing portrayal of victims of crime as total innocents (Viano, 1990). Most scholars have avoided this field altogether for fear of being accused of "blaming the victim," which has been translated into "Do not explore the role of the victim."

Sexual coercion has haunted women for many millennia, paralleling the ways in which dominant cultures enslave, exploit, and destroy weaker ones (Brownmiller, 1975; Herman, 1992). The feminist and civil rights movements have been instrumental in attempting to correct this gross injustice by fighting for equal rights and dignity for all people. Although the feminist and civil rights principles are undebatably just, some have taken them to illogical extremes. There are those who would consider the culpability of a woman dating a man who had previously raped her on a par with that of a victim of child rape.

It is clear that abuse of women by men is unjustifiable under any circumstance, however, it is also important to differentiate between relative degrees of responsibility. To adhere to an ideology that victims are always and completely innocent is absurd. It has yet to be widely understood that by alleviating all women and any victims from all responsibility to predict, prevent, or even unconsciously invite abuse is to reduce them to helpless, incapable creatures—and, in fact, re-victimize them.

In her popular book *The Battered Woman*, Walker (1979) uses Seligman's (1975) theory of "learned helplessness" to explain why women do not leave battering relationships. The popular approach implies that women who are battered, like experimental dogs, have absolutely no choice, no say, and no control over the initiating of and staying in these abusive relationships. In reality, these two situations cannot be compared so easily. There is no doubt that most battered women do not perceive that they have viable and safe options such as shelters, rape counseling, or legal services geared specifically to them. This perception stems from their often realistic fear for their own and their children's lives, grim economic realities, as well as the social, law enforcement, and legal system's high tolerance of wife beating (Gelles & Straus, 1988; Walker, 1979). To use Seligman's model in a battering situation is not only humiliating and degrading to women, but also casts them in the role of the totally helpless victim.

Any analysis assuming that women make choices, contribute to their misfortune, and are neither the only victims nor totally innocent and helpless is seen as blaming the victim, betraying women, and allying with a patriarchal society and sexist men (Caplan & Hall-McCorquodale, 1985; Cook & Frantz-Cook, 1984; Herman, 1992; Sundberg, Barbaree & Marshall, 1991; Walker, 1979; Yollow and Bogard, 1988).

Mental health workers are fully aware of the wide array of self-destructive behavior, such as playing Russian roulette or chicken, drunk driving, smoking, drug abuse, obsessive gambling, self-mutilation, and, of course, suicide. They are aware that some individuals are more prone to being picked on, repeatedly get into trouble, and are more easily victimized than others. Despite this awareness, the psychology of victims is largely an empty field. In order to better understand the dynamics of violent systems, we must first free ourselves from the binds of politically correct thinking. We must dare to expose the cultural and psychological forces that lead to violence and explore the complementary roles that abusers, abused, and bystanders play in such systems.

On Victims and Victimizers

The family has always been of primary importance in many cultures, ideally providing its members with fundamental needs: safety, food, affection, intimacy, and socialization. In fact, conflict is inevitable in families, and violence is all too often pervasive. In their daring analysis of family violence and abuse, Gelles and Straus (1988) asserted: "You are more likely to be physically assaulted, beaten, and killed in your own home at the hands of a loved one than in any place else, or by anyone else in our society." They conclude that "Violence in the home is not the exception we fear; it is all too often the rule we live by" (pp. 18–19).

From a very young age, we are taught not to trust strangers, not to take candy from them, or follow them to their cars. Milk cartons and grocery bags carry pictures of children who have been abducted. The mass media saturates us with stories of innocent victims who have been raped, robbed, and murdered by people unknown. With increasing frequency Americans arm themselves, barricade their homes, and avoid going places for fear of violent crime. The commonly held belief is that victims and vitimizers are strangers to one another, yet it can be argued otherwise.

Although the media, our teachers, and milk cartons tell us that danger lurks "out there," one is more likely to get hurt at home and or in the neighborhood. Homicide statistics shed further light on the relationship between victimizers and victims. They show that at least eighty-eight percent of murder victims in the United States had an ongoing relationship with their murderers. The relationship ranged from being intimate or close friends (twenty-eight percent), relatives (twenty-four percent), and acquaintances and paramours (thirty-six percent). Only twelve percent of the cases involved complete strangers (Jain, 1990; Wolfgang & Ferracuti, 1967). The FBI reports that 1.5 million children are abducted each year, with most (eighty to ninety percent) abducted by a parent in a custody dispute and not by strangers (Gelles & Straus, 1988).

The political arena presents a very similar picture. Enmity increases with the proximity and similarity of the warring parties. Civil wars and wars of liberation are often more brutal than wars between nations, and disputes between countries that share a common border are reportedly bloodier and less likely to be resolved by nonviolent means than international wars between countries that do not share a common border (Keen, 1986; Zur, 1991).

Legal, sociological, and clinical data have shown repeatedly that although most abusers were themselves abused as children, not all abused children become abusers. In cases of domestic violence, research has shown that both perpetrators and victims are likely to come from backgrounds where they suffered or witnessed consistent abuse (Gelles & Straus, 1988; Viano, 1990). Apparently, the line between victims and perpetrators is not all that clear. The abused are likely to abuse or be abused again. Being a victim in early life undoubtedly increases the likelihood of becoming a victimizer, victim, or both in later life.

To sum it up, perpetrators and victims are much more likely to be intimately involved with each other than to be strangers. Abused and abusers can also be embodied in the same person: the initially violated then becomes the violator.

THE PSYCHOLOGY OF THE VICTIM

In order to understand the psychology of the victim, we must understand the major characteristics of a victim and what differentiates victims from nonvictims. Whether the trauma involves domestic violence, sexual molestation, or a hostage situation, the question remains the same: what separates those who overcome their trauma and live life meaningfully from those who suffer at length from acute posttraumatic stress disorder? For example, what separates women who leave abusive husbands from those who do not? Or what separates Vietnam veterans who today live meaningful lives from those who have become drug addicts or live in the mountains as armed survivalists?

The difference between victims and nonvictims who operate within the same social, political, economic, and legal context lies not in external factors, as so often argued. Rather, the difference is in how they view themselves, the world around them, and their relationship to the trauma. We discuss this in the following section, and provide the first comprehensive description of victim psychology.

Characteristics of the Victim

The basic mode of operation of an adult victim is a feeling of helplessness and self-pity, an absent sense of accountability, and a tendency to blame. This mode is consistent with a number of psychological variables. The victim's locus of control is likely to be external and stable. An external locus of control involves belief that what happens is contingent on events outside a person's control, not on behavior or choice. In this context, stable refers to the consistency of the victim's out-of-control feelings rather than the belief that the outcome of events emanates from luck or random events (Rotter, 1971).

Similarly, victims harbor feelings of self-inefficacy, of not being successful in one's life or in affecting one's environment. In line with these characteristics, victims are likely to attribute the outcome of their behavior to situational or external forces rather than to dispositional forces within themselves. Low self-esteem, an internal sense of "badness," and feelings of shame, guilt, helplessness, and hopelessness are integral elements in the psychology of those who perceive themselves as victims.

According to social exchange theory (Worchel, 1984) and behavioral psychology, victims' actions apparently and unexpectedly provide enough rewards and benefits to sustain their behavior as victims. This means that as long as the cost of being a victim is less than its benefit, or when victim behavior is rewarded, the individual will maintain the behavior. Although the costs and suffering of victims are apparent, the benefits are much more subtle and, for the most part, unconscious. They may include the right to empathy and pity, lack of responsibility and accountability, righteousness, and even relief as the "bad self" is punished.

The Victim–Victimizer Dyad

Co-alcoholics are coupled with alcoholics, abusers with abused, masochists with sadists, and victimizers with victims. Roles of the participants in all these dyads are mutually dependent and complementary. The power of these relationships is revealed most clearly in the alcoholic and co-alcoholic relationship and in intimate abusive relationships. When the alcoholic stops drinking, it is not unusual for the relationship to end and for the co-alcoholic to find another "wet" alcoholic. The conclusion is simple: the co-alcoholic needs to control; being the competent, responsible, "morally right" partner outweighs the hardships of living with an alcoholic. Similarly, if a woman in an abusive relationship has a history of abuse by father, stepfather, or former husbands and healing did not occur, she is likely to be attracted to abusive men. As long as she associates love with violence, she will not be attracted to nonabusive men.

Victims need to be in complementary relationships with victimizers. These needs are often manifested in countertransference analysis during psychodynamic psychotherapy. Therapists who work with victims often experience aggressive, violent, or abusive feelings. These feelings, which must never be acted upon, exemplify the power embodied in the unconscious make-up of the victim to evoke victimization.

The victims' identities and (mainly unconscious) needs are connected to low self-esteem, feelings of shame and guilt, low sense of efficacy, belief that they are not in control, and possibly a desire to be punished. Adults who maintain a primarily victim identity will not be attracted to a nonabusive partner. This is not because they are masochists by nature but because cultural and familial influences, which are described in the next section, have shaped them in certain ways.

The Making of a Victim

Are victims made or born? This question is tied to the debate of nature versus nurture and the dialectical balance between destiny and choice. Our basic assumption is that there is no gene for victimhood. Social/political and familial forces are most influential in our lives. Social and political realities are likely to systematically victimize certain groups, which include women, minorities, and the disabled. The familial environment of early childhood is influential in preparing individuals to embrace or reject the role of victim. A single event such as robbery, war, plane crash, or rape does not transform a person into a victim. It takes a certain consistency in the environment to raise a victim (Sykes, 1992).

As the "American dream," the legal system, the rights movement, the recovery movement, and especially co-dependency groups have contributed to the development of a nation of victims, so, too, do politicians, attorneys, and military generals justify their actions through blame in many cases. U.S. foreign policy is based on claims of "self-defense" and blame. America got into the war in Vietnam and sustained forty years of cold war to avoid "becoming a victim" of the spread of communism. Later America felt victimized and threatened by Granada, Noriega, Saddam Hussein, Osama bin Laden, as well as "War Lord" Adid.

Within this political victim–blame climate, a person's journey toward victimhood often starts at home with abuse or abandonment. Those who were abused in childhood internalize shame, guilt, and a low sense of self-worth. They learn to associate love with abuse, intimacy with violation, and care with betrayal. They internalize the message that they are not worthy of love. To make sense of their world or protect their idealistic view of their parents, they believe their own badness caused the abuse and that they must deserve it.

Victims of childhood abuse may become victimizers, victims, or both. The pain and rage from the abuse and betrayal may turn inward or turn onto another person. With external support or internal resiliency, they can avoid becoming a victim or victimizer. When the rage turns inward, a person can become self-destructive (self-mutilating, suicidal, or displaying other self-defeating behaviors) or be destroyed by others (the victim). Destruction by self or others is for them the last means of maintaining a feeling of potency.

Children who were abused received repeated reinforcement in childhood to act as a victim. Often it was the only way to be acknowledged by parental figures. Identification with and imitation of the parents' roles as victims or victimizers may lead to corresponding behavior. If a boy identifies with an abusive father, we can expect him to attempt to repeat the abusive behavior. Similarly, a girl who observes her mother being abused is more likely to engage in such behavior herself (Gelles & Straus, 1988). It is not uncommon for a person to assume both roles and become an abuser as well as a victim.

Social legitimacy of violence and victimization goes far beyond familial battlefields. Television programs, video games, movies, school playgrounds, neighborhoods, and national and international politics all legitimize the use of violence to resolve conflicts. Sunday morning cartoons, interactive video games centering on violence, and the armed invasion of a foreign land all send a clear message that it is acceptable to use force as a means to achieve a goal. When the culturally violent messages complement the familial ones, children who may not have any other frame of reference are most likely to fall into the role of victim and/or victimizer.

Typology of a Victim

The basic assumption of the legal system is that there is one party in a dispute that is guilty and totally responsible for the crime and another party that is totally innocent. In some cases the responsibility is clear, however, in most cases the situation is more complex.

The following is an attempt, based partly on Mendelson's (1974) original formulation, to classify victims according to their relative degree of responsibility and power to control or affect situations. These categories range from total innocence/no guilt to total responsibility/complete guilt.

1. *Not guilty/innocent victim*: This category includes victims who do not share responsibility for the offense with the perpetrators. These are innocent victims who cannot be expected to anticipate or prevent the offense.

   Examples:

   - Children who are sexually or physically abused or neglected.
   - Rape or murder victims when the crime is unforeseen, unprovoked, and perpetrated by complete strangers.
   - Severely mentally ill or disabled adults who are hurt or exploited.
   - Those who suffer a crime while unconscious.
   - Victims of random or rampage shooting.
   - Victims of unexpected natural disasters (e.g., victims of an earthquake in a nonearthquake zone).

2. *Victims with minor guilt*: This category includes victims who with some thought, planning, awareness, information, or consciousness might have anticipated danger and avoided or minimized the harm to themselves. In other words, they could or should have known better.

   Examples:

   - Adult victims of repeated domestic violence in areas where shelters are available (after patterns are established and behavior is no longer unpredictable).
   - Marital rape victims after the first few episodes (when the pattern has been established and it is no longer a surprise).

- Women who are raped after choosing to get drunk. Their minor responsibility is electing to become completely helpless and at the full mercy of others in a situation that has the potential to be dangerous.
- Adults who were victimized by being in the wrong place at the wrong time in situations where with some awareness, preparation, and caution they could have prevented the assault.
- Jews who suffered during the Holocaust. They, of course, are not responsible for the evils of the Nazis, but they could have resisted more, been less cooperative, and not gone like lambs to the slaughter. They could have read the situation better and left in time, as forty percent of them did.

3. *Victims who share equal responsibility with the perpetrators:* This category includes victims who share equal responsibility with the offender for the harm inflicted on them. These are people who are conscious and aware of the situation and choose to be part of it. They are not caught by surprise, and common sense could have anticipated the damage that occurred.

Examples:

- Co-alcoholics, co-addicts after the initial phase of their relationship (when it has been clearly established that the partner is an addict).
- A man who contracts a sexually transmitted disease from a prostitute.
- Victims who seek out, challenge, tease, or entice the perpetrator.
- Willing participants in a game of chicken, a gun duel, or a double suicide.

4. *Victims who are slightly more guilty than the offender:* This category includes victims who are active participants in an interaction where they are likely to get hurt. The victim seeks the damaging contact, and the offender can easily withdraw from the situation. In this category the offender is less responsible for the damage than is the victim.

Examples:

- An abusive husband who is killed by his battered wife. He is primarily responsible, but the abuse must also be viewed as an interaction and some responsibility shared by the couple.
- Drunk people who harass sober bystanders and get hurt.

- Gay bashers who get hurt.
- Cult members who willingly enter a cult as adults and then are brainwashed and harmed (i.e., Jonestown, Waco).
- Citizens who passively collude in their country's atrocious acts and get hurt by the armies of other countries (i.e., politically inactive German civilians who did not fight the Nazi regime and were killed in allied army attacks).

5. *Victims who are exclusively responsible for their victimization:* This category includes victims who initiated the contact and committed an act likely to lead to injury. In such cases, the one who inflicts the damage is not guilty, acting in pure self-defense or as his or her position dictates. This category is reserved for legally and clinically sane adults.

Examples:

- Rapists who are killed by their complete-stranger victims in self-defense.
- Mercenaries who are wounded or killed.
- People who smoke and get lung cancer.
- People who commit suicide and are not mentally ill. (Mentally healthy and competent individuals can choose to commit rationally planned suicide for which they bear full responsibility.)

These categories represent an attempt to differentiate the many guises of victimhood. They comprise a controversial, inconclusive, and incomplete grid for determining guilt or responsibility. Although not accounted for in the above categories, demographic, cultural, and personal variables are nevertheless crucial for the assessment of guilt and responsibility. Evaluating the degree of responsibility entails the following parameters.

- *Ethnicity*: Minorities are more disposed to victimization than those in the majority.
- *Gender*: Women are more disposed to victimization than men.
- *Socioeconomic status:* The poor are more disposed to victimization than the rich.
- *Physical attributes:* Less attractive people are seen as weaker and thus are more prone to victimization than those who are attractive.
- *Mental status:* The mentally ill are perceived as dysfunctional and are more prone to victimization than the healthy.

- *Familial background:* The abused and neglected are more prone to victimization than those who are loved and nurtured.
- *Cultural values:* People in cultures that promote violence are more prone to victimization than those in cultures that promote harmony.

MOVING FROM BLAME TO HEALING

As violence begets violence, so does blame beget blame. Blaming men, women, minorities, the rich, or the poor keeps the race for victim status alive. An individual or group can win the battle and become the victim of the year, yet lose the war. Behavior based on blame and lack of accountability is the very reason that victims may continue to get hurt, injured, and abused. It is apparent that the blame approach is ineffective in resolving the problems of violence and in shielding the victim from further victimization or protecting future generations from continuing the cycle of abuse.

The systems analysis approach offers an alternative (Bateson, 1979; Laszlo, 1976). Applied to victimization, systems analysis is concerned with the ways the dynamics of victimization develop, how they escalate toward violence, and how they might be shifted toward a nonviolent resolution. This approach is not concerned with who is right and who is to blame. Instead, it offers ways to intervene that have the potential to stop the patterns of violence.

Applying systems analysis to victimization gives rise to the following assumptions.

- Victimization, like violence, is not genetically programmed.
- Victimization happens within a context of relationship and a certain environment or culture. Hence, each participant's behavior must be understood within the framework of the relationship and its legal, economical, political, and social context.
- Participants in the victims–victimizers–bystanders dynamic assume, mainly unconsciously, mutually dependent and complementary roles.
- Intervention or change in the system can be initiated at any time, by any participant. Any change in behavior by one of the participants is likely to affect the behavior of the others and may lead to a different outcome.
- Interaction within the victimizer–victim environment can lead to violence or to other options, including nonviolent or peaceful

resolution. The nonviolent options will alter the victim and victimizer roles and may include termination of the relationship.

- Cultures can promote victim–victimizer, violent, or blame systems, or they can foster respectful relationships among their members who, in turn, commit to resolving conflicts in a nonviolent manner.

The cornerstone of the systems analysis approach is to view the different roles in victim systems (i.e., the abuser, abused, and bystander) as mutually dependent. The psychology of abusers (Beasley & Stoltenberg, 1992; Viano, 1990) and bystanders (Lantane & Darley, 1970) has been thoroughly explored, however, systems analysis also demands an examination of the generally ignored role of victim.

Victimization is a complex phenomenon and any inquiry or therapy must include multiple approaches or perspectives. Therapists should explore five types of considerations, all equally important, when they work with a victim system.

1. The nature of the interaction among victimizers, victims, and the environment (including bystanders) requires scrutiny. It is of utmost importance that no finger of blame be pointed at the victimizer or the victim.
2. The therapist must approach the individual victim with empathy and attempt to understand the current self-destructive behavior in light of the victim's past and evolution.
3. The therapist must assess the victim's level of consciousness, sanity, and ability to plan and control behavior.
4. Cultural and subcultural factors present since childhood—such as race, economic status, and gender—must be taken into account.
5. The therapist must consider the cultural context as revealed through the legal, educational, and political systems, as well as the media and popular trends.

The therapist applying these clinical guidelines to a case of domestic violence where the husband is the abuser must first understand the interplay between husband and wife and how their behaviors contribute to the maintenance and escalation of violence. The therapist should blame neither the abusive husband nor the battered wife but focus on the destructive system they both have developed and maintain. The behavior of both victim and abuser must be empathetically understood within the context of their familial history, with special attention given to the history of abuse and abandonment.

Subsequently, the woman's mental, intellectual, physical, and economic resources must be assessed. If necessary, protection should be provided accordingly and/or immediately. The therapist must then seek to understand how gender, race, and other factors such as disability apply to the couple's system of violence. Finally, the therapist must determine how the culture and subculture within which the couple operates (including the criminal justice system, economic and community resources, etc.) contribute to, collude with, and perpetuate the system of violence.

Only when the therapist understands these components and uses the system theory (often in conjunction with other theoretical orientations) is intervention likely to be effective. Whether the therapist works with individuals or the whole system, the most immediate task is to prevent imminent violence. The long-term goal must be to help the patient—whether victim, victimizer, or bystander—assume a new role and new behavior.

When working with the victim individually, the therapist must walk the fine line between empathy and collusion. Without assigning blame, the therapist's goal is to move the victim from blame to responsibility, from helplessness to accountability, and from hopelessness to empowerment. Victims need to develop an understanding of how they contribute to their own victimization. While acquiring a cohesive sense of self, victims must be helped to feel better about themselves, raise their self-esteem, and work through the legacy of their childhood abuse. Therapy must enable victims to break the dangerous and painful link between love and abuse while helping them to realize that they deserve the same respect and dignity as any other human being.

CONCLUSION

Understanding types, origins, and mode of operation of victims will allow therapists and nontherapists alike to recognize, prevent, and intervene in violent systems, enabling all participants to live better lives. For this to occur, victims must be helped to overcome their feelings of helplessness, hopelessness, and low self-esteem. They must not focus on blame, and they must avoid moral self-righteousness. Victims have to believe that they have a say in what happens to them and learn to overcome their victim patterns. The healing process should empower them to become conscious contributors to the unfolding of their lives, which can become dignified and meaningful.

REFERENCES

Bateson, G. (1979). *Mind in Nature*. New York: Dutton.

Beasley, R. & Stoltenberg, D.C. (1992). Personality characteristics of male spouse abusers. *Professional Psychology: Research and Practice, 23*(4), 310–317.

Brownmiller, S. (1975). *Against Our Will: Men, Women, and Rape*. New York: Simon & Schuster.

Caplan, L.P. & Hall-McCorquodale, T. (1985). Mother blaming in major clinical journals. *American Journal of Orthopsychiatry, 55*(3), 345–353.

Cook, D. & Frantz-Cook, A. (1984). A systematic treatment approach to wife battering. *Journal of Marital and Family Therapy, 10,* 83–93.

Etzioni, A. (1987). *A Responsive Society*. San Francisco: Jossey-Bass.

Gelles, R.J. & Straus, M.A. (1988). *Intimate Violence*. New York, Simon & Schuster.

Herman, J.L. (1992). *Trauma and Recovery*. New York: Basic.

Hughes, R. (1993). *Culture of Complaint: The Fraying of America*. New York: Oxford University Press.

Jain, R.S. (1990). The victim–offender relationship in family violence. In E. Viano (Ed.), *The Victimology Handbook* (pp. 107–111). New York: Garland.

Kaminer, W. (1992). *I'm Dysfunctional, You're Dysfunctional*. New York: Addison-Wesley.

Keen, S. (1986). *Faces of the Enemy*. New York: Harper and Row.

Keen, S. (1991). *Fire in the Belly: On Being a Man*. New York: Bantam.

Lantane, B. & Darley, J.M. (1970). *The Unresponsive Bystander: Why Doesn't He Help?* Englewood Cliffs, NJ: Prentice-Hall.

Laszlo, E. (1976). *The System View of the World*. New York: George Braziller.

Mendelson, B. (1974). The origin of the doctrine of victimology. In L. Drapkin & E. Viano (Eds.), *Victimology*. Lexington, KY: Lexington Books.

Ochberg, F.M. & Willis, D.J. (Eds.) (1991). Psychotherapy with victims. *Psychotherapy 28*(1).

Rotter, J.B. (1971, June). External and internal control. *Psychology Today,* 37–42, 58–59.

Russel, D.E.H. (1984). *Sexual Exploitation: Rape, Child Sexual Abuse, and Workplace Harassment*. Beverly Hills, CA: Sage.

Ryan, W. (1971). *Blaming the Victim*. New York: Vintage.

Schaef, A.W. (1986). *Co-Dependency: Misunderstood–Mistreated*. New York: Harper & Row.

Seligman, M.E.P. (1975). *Helplessness: On Depression, Development and Death*. San Francisco: W.H. Freeman.

Sundberg, S.L., Barbaree, H.E., & Marshall, W.L., (1991). Victim blame and the disinhibition of sexual arousal to rape vignettes. *Violence and Victims, 16,* 103–120.

Sykes, C.J. (1992). *A Nation of Victims: The Decay of the American Character*. New York: St. Martin's.

Tavris, C. (1993, January). Beware the incest survivor machine. *New York Times,* Book Review, 1, 16–18.

Viano, E. (Ed.) (1990). *The Victimology Handbook*. New York: Garland.

Walker, E. (1979). *The Battered Woman*. New York: Harper & Row.

Wolfgang, M.E. & Ferracuti, F. (1967). *The Subculture of Violence*. New York: Barnes & Noble.

Worchel, S. (1984). The darker side of helping. In E. Staub et al. (Eds.), *The Development and Maintenance of Prosocial Behavior*. New York: Plenum.

Yollow, K. & Bogard, M. (Eds.) (1988). *Feminist Perspectives in Wife Abuse*. Beverly Hills, CA: Sage.

Zur, O. (1989). War myths. *Journal of Humanistic Psychology, 29,* 297–327.

Zur, O. (1991). The love of hating: Exploring enmity. *History of European Ideas, 13,* 345–369.

Zur, O. and Glendinning, C. (1987). Men/women–war/peace: A systems approach. In M. Macy (Ed.), *Solution for a Troubled World* (pp. 107–121). Boulder, CO: Earthview.

4

HOMOPHOBIA: CONCEPTUAL, DEFINITIONAL, AND VALUE ISSUES

William T. O'Donohue and Christine E. Caselles

Homophobia is a potentially important construct, given the significant amount of violence and other violations of rights that homosexuals experience and the reactions that the relatively recent complexities of AIDS have evoked toward homosexuals and homosexuality. In this chapter, we examine the historical context that contributed to homophobia's emergence. We also explore whether, like past psychiatric definitions of "homosexuality," it implicitly and somewhat ironically contains an illegitimately pejorative evaluation of certain open and debatable value positions. We also review extant measurement instruments of homophobia to assess their psychometric adequacy.

Special attention is paid to the concurrent content and construct validity of their psychometric properties, critical for determining exactly what is being measured. This chapter also offers several proposals for theory development and construct definition in the domain of reactions to homosexuals and homosexuality.

A BRIEF HISTORY OF HOMOSEXUALITY

In 1973, by a vote of 5,854 to 3,810, the diagnostic category of homosexuality was eliminated from the *Diagnostic and Statistical Manual of Mental Disorders* (DSM) of the American Psychiatric Association (Bayer, 1981). In the first edition of the DSM, homosexuality was included as one of the sexual disorders classified among the Sociopathic Personality Disorders by the American Psychiatric Association (1952). Sociopathic disorders were characterized by a lack of distress or anxiety despite the presence of severe pathology. This allowed homosexuality to be classified as a mental disorder, despite the homosexual's possible satisfaction with his or her sexual orientation.

In the second edition of the DSM (APA, 1968), homosexuality was reclassified as a sexual deviation among the nonpsychotic disorders. The category of sexual deviation includes individuals whose sexual interests are directed toward objects other than persons of the opposite sex, toward acts not usually associated with coitus, or toward acts involving coitus under bizarre circumstances. It was noted that although these individuals may be disturbed by their sexual behavior, they are unable to substitute "normal sexual behavior."

In 1973, when homosexuality was eliminated from the DSM, the third edition of the manual contained the diagnosis of ego-dystonic homosexuality (American Psychiatric Association, 1973), which described individuals with a sustained pattern of overt homosexual arousal that is unwanted or distressing, accompanied by a desire to acquire heterosexual arousal. (It is interesting to note that in the ninth edition of International Classification of Diseases (World Health Organization, 1980) homosexuality is still classified as a disease.)

Writing about the 1973 decision and the dispute that surrounded it, Bayer (1981) contended that these changes were produced by political rather than scientific factors. Bayer argued that the revision represented the APA's surrender to political and social pressures, not new data or scientific theories regarding human sexuality. Bayer describes one instance in 1972 in which the New York Gay Activist Alliance organized a protest during a conference of the Association for the Advancement of Behavior Therapy. The protesters called for "an end to the use of aversion techniques to change the natural sexual orientation of human beings" (p.115). These views were explicated in a flier entitled "Torture Anyone?" A group of the activists gained access to one of the conference rooms during a presentation in front of a large audience that included Dr. Robert Spitzer, then a member of the APA's Nomenclature Committee. This was the first time Spitzer had been confronted with homosexuals demanding changes in psychiatry's conceptualization of homosexuality. Apparently, impressed by the passion and arguments of the protesters, Spitzer arranged for a formal presentation of their views to the Nomenclature Committee.

Consistent with the political and social climate of the United States during the second half of the 1960s, the issue of homosexuality became politicized. There was a movement by an increasing number of gay activists to promote the civil and political rights of homosexuals inasmuch as homosexuality was beginning to denote minority status with regard to political and civil rights rather than a category of deviance. Psychiatry, which had previously defined homosexuality as a disease and diagnosed homosexuals as mentally ill, was considered a formidable but politically and strategically important obstacle in the struggles of homosexuals for social and political status. In the late 1960s, homosexuals in the United States forged a potent movement to depathologize homosexuality.

The movement explicitly adopted the views of Thomas Szasz (1961, 1965, 1970), who criticized a neutral conceptualization of mental illness and exposed and cautioned against the role of the psychiatric profession in coercively promoting or attacking various values, aesthetic preferences, and political positions. This attraction to the views of Szasz on the part of gay activists was somewhat selective in that Szasz (1965, p. 124) had also stated,

> Ever since the Freudian revolution, and especially since the Second World War, it has become intellectually fashionable to hold that homosexuality is neither a sin nor a crime but a disease. This claim means either that homosexuality is a condition somewhat similar to ordinary organic maladies, perhaps caused by some genetic error or endocrine imbalance, or that it is an expression of psychosexual immaturity, probably caused by certain kinds of personal and social circumstances in early life. I believe it is very likely that homosexuality is, indeed, a disease in the second sense and perhaps sometimes even in the stricter sense. Nevertheless, if we believe that, by categorizing homosexuality as a disease, we have succeeded in removing it from the realm of moral judgment, we are in error.

However, Szasz also argued that the language of the mental health professions can falsely appear to de-ethicize and de-politicize what are essentially moral, aesthetic, and political issues in human relations and personal conduct. In some of his more extreme statements, Szasz

(1970) stated that much of what passes as psychiatry and behavioral science is force and fraud, which function to oppress and coerce individuals who express unacceptable ideas. Thus, gay activists also took Szasz to be saying that when the psychiatric profession defined homosexuality as a mental illness, it was attempting to use the language of science to obscure and condemn a set of what are essentially value positions. This ultimately had the effect of illegitimately abridging the autonomy and civil rights of homosexuals.

Shortly after the nosological revision, there was a significant shift in the focus of research related to homosexuality. Rather than focus on the "etiology" and "cure" of homosexuality, theorists and researchers in psychology began to suggest that negative attitudes toward homosexuals, rather than homosexuality itself, cause many of the difficulties that homosexuals face (Smith, 1971). Many of these researchers rejected what they referred to as the "victim analysis," and redirected their empirical pursuits toward the possible victimizers, more specifically, toward the attitudes of nonhomosexuals toward homosexuals and homosexuality (MacDonald, Huggins, Young, & Swanson, 1972). Homosexuality was now regarded as a normal, healthy, lifestyle choice. Thus, new questions arose: what are the etiology and associated features of individuals who have negative attitudes and reactions toward homosexuals and homosexuality? What is the cure for this attitude?

In 1972, Weinberg coined the term "homophobia" to describe "the dread of being in close quarters with homosexuals" (p. 4). Weinberg maintained that an individual who displays deeply negative attitudes toward homosexuals should not be considered mentally healthy. Much subsequent research on attitudes of nonhomosexuals toward homosexuals and homosexuality has used this construct. Hudson and Ricketts (1980) reported that between 1971 and 1978, at least thirty-one studies were published that investigated attitudes of nonhomosexuals toward homosexuality. A computer-based literature search using the topics "homosexuality and attitudes" and "homophobia" yielded at least 539 additional articles examining attitudes and reactions toward homosexuality between 1979 and 1991.

PROBLEMS IN THE DEFINITION OF "HOMOPHOBIA"

It appears that during the past two decades, the term homophobia has been generalized to denote any negative attitude, belief, or action toward homosexuals (Haaga, 1991; Fyfe, 1983). Fyfe suggested that homophobia might operate on different levels: (1) cultural homophobia, which maintains traditional sex role distinctions; (2) attitudinal homophobia, a set of fixed negative attitudes toward homosexuals; and (3) homophobia as a personality dimension. This "trait" is taken to be correlated with rigidity, authoritarianism, conservatism, and intolerance for ambiguity and deviance. Other variants of the more general definition of homophobia include Colin's (1991) description of homophobia as any antihomosexual bias and discriminatory behavior.

There were still other definitional attempts. Morin and Garfinkle (1978) characterized the homophobic as an individual who does not value a homosexual lifestyle equally with a heterosexual lifestyle. Other researchers have defined homophobia in terms of some behavioral referent. For example, one study considered discrimination against individuals wearing progay paraphernalia to be a manifestation of homophobia (Colin, 1991). Bell (1991) considered homophobia to be the equivalent of homonegativity, which refers to any negative feelings or thoughts about homosexuals or homosexuality. Reiter (1991) defined homophobia as antihomosexual prejudice, a complex phenomenon whose roots have been traced to a cultural context.

Although one is free to stipulate any meaning for any word, avoiding serious problems in communication requires a consensus regarding a term's meaning and reference. One option is to take homophobia as representing a narrow and etymologically based concept: "an irrational fear and avoidance of homosexuals and homosexuality." This is a strategy followed by MacDonald (1976, p. 23) who defined homophobia as an "irrational, persistent fear or dread of homosexuals." This definitional strategy, of course, parallels the DSM-III-R's diagnostic criteria of simple phobia and suggests that homophobia may be similar to other phobias, for example, claustrophobia, arachnophobia, and so on. Whether this similarity is sufficient to warrant its inclusion in the DSM as a mental disorder is another question. However, a significant advantage of this option is that it appears to capture at least a subset, and possibly an important subset, of the negative reactions toward homosexuality and homosexuals that have motivated previous usage of this word.

How are we to understand the lack of clarity and consistency in the use of "homophobia?" Szasz (1970, p. 49) raises an interesting possibility:

> Language has three main functions: to transmit information, to induce mood, and to promote action. It should be emphasized that conceptual clarity is required only for the cognitive, or information-transmitting, use of language. Lack of clarity may be no handicap when language is used to influence people; indeed, it is often an advantage.

In a subsequent section of this chapter, we take the position that homophobia does make a pejorative reference to certain open moral questions. Thus, the ambiguity surrounding this term has functioned to help hide what might be more controversial should it be explicated: that the construct of homophobia might be used to influence individuals to react differently toward homosexuals and homosexuality by condemning certain sets of negative reactions.

As intelligence might be what intelligence tests measure, so might homophobia be what homophobic scales measure. This is an important point, for it is possible that scales might not actually measure what they purport to measure. In the next section we closely examine the psychometric properties of scales purporting to measure homophobia in an attempt to discern more accurately what is measured by these scales.

Measuring Homophobia

One of the earliest attempts to measure homophobia consisted of an effort to discover psychosocial correlates of individuals reporting negative attitudes toward homosexuals (Smith, 1971). Smith developed a twenty-four-item self-reporting questionnaire, which consisted of a nine-item Homophobia Scale (H-scale) and fifteen items assessing attitudes related to a diverse set of topics, such as patriotism, materialism, sexuality, religion, and traditional sex roles. Examples of these items include: "There is nothing wrong with a man being passive when he feels like it," "Blacks are asking for too much too soon," and "A belief in God is not important to the maintenance of morality."

Smith conceded that the questionnaire did not truly represent a "scale" because it used a forced-choice response format rather than a continuum. The H-scale contained questions that addressed a person's legal and moral attitudes toward homosexuals. Examples include: "Homosexuals should be locked up to protect society," "I would be afraid for a child of mine to have a teacher who was a homosexual," and "Homosexuals should not be allowed to hold government positions." There were also a number of items that assessed an individual's personal comfort with homosexuality: "I find the thought of homosexual acts disgusting," "If a homosexual sat next to me on the bus, I would get nervous," and "It would be upsetting for me to find out that I was alone with a homosexual."

The questionnaire was administered to a group of undergraduate psychology students. Of the ninety-three returned questionnaires, those with the twenty-one highest and twenty-one lowest scores on the

H-scale comprised the homophobic and nonhomophobic groups. Differences between these two groups' responses to the other items were reported. The results were interpreted as being indicative of the "personality profile" of the homophobic. Smith suggested that the homophobic personality may be authoritarian, sexually rigid, and status conscious.

The psychometric properties of the H-scale and the remaining items were not reported in this study. It appears that no reliability measures of the H-scale or the measures of the personality variables were obtained. Moreover, it is unclear whether using the twenty-one lowest scores constituted an adequate method of determining cutoff scores for categorization. It is possible that this group might have had a truncated range and not scored in a sufficiently extreme manner to warrant classification as either "homophobic" or "nonhomophobic."

Thus, Smith's H-scale (1971) is a psychometrically questionable measure of homophobia. If psychometric properties were evaluated, they were not reported by the author. There were no established norms or acceptable validity criteria for the H-scale; rather, arbitrary cutoffs were designated based on the twenty-one lowest scores in the sample.

Lumby (1976) converted Smith's H-scale to a Likert index, with ratings from 1 ("strongly disagree") to 5 ("strongly agree"), and conducted a study that purportedly assessed the validity of the measure. Lumby assumed that if the H-scale actually measured homophobia in nonhomosexuals, there would be significant differences between the responses of homosexuals and those of heterosexuals. The glaring flaw in the logic of this assumption is that although any valid measure of homophobia would be expected to discriminate between homosexuals and heterosexuals, it does not follow that a measure that discriminates between these two groups necessarily is a valid measure of homophobia. In fact, all that could be concluded from such a measure is that certain response patterns correlate positively or negatively with heterosexuality. Moreover, some writers have subsequently claimed that often homosexuals themselves are internalized homophobics. If this is true, it further vitiates the logic of this research.

The results of this study indicated that all homophobic items significantly discriminated between homosexuals and heterosexuals. Lumby, however, reported that the scale cannot be considered a valid measure of homophobia because it failed to meet the minimal Guttman Scalogram requirements. This finding was attributed, in part, to the ambiguity and awkwardness of the wording of many items. Lumby suggested that large numbers of items relevant to homophobia should be generated and validated so that a valid homophobia scale could be produced.

Although Lumby remedied the difficulties resulting from Smith's (1971) forced-choice format, his Likert index does not represent a significant improvement in the measurement of homophobia. Lumby's attempts to validate the scale by using a homosexual comparison group are an inadequate approach to ascertaining validity. Moreover, the author presented no reliability data concerning the scale, which if taken as reliable preliminary to validity studies sets the upper limit on validity (Anastasi, 1988).

The most widely used measure of homophobia was constructed by Hudson and Ricketts (1980). These researchers attempted to combine items that assessed attitudinal dimensions of homophobia, as well as affective components of the homophobic response. The scale, titled the Index of Homophobia (IHP), consists of twenty-five items with a Likert response scale. Possible scores range from 0 to 100 and indicate in which of four categories the individual resides: "high-grade homophobic" (75 to 100), "low-grade homophobic" (50 to 75), "low-grade nonhomophobic" (25 to 50), and "high-grade nonhomophobic" (0 to 25).

An evaluation of the content of the IHP reveals that the items are concerned primarily with an individual's "comfort" concerning proximity to and involvement with homosexuals. Examples of items on this scale include: "I would feel comfortable working closely with homosexuals," "I would enjoy attending social functions at which homosexuals were present," and "If a member of my own sex made a pass at me, I would feel flattered." The wording of most of these items seems to imply that in order to achieve a nonhomophobic rating one needs to have some positive affective response toward proximity to and the company of homosexuals rather than holding a neutral attitude.

In fact, if an individual responded "neither agree, nor disagree" to all of the items, his or her score would result in the label "high-grade homophobic." This scoring procedure appears flawed, inasmuch as consistently neutral responses might be expected of individuals who do not harbor negative attitudes toward homosexuals but do not seek out or prefer the company of homosexual individuals. Although an indifferent stance as described is definitionally inconsistent with homophobia, the IHP would classify this individual as a high-grade homophobic.

The IHP represents a psychometric improvement over previous measures of homophobia in that validity and reliability measures were reported. It is probably these qualities that resulted in the widespread usage of the IHP in research settings. The authors report sound measures of the IHP's internal consistency (e.g., a coefficient alpha of .901 and a standard error of measurement of 4.75), however, there has been no evaluation of the temporal stability of the IHP (e.g., test–retest measures). Because homophobia is usually considered as a trait, this is a serious problem. A measure's construct validity is dependent on its ability to yield consistent measures of the trait under inspection. If an instrument fails to produce consistent results over time, this may indicate that the instrument is not actually measuring the stable trait it purports to measure but, rather, is heavily susceptible to random variation. Alternatively, inconsistency may indicate that the construct being measured may actually be unstable over time.

In addition to being constrained by the inadequacy of the reliability data provided for the IHP, the issue of the scale's validity has other serious problems. Essentially, its validity is predicated on inferences that may be unfounded. For example, Hudson and Ricketts (1980) purportedly ascertained the construct validity of the IHP using several criteria variables. The first problem with their approach to construct validity is that all of the criteria variables were scores on self-report instruments. This single-method approach to construct validity is inadequate (Anastasi, 1988).

Furthermore, an examination of the self-report measures used to validate the IHP reveals that there are flaws with these criteria measures. According to Hudson and Ricketts, the criteria that best support IHP's validity are scores on the Sexual Attitudes Scale (SAS). The SAS is reportedly a valid and reliable measure of an individual's sexual conservatism or liberalism and taps an individual's beliefs about the "expression of human sexuality." Hudson and Ricketts reported that the IHP and SAS scores had a correlation of .53, which was significant at the $p < .0001$ level. The problem with interpreting this correlation as an indication of construct validity is that it possibly demonstrates nothing more than a significant correlation between sexual conservatism and higher scores on the IHP.

At best, this is a demonstration of convergent validity, which is incomplete in the absence of any indication of the discriminant validity of the IHP. In other words, if the IHP does nothing more to discriminate individuals than the SAS, what qualifies it as a measure of anything more than sexual conservatism? A more serious criticism is why sexual conservatism should be regarded as a criterion for homophobia. Homophobia is typically construed to be a pathological state, although it is not at all clear that traditional views regarding sexual behavior are pathological.

Hudson and Ricketts' second measure of construct validity proved to be even less adequate than the SAS. The authors inferred that high levels of homophobia are "likely to be a signal that the person has experienced social learning and training that would make them more susceptible to personal problems and difficulties with interpersonal relationships" (1980, p. 364). No independent research is cited to support this statement, nor does any appear to exist. Therefore, Hudson and Ricketts' assertion that correlations between difficulties in certain areas and high scores on the IHP support the construct validity of the IHP is unfounded.

The psychometric qualities of this measure appear even bleaker when one notes the measure of "the severity of an individual's problems in 20 different areas" that was employed. Hudson and Ricketts did not report any reliability of validity measures or any information concerning the derivation of this scale. It might reasonably be assumed, then, that the scale was constructed for the purpose of validating the IHP and was not subjected to reliability or validity tests. Moreover, when, contrary to their predictions, they found that homophobia was negatively correlated with a subset of problems on this scale that they thought reflected interpersonal difficulties, they decided, in an ad hoc manner, that this part of the scale did not adequately measure the construct of interpersonal problems. It is interesting that this did not cause them to alter their interpretation of the "confirmation" of a positive correlation of homophobia and other noninterpersonal psychological problems that were measured by the same device.

Another major flaw with the procedures used to validate the IHP is the sample used. At least 50 percent of the sample was of Asian descent: 35 percent Japanese, 9.7 percent Chinese, and 7 percent Filipino. This raises a serious question as to whether the findings reported in this study can reliably be generalized to a non-Asian population.

Hudson and Ricketts emphasized the content validity of the IHP as a tremendous asset of the scale. Expanding on Weinberg's (1972) definition of homophobia, Hudson and Ricketts proposed that homophobia is a construct that includes the personal affective responses—including disgust, anxiety, aversion, discomfort, fear, and anger—related to any contact or involvement with homosexuals. Presumably, the scale is designed to exclude judgments and personal decisions regarding the moral, legal, and social desirability of homosexuality. However, by the author's own admission, four of the twenty-five items deal with personal decisions, moral judgments, and preferences. The authors minimize the importance of the four items that do not support the content validity of the IHP. Considering that these items represent almost twenty-five percent of the total items, their contribution in detracting from the validity of the scale may be significant. Because the scoring procedure of the IHP results in categorizing the individual into one of four groups, each with a range of twenty-five points, these four items alone can result in inaccurate classification. If an individual answered each of these four items with an extreme response, it is probable that the twenty points lost or gained would result in a change in classification.

An evaluation of the content validity of a scale involves an analysis of both the denotative meanings of the words in items and a thorough consideration of the connotative values of the items. This becomes particularly crucial when the items involve terms with controversial histories and rich connotative implications. Terms such as "homosexual," "gay bar," "sexual advances," and "working closely with a homosexual" are associated with a variety of images and meanings.

For example, the term "homosexual," defined as "one who feels romantic love for persons of the same sex," may have connotative meanings that refer to sexual activities. Some individuals may have certain negative aesthetic or moral reactions to these activities. Therefore, when an individual responds affirmatively to the item, "I find the thought of homosexuality disgusting," it is possible that this is a response based on the connotative meanings of the word (males who more frequently than heterosexuals engage in "fist-fucking," in high magnitudes of promiscuity, and who insert rodents in rectums), which may or may not be valid. Thus, another problem in measurement involves the various interpretations and connotations that may be associated with key words.

Overall, the developers of the IHP used a somewhat more empirical and psychometrically sophisticated approach than previous researchers who produced instruments to measure homophobia. The internal consistency of the scale was evaluated, and some validation issues were addressed by the researchers. However, significantly more research is needed before conclusions can be made about the reliability and the validity of inferences from this scale. Questions remain about whether this scale actually measures homophobia or a reaction to homosexuality.

Prior to the development of the IHP, Millham, San Miguel, and Kellogg (1976) conducted what appears to be the most methodologically sound investigation of attitudes toward homosexuality. These researchers developed a questionnaire consisting of thirty-eight items designed to survey a broad range of attitudes and beliefs toward homosexuality. Items included statements pertaining to emotional reactions to homosexuals, the legal status of homosexuals, the mental health of homosexuals, acceptance of stereotypes about homosexuals, and moral and ethical aspects of homosexuality. Responses were in a true–false format. All items were duplicated to refer separately to male and female homosexuals.

The 76 items were administered to a pool of 795 subjects drawn from a population of undergraduate psychology students. A factor analysis performed on the data resulted in the emergence of six discrete factors, which are presented in Table 4.1

It is interesting that the "personal anxiety" factor, which the researchers believe corresponds with other researchers' definitions of homophobia, accounts for only ten percent of the variance in attitudes toward male

TABLE 4.1 Factors Obtained on the Homosexuality Attitudes Scale % Variance

Factor Label	Description of Factor	Male Target	Female Target
Repressive–dangerous	The belief that homosexuals are dangerous and the belief that homosexuals should be subject to social and legal restrictions not imposed on other members of society	55.6	14.4
Personal anxiety	Experience of anxiety in the presence of homosexuals, disgust, avoidance of homosexuals	10.1	52.7
Preference for female over male homosexuals	The opinion that female homosexuals are preferable to male homosexuals	12.7	11.5
Cross-sex mannerisms	The belief that homosexuals manifest certain characteristics of the opposite sex	4.1	6.2
Moral reprobation	The belief that homosexuality is sinful and wrong	4.5	4.9
Preference for male over female homosexuals	The opinion that male homosexuals are preferable to females	6.7	3.2

homosexuals. Examples of items that hinge on this factor are listed below.

1. Male/female homosexuals are sick.
2. It would be very easy for me to have a conversation with someone whom I knew to be a male or female homosexual.
3. I would like to have male homosexual friends.
4. Male homosexuality is a perversion.
5. Male homosexuals should be allowed to teach young children.

We discuss issues related to the implicit value positions associated with this construct later in the chapter. At this point, it is important to note that most of these items appear to refer manifestly to debatable value positions and judgments.

Another important finding of this study was the large variances in each factor for both male and female homosexuals. For example, the repressive-dangerous factor accounted for the most variance (55 percent) in attitudes toward male homosexuals, whereas the personal anxiety factor accounted for the most variance (52.7 percent) in attitudes toward female homosexuals. The implications of this finding may be that attitudes toward male and female homosexuals differ in fundamental ways, a distinction overlooked by researchers investigating homophobia.

Overall, this study suggests that attitudes and reactions to homosexuals are multidimensional. The orthogonality of the personal anxiety factor to factors involving beliefs about the legal status of homosexuals suggests that it is inaccurate to infer that personal discomfort and anxiety related to homosexuality underlie biases or prejudices against homosexuality. This may imply that what researchers are terming homophobia may involve a personal preference.

Perhaps the most serious psychometric flaw involving the validation of all scales of homophobia is the absence of a pre-existing, behaviorally referenced criterion group. The validation of the homophobia instruments examined involved a criterion group designated by scores on measures of some construct that was believed to be related to homophobia, such as sexual conservatism, religiosity, or maladjustment. This defect might have been remedied by using a criterion group such as individuals who have engaged in hate crimes against homosexuals.

Thus, given the numerous psychometric problems with each of these scales, many of the inferences researchers make based upon instruments designed to measure the homophobia construct are invalid. In a particularly illustrative example, Stark (1991) found that individuals who hold traditional views pertaining to gender roles tend to show higher levels of homophobia as measured by the IHP. On this basis, Stark concluded that traditional gender roles have negative ramifications in society. Based on the psychometric properties of the IHP, Stark's conclusion is an invalid and potentially dangerous one. What is of particular concern is that this exemplifies how a positive correlation with homophobia is taken to be a marker of other attitudes and behaviors that are undesirable.

Value Issues in Homophobia

We now examine whether value issues are contained in the construct of homophobia, first by using the most narrow and empirical definition of homophobia, that is, "an irrational fear and avoidance of homosexuals." We then show how the conclusions reached from this definition apply to the more general definitions of homophobia given above.

Although the measurement of fear and avoidance is an empirical matter (e.g., Nietzel, Bernstein, & Russell, 1988), deciding whether these are irrational is not. It is obvious that it is not irrational to fear and avoid some things, for example, murderers, rapists, attack dogs, and malfunctioning airplanes. But is it irrational to fear and avoid homosexuals and homosexuality? We claim that this is partly a value question, because the moral status of homosexuality is an open question. Our argument is based on the following logic: if there is at least one argument (and we see several) that concludes that homosexual behavior is morally impermissible, and if this argument is not obviously unsound, then the moral status of homosexuality is an open moral (value) question.

Thus, we claim that it is reasonable, and perhaps even to be expected, for individuals who actually believe a version of one of these arguments to behave in a manner that is avoidant and fearful. That is, it is not irrational for an individual who believes that an act is immoral to want to avoid people who behave in such a manner and to become anxious in the presence of such people or such acts. Similar considerations hold for abortion, euthanasia, and anti-Semitism. For those who consider these acts immoral, it is not irrational to want to avoid abortionists or Nazis and to become anxious around them.

It is important to point out that this is not to say that we take any argument for the moral impermissibility of homosexuality to be sound or that we feel these arguments have more merit than the relevant counterarguments (e.g., see Ruse, 1988, for an excellent critical response to some of these arguments). However, the points made by Szasz and often embraced by gay activists hold here: that certain value, moral, aesthetic, and political questions and positions in a free society should not be closed and suppressed by mental health professionals and behavioral science research. The moral status of homosexuality is one of these.

There are readily available arguments for the moral impermissibility of homosexual acts that are not obviously unsound. Historically, in both Western and non-Western cultures, the majority of cultural institutions has argued against the morality of homosexuality (Batchelor, 1980). Various religious arguments hold that God has revealed in various ways (e.g., the burning of Sodom or direct divine pronouncements) that homosexual acts are morally impermissible. Given that this is the position of a vast number of religions (Roman Catholicism, many conservative Protestant churches, as well as the Jewish and Islamic faiths), and given the number of individuals professing these faiths, it would seem that this is a commonly held argument. Again, we invoke the Szaszian point that it is not the proper role of mental health professionals and behavioral scientists to judge as abnormal or irrational a belief in God and specific beliefs regarding what God has revealed. These are properly open issues that citizens of a free society should debate and decide upon, free of the interference of the mental health profession's attempts to make either ethical position a mental health issue.

There are other secular arguments concerning the immorality of homosexuality. Kant (1963, p. 170, as quoted by Ruse, 1988), for example, thought that homosexual acts violate the categorical imperative:

> A second *crimen carnis contra naturam* [immoral acts against our animal nature] is intercourse between *sexus homogenii*, in which the object of sexual impulse is a human being but there is homogeneity instead of heterogeneity of sex, as when a woman satisfies her desire on a woman, or a man on a man. This practice too is contrary to the ends of humanity; for the end of humanity in respect of sexuality is to preserve the species without debasing the person; but in this instance the species is not being preserved (as it can be by a *crimen carnis secundum naturam*), but the person is set aside, the self is degraded below the level of the animals, and humanity is dishonored.

This argument, based on a natural law account of ethics, and similar natural law arguments concerning the immorality of homosexuality are given by Plato's laws and Aquinas (1968) and by more modern ethicists such as Ruddick (1975).

Utilitarian arguments can reach similar conclusions concerning the moral impermissibility of homosexuality if we postulate that the net effects of homosexual practices (e.g., failure to reproduce, increasing exposure to social sanctions, increased health risks especially in the time of AIDS, etc.) are negative relative to the positive consequences of homosexuality and relative to the net effects of heterosexual practices. Of course, these possible empirical consequences are quite debatable. The point is not that these actually have been proven true, but simply that these are open possibilities.

Thus, we conclude that ethical arguments exist that take homosexuality to be morally wrong and that are not obviously unsound.

PROPOSAL FOR A BEHAVIORAL SCHEMA

Interest in homophobia seems to emanate from a broader interest in general reactions to homosexuals and homosexuality. Thus, conceptual clarity would be gained by clearly delineating the domain of reactions to homosexuals and homosexuality, how elements of this domain may constitute higher-order constructs, and the interrelationships between subsets of this domain.

A schema of the domain of reactions to homosexuality and homosexuals is contained in Table 4.2. We propose that there are three broad types of reactions to homosexuality and homosexuals: emotional, intellectual/cognitive, and behavioral reactions. By emotional reactions we mean an involuntary reaction pattern that includes physiological changes, expressive behaviors, and states of feeling (Wortman & Loftus, 1988). These emotions may be negative (e.g., anxiety, disgust, anger), positive (e.g., love, happiness), or more neutral (e.g., curiosity). Intellectual reactions are cognitive products such as belief in certain propositions, arguments, or factual memories. These may be further divided into moral beliefs (e.g., "Homosexuality is morally permissible because God created us all as equals and loves us equally"), aesthetic beliefs (e.g., "Sodomy is aesthetically negative"), political beliefs (e.g., "Homosexuals should have the same rights as anyone else"), and general knowledge categories (e.g., "Homosexuals are more likely to contract AIDS than heterosexuals"). These may be true or false or sound or unsound in some normative sense, but what is relevant here is whether someone actually holds these beliefs. The last category is behavioral reactions, which may be defined as responses involving striated muscles such as avoidance, approach, aggression, and so on. It

TABLE 4.2 Reactions to Homosexuals and Homosexuality

Emotional	Intellectual	Behavioral
Negative	Moral Evaluations	Positive
1a. Anxiety	2a. Homosexuality is morally permissible.	3a. Approach
1b. Disgust	2b. Homosexuality is morally impermissible.	Negative
1c. Discomfort	Aesthetic Reactions	3b. Avoidance
	2c. Homosexuality is aesthetically pleasing.	3c. Aggression
Positive		
1d. Sexual arousal	2d. Homosexuality is aesthetically displeasing.	
1e. Love	Political Reactions	
1f. Comfort	2e. Homosexual partners should be given legal rights.	
	2f. Homosexual partners should not be given legal rights.	
Neutral		
1g. Curiosity	Nonevaluative Beliefs	
	2g. Homosexuals are promiscuous.	

Examples of Conclusions:
(1a) + (3b) − [intellectual reactions] = homophobia
(3c) = antihomosexual disorder
(1a) + (3b) + (2b) = moral stance

should be noted that these may also need to be subclassified by gender, that is, reactions to male and female homosexuals may be different.

From this domain certain combinations of reactions can be isolated and combined to form what might prove to be useful constructs. For example, we propose that an irrational fear of homosexuality and homosexuals can be defined as the emotional reaction of fear, plus the behavioral reaction of avoidance, in the absence of the intellectual reaction of negative moral or aesthetic arguments. This might be taken as homophobia. On the other hand, fear and avoidance in the presence of intellectual reactions that include negative moral arguments might, for example, simply be called a reaction based on a moral stance and, hence, rational. The presence of a reasonable argument makes the response rational and hence not phobic (which requires an irrational reaction). Criminal behavior toward homosexuals might be defined by behavioral reactions such as aggression. Whether such aggression is simply a criminal violation or whether it is also a mental disorder is a debatable question.

An important advantage of explicating this behavioral domain is that positive reactions to homosexuality and homosexuals are also recognized. In the existing literature, positive reactions have been given little attention. In fact, in the homophobic literature the only way positive reactions can be identified and expressed is negatively; that is, one is not homophobic. However, this does not do justice to the full range of potentially positive reactions. This schema allows the study of a number of positive reactions, such as love, sexual attraction, approach, and so on.

Finally, by attempting to explicate the major reactions to homosexuals and homosexuality, this schema can serve as a useful heuristic for the investigation of the interrelationships between these variables. For example, one can investigate whether those who are aggressively against homosexuals become sexually aroused to homosexual stimuli (as certain psychoanalytic theories might predict) or whether what we have defined as antihomosexual disorder is related either to homophobia or to a moral/political stance as detailed above.

CONCLUSION

Existing psychometric measures of homophobia have been inadequate and therefore it is not clear currently whether this construct can be accurately measured. The development of the construct of homophobia appears to be in its infancy. It is of paramount importance to establish a consensus on a clear univocal definition of this term. A family of related terms could range from the very general (e.g., "homonegativity"), referring to any negative attitude or behavior, to the more specific. In addition, it could carve out subsets of this domain such as homophobia (e.g., an irrational fear and avoidance) or homoaggressiveness (e.g., individuals who commit illegal acts that hurt homosexuals). Because the interrelationships of these constructs pose important empirical questions, psychometrically sophisticated work needs to be done to develop better measures. It is essential that such research also encompass positive reactions toward homosexuals and homosexuality and the possibility of different reactions to male and female homosexuality.

Moreover, given that social scientists have not yet disproved certain normative (i.e., theological or moral) claims and arguments, care must be taken not to make a mistake similar to that which was made in the concept of homosexuality as a disease. It is most unfortunate when scientists attempt to pass implicit or explicit pejorative evaluations of individuals holding certain open and debatable value positions as part of their science.

REFERENCES

American Psychiatric Association (1952). *Diagnostic and Statistical Manual of Mental Disorders*. Washington, DC: American Psychiatric Association.

American Psychiatric Association. (1968). *Diagnostic and Statistical Manual of Mental Disorders*. Washington, DC: American Psychiatric Association.

American Psychiatric Association. (1973). *Diagnostic and Statistical Manual of Mental Disorders*. Washington, DC: American Psychiatric Association.

Anastasi, A. (1988). *Psychological Testing*. New York: Macmilllan.

Aquinas, St.T. (1968*). Summa Theologiae, 43, Temperance*. (T. Gilby, Trans.). London: Blackfriars.

Batchelor, E. (Ed.) (1980). *Homosexuality and Ethics*. New York: Pilgrim.

Bayer, R. (1981). *Homosexuality and American Psychiatry*. New York: Basic.

Bell, N. (1991). AIDS and women: Remaining ethical issues. *AIDS Education and Prevention, 1*, 22–30.

Colin, G. (1991). The effects upon helping behavior on wearing pro-gay identification. *British Journal of Social Psychology, 30*, 171–178.

Fyfe, B. (1983). "Homophobia" or homosexual bias reconsidered. *Archives of Sexual Behavior, 12*, 549–554.

Haaga, D. (1991). "Homophobia?" *Journal of Social Behavior and Personality, 6*, 171–172.

Hudson, W. & Ricketts, W. (1980). A strategy for the measurement of homophobia. *Journal of Homosexuality, 5*, 357–372.

Kant, I. (1963). *Lectures in Ethics*. (L. Infield, Trans.). New York: Harper & Row.

Lumby, M. (1976). Homophobia: A quest for a valid scale. *Journal of Homosexuality, 2*, 39–47.

MacDonald, A. (1976). Homophobia: Its roots and meanings. *Homosexual Counseling, 3*, 23–33.

Macdonald, A., Huggins, J., Young, S., & Swanson, R. (1972). Attitudes toward homosexuality: Preservation of sex morality or the double standard? *Journal of Consulting and Clinical Psychology, 40*, 161.

Millham, J., San Miguel, C., & Kellogg, R. (1976). Factor analytic conceptualization of attitudes toward male and female homosexuals. *Journal of Homosexuality, 2*, 3–20.

Morin, S. & Garfinkle, F. (1978). Male homophobia. *Social Issues, 34*, 29–47.

Nietzel, M.T., Bernstein, D.A., & Russell, R.L. (1988). Assessment of anxiety and fear. In A. S. Bellack & M. Hersen (Eds.), *Behavioral Assessment*. (3d ed., pp. 280–312). New York: Pergamon.

Reiter, L. (1991). Developmental origins of anti-homosexual prejudice in heterosexual men and women. *Clinical Social Work Journal, 19*, 163–175.

Ruddick, S. (1975). Better sex. In R. Baker & F. Elliston (Eds.), *Philosophy and Sex* (pp. 83–104). Buffalo, N.Y.: Prometheus.

Ruse, M. (1988). *Homosexuality: A Philosophical Inquiry*. Oxford: Basil Blackwell.

Smith, K. (1971). Homophobia; A tentative personality profile. *Psychological Reports, 29*, 1091–1094.

Stark, L. (1991). Traditional gender role beliefs and individual outcomes: An exploratory analysis. *Sex Roles, 24*, 639–650.

Szasz, T.S. (1961). *The Myth of Mental Illness*. New York; Hoeber-Harper.

Szasz, T.S. (1965). Legal and moral aspects of homosexuality. In J. Marmor (Ed.), *Sexual Inversion*. New York: Doubleday.

Szasz, T.S. (1970). *Ideology and Insanity*. New York: Doubleday.

Weinberg, G. (1972). *Society and the Healthy Homosexual*. New York: St. Martin's.

World Health Organization (1980). *International Statistical classification of diseases and related health problems* (9th Revision). Geneva, Switzerland: Author.

Wortman, C.B. & Loftus, E.F. (1988). *Psychology* (3d ed). New York: Knopf.

Section B
Mental Healthcare Economics

5

EXPANDING A SHRINKING ECONOMIC BASE: THE RIGHT WAY, THE WRONG WAY, AND THE MENTAL HEALTH WAY

Nicholas A. Cummings

Psychology had just become the nation's preeminent psychotherapy profession when managed care decimated its independent solo practice. Long-term therapy, the economic mainstay of the independent practice of psychology, was curtailed. Psychoanalysts suffered the most, but all psychotherapists saw their practices spiral downward. Social workers suffered least because they assumed most of the referrals. However, fee scales changed accordingly, reflecting master's-level rather than doctoral-level reimbursement. In other words, doctoral psychologists were earning roughly the same as master's-level practitioners, whose ranks (social workers, marriage/family therapists, counselors, etc.) had grown exponentially, far exceeding demand. Psychologists who had been in practice for a decade or more reported as much as a fifty percent decline in their incomes beginning in the early and mid-1990s. Those who maintained their approximate income levels worked many hours, seeing more patients for a smaller fee. Others took salaried jobs, left psychology entirely, or took early retirement.

There have been exceptions, of course. Some psychologists mastered the art of managed care and are doing better than ever, and others carved profitable niche practices for themselves. Certain localities have been less affected, usually because fewer practitioners reside there. California is a favorite residence of psychotherapists, and it is estimated there is a twenty to twenty-five percent surplus of practitioners (California Psychological Association, 2002). On the other hand, Hawaii provides an extraordinary example of psychologists still flourishing, primarily because social workers, who are not licensed there, are ineligible for almost all third-party reimbursement.

In the main, however, psychotherapy as a profession has responded to the too-many-therapists-seeing-much-fewer-patients phenomenon by labeling an increasing number of ordinary persons as patients. This is a pseudoeconomic expansion of a shrinking base, and seems to have temporarily hoodwinked third-party payers and even the legal system. Seemingly well-meaning and perhaps unconscious, this subterfuge follows a simple formula: first you devise a treatment, and then invent a "syndrome" requiring that treatment. Once the syndrome is in the American Psychiatric Association's *Diagnostic and Statistical Manual* (DSM), insurance and government reimbursement follow.

We have already witnessed some backlash, the most far-reaching example being opposition to the so-called recovery of repressed memories of incest. While the special task force appointed by the American Psychological Association (APA) to formulate guidelines for practitioners remained paralyzed by internal political wrangling, the courts settled the matter. They had spent almost a decade sending fathers to prison on questionable testimony, followed by a decade of releasing these same fathers from prison. Practitioners involved lost licenses to practice or received other sanctions, leading one of the outstanding proponents to declare, "Even if you uncover repressed incest memories, keep your mouth shut because it's too dangerous to say anything" (Brown, 1999).

Most practitioners today believe that third-party reimbursement, which made the independent practice of psychotherapy economically feasible, has always been there. They are unaware that the practice of psychotherapy by psychologists is a creation of the past fifty years, since World War II. They are also ignorant of how a sound economic base was developed and how these same principles are applicable during the current economic crisis. Thus, before addressing current pseudoeconomic aspects, it might be well to offer a brief review of how a solid psychotherapy economy was created where absolutely no economic base had existed.

A BRIEF ECONOMIC RETROSPECTIVE

Prior to World War II, there were a few dozen independently practicing psychologists scattered throughout the United States. Most were women with master's degrees who limited their practices to children. Somehow in the eyes of male-dominated psychiatry, "spinsters" [sic!] seeing only children did not pose the threat to their practices that they ascribed to doctoral-level male psychologists seeing adults. World War II changed all that. General William Menninger, chief psychiatrist of the U.S. Army and co-founder with his brother Karl of the celebrated Menninger Clinic in Topeka, concluded that protracted and even life-long psychological illnesses resulting from battle neuroses could be avoided by having frontline treatment in the battlefield itself. Most psychiatrists at the time were elderly with thick German accents, so Menninger utilized brand-new medical graduates who had not even served their internships and who had been given a few-hour crash course in psychiatry. He also tapped psychologists, who at the time were mostly academicians, and near the end of the war included graduate social workers. These became our battalion aid station psychotherapists, situated just behind the front lines.

The psychologists and social workers thus recruited rose brilliantly and bravely to the occasion, so impressing the government that after the war both the Veterans Administration (VA) and the National Institute of Mental Health (NIMH) provided training stipends for psychologists and social workers, as well as for psychiatry. Graduate departments of psychology and schools of social work took advantage of liberal funding to create doctoral programs in clinical psychology and master's programs in psychiatric social work. Students flocked to both, and a pool of professionals was created almost overnight.

These trained psychologists quickly became disenchanted with the psychiatric dominance in our public and private institutions and flocked to independent practice, whereas social workers, who seemed to chafe less, remained in these institutions. This was during the late 1940s and early 1950s, in which there was no licensing, third-party reimbursement, malpractice insurance, or public recognition of psychologists. The postwar demand for psychotherapy was enormous. Patients were willing to pay out of pocket, but they sought psychiatrists and often cancelled their appointments upon learning the doctor was a psychologist. Psychologists ingeniously solved this by associating with psychiatrists, who had more patients than they could possibly see. Psychologists took psychiatrists' overflow, and both prospered.

Responding to public demand during the late 1950s, health insurance began to cover "psychiatric illness." However, only psychiatrists were reimbursed. Initially, psychiatrists billed for the services of psychologists associated with them, but it was not long before this was outlawed. Psychologists were in danger of being left out of independent practice. Realizing that this would signal the end of nonmedical psychotherapists, the Dirty Dozen—actually fourteen psychologist–activists, so named because of their guerilla tactics—began their thirty-year crusade to create and insure the autonomous practice of psychology. Led fearlessly by Rogers Wright, joined by Nick Cummings and twelve other colleagues, they fought the APA, which by that time had instructed its members not to associate with psychologists, and the APA, which opposed its members entering independent practice. The Dirty Dozen also sought to persuade a reluctant insurance industry, which believed that increasing the number of practitioners to include psychologists would inflate its costs. This heroic saga has been extensively chronicled (Wright & Cummings, 2001), as have been the successes of social workers and other master's-level practitioners who some quarter of a century later followed the trail blazed with great difficulty and ingenuity by psychology (Cummings, 1990, reviews how in three decades psychology forged a sound economic base from absolutely nothing).

After years of proving the value of psychology in the ultimate marketplace—patients willing to pay out of pocket—the advent of insurance and government reimbursement intensified the value of psychological services. However, when managed care began eroding psychology's economic base, most psychologists suffered from economic illiteracy (Cummings, 2002) and did not know how to create a viable, clinically driven system in response to the industrialization of healthcare. They were unable to heed the warnings that were enunciated early in the 1980s, and control of psychotherapy sadly slipped from the clinicians to business interests.

SYNDROMES TO THE RESCUE

Still suffering the effects of economic illiteracy, and floundering as it tried to meet the challenges of the industrialization of healthcare, psychology took to fabricating an expanded economic base by inventing syndromes and their treatment. Some of these syndromes fade rapidly, whereas others are more enduring. Those that succeed proceed through a series of alliterative definitions that continue to expand the number of persons that can be subsumed under the rubric of psychological disorders. Before visiting some of these inventions, let us contemplate a tongue-in-cheek boilerplate that frighteningly mirrors the real activity that continues to take place.

Employee Ennui Disorder (EED): A Formula and a Template

Symptoms. Persons manifesting EED hate Monday mornings and are jubilant on Friday afternoons. They hate the boss, resent their supervisors, and engage in workplace gossip, especially around the water cooler. They are instrumental in spreading rumors and enlarging their scope. They are frequently and even chronically late for work, and often sneak out early at the end of the workday. Such individuals are prone to stretch out lunch hours and coffee breaks. They have been known to read and send personal e-mails on the company computer, and severe cases even play computer games on company time. They are victimized because they are invariably and unfairly passed over for promotion.

Prevalence. Statistics vary, but NIMH speculates EED may affect as many as 100 million Americans. The disorder affects men and women equally, according to human resource directors and employee assistance counselors. Several surveys have been published, ranging from a low of 5 million in those conducted by the Republican National Committee to a high of 150 million in numbers reported by labor unions.

Treatment. Treatment includes a combination of individual and group psychotherapy, augmented by antidepressant medications. Severe cases may require several periods of paid sick leave dispensed over the course of treatment. Care must be exercised not to encourage the client to get a different job, as this would only mitigate the fact that the entire employment system is worker exploitative and antithetical to mental health. Also, the therapist must be wary of a spontaneous burst of ambition and discourage it, as this may be nothing more than a flight into health.

Course. The disorder begins with mild symptoms but once manifested progresses rapidly in severity. Thus, early intervention is important. It can be highly contagious, infecting large groups within an employment setting. Recovery is complicated by low self-esteem. Guided imagery encouraging increased self-esteem and the overcoming of learned helplessness aids in recovery. EED is exacerbated by difficult economic times or an unsympathetic boss. Company restructuring is a known pathogen. If EED is not treated, it can progress to unemployment, then to nonemployability, and eventually to homelessness.

EED of Childhood and Adolescence. This disorder is expandable to include children and adolescents. The symptoms are only slightly adjusted for age: for example, a distaste for household chores, making one's bed, cleaning one's room, doing homework, and even going to school. Without treatment, the disorder will progress to truancy, dropping out of school, delinquency, and even running away from home.

Discussion. Practitioners like this syndrome because it creates a treatable and therefore reimbursable disorder. Clients (patients) like this syndrome because it eliminates such victim-blaming pejoratives as lazy, oppositional, lacking ambition, unemployable, and indolent. Everybody likes this syndrome because it is politically correct.

Palmer Economics. Inventing disorders in this fashion befits "Palmer economics," so named by this author after the founder of chiropractics. In the first half of the twentieth century, chiropractors had only one treatment tool: spinal column manipulation and realignment. The Palmer method, as it was known, kept expanding the number of diseases and illnesses that were ostensibly caused by spinal column misalignment. Psychotherapists can learn much from Palmer economics. First, be sure the new disorder will fit treatment methods readily available to psychotherapists, even if these have never been shown to be applicable. Second, create the syndrome out of groups of symptoms, citing prevalence and avoiding all evidence-based research and extensive clinical experience. If you imply neurological or central nervous system involvement, be careful to downplay as unimportant the lack of evidence of cellular changes. Be quick to accuse skeptical scientists and experienced professionals of a lack of compassion in wanting to deny treatment to these needy patients.

With this formula and template in mind, let us now look at a variety of questionable disorders that currently are being treated, avoiding such past legal debacles as recovered repressed memories of incest and staying away from looming failures such as nonattachment syndrome treated by rebirthing (there have already been arrests and prosecutions in Colorado), treatment of those abducted and sexually abused by space aliens (the Harvard psychiatrist promoting and conducting this therapy has been unflatteringly described), and multiple chemical sensitivities (a fad that peaked several years ago but not before Marin County, California, banned the wearing of perfume at public gatherings).

As did the foregoing fictitious EED scenario we presented, all the "real" syndromes and disorders we examine in this chapter have some basis in fact. However, in keeping with the mental health trend to greatly expand the pool of patients requiring psychiatric or psychological treatment, these disorders—which affect a circumscribed number of people—have become overblown, popularized, and politically correct "mini-epidemics."

Attention-Deficit/Hyperactivity Disorder (ADD/ADHD)

Subtle learning disabilities of childhood requiring psychological evaluation, special classes, and even medication have been recognized since the 1960s. Originally, stringent requirements had to be met before a diagnosis could be made. Often the diagnosis brought with it the recommendation for stimulant medication (e.g., Ritalin), and child psychiatrists and pediatricians were reluctant to unnecessarily medicate children before being convinced that a treatable disorder existed. In the last several decades, however, there has been a steady erosion of these rigorous criteria, and when the APA (1994) revised the criteria in the DSM-IV-R for diagnosing ADD/ADHD, the number of children who qualified literally quadrupled.

The consequent explosion in the number of children (including preschoolers) diagnosed as ADD/ADHD caused off-label prescribing of drugs to skyrocket. Alarms were sounded by many psychiatrists and pediatricians concerned with the potentially damaging effects on the rapidly changing yet immature central nervous systems of adolescents, children, and especially preschoolers. A special White House Conference was convened (Zito et al., 2000; Rabasca, 2000). The conference recommended caution in medicating and called for prospective community-based, multidimensional outcome studies. This White House Conference has been all but forgotten in the wake of the relentless increase in reliance on medication for children and adolescents over less invasive treatments.

It is assumed that in ADD/ADHD some form of cerebral malfunctioning exists. Yet in spite of extensive investigations, no biological component has ever been found (Brokaw, 2000). If there ever was a neurological component in the strict diagnoses made several decades ago, the current patient pool has been so adulterated with hordes of questionable diagnoses that perhaps less than five or ten percent of those diagnosed exhibit even the slightest hint of biological etiology.

The current diagnosis of ADD/ADHD is rendered from a pure description of an array of symptoms, with no scientific corroboration. It is a stellar example of the descriptive psychiatry that dominated the nineteenth century and resulted in such invasive, nonevidence-based procedures as the spinning chair, dunking in an icy pond, and the "Scotch douche." The almost universal use of Ritalin or its newer alliterations is the twentieth century equivalent.

In spite of advances in molecular biology, genetics, and neuroscience, the practice of psychiatry continues to be essentially a descriptive practice. For example, SARS (severe acute respiratory syndrome) so resembles influenza that it was indistinguishable until physiological tests were developed. No such definitive tests exist for the currently overused diagnosis of ADD/ADHD. Yet on a purely descriptive level, with arbitrarily collected symptoms and no demonstrable neurological concomitants, psychiatry not only renders diagnoses but also prescribes drugs with unknown long-term consequences, especially to developing organisms.

Cummings and Wiggins (2001) accessed the electronic records of the 168,113 children and adolescents treated during a four-year period in a national prepaid healthcare plan. Of these, sixty-one percent of the boys and twenty-three percent of the girls had been diagnosed ADD/ADHD and placed on medication prior to referral for psychological treatment. The health plan had an extensive behavioral treatment benefit for such cases, and without imposed limits it averaged 6.3 sessions with the child or adolescent and 10.9 sessions with the parents.

Because of the noted absence of fathers in this child/adolescent population, a strong effort was made to pair the patients with male therapists who related well with this patient population. The approaches were behavioral, with special attention paid to developing positive relational attachment to a male figure. At the end of the treatment episode, only eleven percent of the boys and two percent of the girls remained on medication, despite the very strict criterion for ceasing the medication: the complaining entity (parent, school, juvenile justice system, etc.) had to agree that the child/adolescent was doing so well that medication was not needed. Follow-up revealed that relapses requiring resumption of medication amounted to less than one percent of this population. (See chapter 7 for details on this study and ADHD.)

The authors (Cummings & Wiggins, 2001) conclude that (1) either there is an overdiagnosis of ADD/ADHD, or (2) these conditions are far more amenable to behavioral interventions than heretofore has been acknowledged. They question the cerebral malfunctioning theory as it is applied to the currently inflated and criteria-diluted population of patients, and suggest that social forces may be major contributors. Among these social forces are: the absence of positive father role models; the presence of a revolving door for negative male role models brought into the home; poor parenting; the need for order in the classroom when teachers are severely curtailed in meting out discipline; a declining appreciation in our culture of what constitutes normal boy behavior (see also Pollock, 2000); the medicalization of psychiatry, with its emphasis on medication over behavioral therapies; and the propensity to seek a medical (a politically correct stance of "don't blame the victim") etiology over behavioral concomitants.

Crowded, unruly classrooms produce impatient teachers who pressure parents to seek medication for their children. Harried single moms, frantically trying to raise their children and maintain a job, are not prone to understand annoying boyish behavior, no matter how typical it is. The behavioral interventions we cited were effective in a very large sample. However, they were not politically correct in that they emphasized the deficit of a male role model. Medication, on the other hand, is as politically correct as it is overused. The authors concluded that if given the current climate in the era when they were growing up both of them would have been put on Ritalin, to say nothing of some of the most successful and productive male members of our society.

Organized psychiatry has remained silent regarding the overuse of medications with children and adolescents, understandable when one realizes that medication and hospitalization have remained that profession's sole armamentarium now that it has largely given up what it disdainfully calls "talk therapy." Psychology's equivalent silence is puzzling, inasmuch as it does not prescribe medications, derives no financial gain from the expansive drug industry, and remains the preeminent psychotherapy profession. Furthermore, psychologists have done most of the research indicating that in many instances psychotherapy is superior to psychotropic medication (e.g., Antonuccio, Danton, & DeNelsky 1999). Only recently has an organized voice been raised. Writing as the president of the APA's Division of Clinical Psychology in her front page President's Column, Willis (2003) asks with alarm, "The Drugging of Young Children: Why Is Psychology Mute?"

Were it not for the importance of the many unanswered questions, much of this activity would resemble the theater of the absurd. This is especially true of the multimillion-dollar media campaign launched to promote questionable syndromes and their even more questionable drug treatment. A television commercial extensively aired by Lilly during the summer of 2003 shows a woman whose mind is wandering while she and her business colleagues are ostensibly discussing a matter around the conference table. Suddenly the boss calls upon her, and she is at a loss to respond. An authoritative voice then injects the thought that if this happens to you, you may have adult ADD. One might ask whether daydreaming during a boring meeting might not be more reflective of employee ennui syndrome.

Dissociative Identity Disorder (DID)

Along with ADD/ADHD, dissociative identity disorder (DID) is one of the most entrenched, and most controversial, diagnostic categories in the DSM-IV. As an octogenarian in his fifty-fifth year as a psychologist, I saw the trickle and then explosion of both ADD/ADHD and DID. Originally called multiple personality disorder (MPD), the latter received a polishing and renaming in the DSM-IV, setting the stage for a mini-epidemic. Again, social forces—this time in the form of pop culture—more than the professions, set the stage for the popularization and glamorization of DID. However, the mental health professions did not hesitate to seize the opportunity to expand the number of prospective clients.

Every good clinician knows that dissociation (or, more specifically, dissociative phenomena) not only exists, but is prevalent and highly subject to suggestion. It was discovered by the nineteenth century French neurologist Pierre Janet. Freud questioned multiple personality as a diagnostic entity and favored the view that it was one form of dissociation that accompanied hysteria or other diagnostic entities. Morton Prince in 1905 popularized his case of "Miss Beachamp," but DID remained rare. There were only seventy-nine documented cases until the latter half of the twentieth century (Lilienfeld & Lynn, 2003).

In 1959, Hollywood released the movie *The Three Faces of Eve,* based on a popularized book by two psychiatrists (Thigpen & Cleckley, 1957). Joanne Woodward, who starred as Eve, won the Academy Award, subsequently married Paul Newman, and became an American idol. During that time I was chief psychologist at Kaiser Permanente in San Francisco, implementing the nation's first comprehensive prepaid psychotherapy benefit. Suddenly we were blindsided by a plethora of DID (then MPD) cases, all of them women. We hypothesized that this disorder must be far more prevalent than was thought in the era without mental health benefits, and that the prepaid benefits were revealing the true figures. We contacted Cleckley and learned to chart the various personalities of our patients. Three years later I found myself sitting next to Cleckley at a professional luncheon and asked how "Eve" was doing. I had noted that at the end of his book the number of personalities had grown from three to eleven. He replied that she was now up to 26 personalities and shrugged off my dismay, saying that everything was going according to treatment plan.

Feeling hoodwinked and considerably chastened, my staff and I began rethinking the entire disorder. We noted that all of our MPDs were somewhat shallow young women who worshipped the celebrated star of *The Three Faces of Eve*. Furthermore, they were borderline personalities, patients with known propensities for dissociation, faddism, and a desire to mimic whatever seemed to interest the therapist. The more extensive our charting of these multiple personalities, the more they flourished and increased in number.

We decided to reverse the process, and arrived at an intervention. We advised the next new patient who manifested the emergence of a new personality during a session that we were terminating the interview because "psychotherapy is a special patient–therapist relationship and no third person is allowed to intrude." The therapist then stood and walked toward the door, signaling that the session was over. Invariably the new "person" would disappear, never to return again. We then would resume what we should have been doing all along: treating the borderline personality disorder.

We employed this intervention through hundreds of psychotherapists we trained in the method, first at Kaiser Permanente and then nationally at American Biodyne, with none other than positive results that facilitated, rather than distracted, the therapeutic process. By the time the next epidemic of DID (then still called MPD) swept the land following the popularization of the novel and TV movie *Sybil* in the mid-1970s (Schreiber, 1973), we were more than prepared for the explosion. And we were not surprised when it was exposed by Sybil's backup therapist that her main psychiatrist produced the multiple personality phenomenon by constant suggestion (see Lilienfeld & Lynn, 2003, for a recounting of Herbert Spiegel's assertion).

A test of this therapeutic strategy occurred in 1987 when it was discovered that American Biodyne's small center in New Albany, Indiana (near the Kentucky border) had more diagnosed MPDs than the entire national system covering 14.5 million lives. The director of the center argued that this was a backwoods community in which dissociation was common. However, shortly thereafter he was transferred to Orlando, Florida, far from a backwoods community, and that center suddenly was inundated with MPDs. In subsequent meetings it became apparent that this well-intentioned psychologist was inadvertently fostering MPD without being aware of doing so. He expressed amazement at how the subtlest suggestive cues were readily picked up by his patients.

Surveys of clinicians indicate that numerous professionals are deeply skeptical that DID actually exists (Lilienfeld & Lynn, 2003), and prevailing theories as to its etiology have been questioned (Cormier & Thelen, 1998; Dell, 1988; Pope, Oliva, Hudson, Bodkin, & Gruber, 1999). Yet after celebrities such as Roseanne Arnold announced they suffer from DID and thus glamorized it, the number of cases grew from 79 in 1970 to 40,000 by the late 1990s (Marmer, 1998). The complaints by those affected also have changed with the pop culture. Before *Sybil* the mean number of multiple personalities reported was 3, whereas after the movie the mean rose to 16 (Acocella, 1998). *Sybil* fostered the idea that child abuse was the basis of DID. Whereas before the airing of the TV movie very few cases reported child abuse, after *Sybil* a substantial number of cases reported a history of child abuse. What had been a rarity was catapulted into the typical case (Spanos, 1996).

Research has determined that different psychophysiological states can exist among the several personalities (called alters) of the same person, and this is often proffered as evidence that these alters truly exist. These include differences in brain wave activity (Ludwig, Brandsma, Wilbur, Bendefeldt, & Jameson, 1972), markedly different respiration rates (Bahnson & Smith, 1975), and differences in skin conductance response (Brende, 1984). Any skilled hypnotist knows that altered states, along with unique psychophysiological changes, can be induced in hypnotized individuals rapidly, interchangeably, and with little difficulty. If, indeed, these are dissociative states, such psychophysiological differences are to be expected and are hardly evidence of anything beyond common phenomena found in dissociation. Hypnosis and self-hypnosis can induce all of this.

While the controversy continues among psychologists, the landscape is becoming more ludicrous, with psychologists defying common sense. In 2001, I was asked by an insurance company to review the case of a psychologist toward whom fraud charges were being contemplated. Unbeknown to the third-party payer, the psychologist was seeing the same DID patient five times a week (although authorized only for weekly sessions) but billing each as five different patients, using their DID names in the billing. She insisted this was proper as she was treating the multiple personalities as separate individuals.

In 2002 a woman filed rape charges against a man after she had consented to sex. It seems that during the sex act one of her nonconsenting personalities emerged and was traumatized. This particular personality claimed to be prudish and characterized the consenting personality as promiscuous. The court suffered through the ridiculous spectacle of two personalities of the same woman testifying against each other (one asserting mutual consent, the other charging rape) on the stand, and the further spectacle of psychologists lining up on both sides to give testimony that had no scientific basis whatsoever.

In 2003 a criminal contested his arrest because his Miranda rights were read to a personality other than the one that had committed the crime. Again, psychologist "experts" vied on the witness stand as to who could be the biggest fool. Truly we have attained the theater of the absurd.

Depression

The DSM-IV (APA, 1994) lists a number of depressive disorders and depressive states, but depression can be thought of as a nearly ubiquitous phenomenon, potentially accompanying any condition, physical or psychological. For example, it is not surprising that as many as seventy percent of patients with chronic physical conditions (e.g., arthritis, asthma, emphysema, etc.) are sufficiently depressed to warrant a secondary diagnosis of depression (see Cummings, O'Donohue, & Ferguson, 2002, for a summary of this extensive research). The specific depressive disorders listed in the current DSM include bipolar disorder, major depression (mild, moderate, or severe, with or without psychosis), dysthymia (chronic depression of two years or more), adjustment disorder with depression, and, so as to leave no stone unturned, depression not otherwise specified (NOS).

It might be assumed that this enormous pool of potential patients would suffice, but not so. There is currently an unprecedented drive to claim just about every normal mood alteration associated with daily living as a treatable depression. The press is replete with surveys conducted by self-proclaimed organizations purporting to show that healthcare is missing, and therefore not treating, most of the cases of depression. This campaign has been joined by a number of celebrities, including the well-meaning Tipper Gore, spouse of the former vice-president of the United States. No one questions the sincerity of these celebrities, who doubtlessly have suffered severe depression, but this is hardly the scientific evidence needed to declare the ubiquitous state of recurring "blues" a syndrome requiring psychiatric or psychological treatment.

Spurring this drive is the emergence of the new antidepressant medications, particularly the serotonin reuptake inhibitors (SSRIs), huckstered in a multimillion-dollar media blitz by the pharmaceutical industry. The message is simple: why not take a pill for the Monday morning blues (or some other such annoyance)? In response to these seductive advertisements, patients demand of their primary care physicians (PCPs) prescriptions for even the most common or trivial mood alterations.

Feeling pressured, but reluctant to overly medicate their patients, PCPs prescribe minimal dosages, resulting in many unnecessary prescriptions and the undermedication of those who really do need to be medicated and could benefit from an appropriate dosage. Thus, depression has earned the appellation "the common cold of psychiatry" (Cummings, 2002), recalling the era that followed the advent of antibiotics, in which patients began demanding antibiotics for the common cold. Patients still continue to demand and receive them, despite universal belief that antibiotics are completely ineffective against viruses. Our misuse of antibiotics has also given rise to superviruses that are proving resistant to all but the most potent antibiotics available.

To be on the safe side, PCPs refer many of the patients demanding psychotropic medications to psychiatrists, resulting in an economic boom for that profession. Psychiatrists, who have deemed "talk therapy" obsolete, are more than willing to prescribe liberally. Psychotherapy for depression (and other conditions giving way to pharmacological treatment) is dwindling, resulting in a surplus of psychotherapists in most locales. On the other hand, getting an appointment with a prescribing psychiatrist requires two to four weeks. Twenty years ago psychiatry was economically beleaguered, residencies were going begging, and some psychiatrists, such as the futurist Stanley Lesse (1982), were predicting the demise of their profession. Suddenly psychiatry is at the top of the psychopharmacology dispensing chain and is determined to thwart the concerted efforts of psychologists to participate in the boom by attaining prescription authority.

The accelerated dispensing of newer psychotropic drugs constitutes the greatest economic expansion of mental health in decades, and there seems to be no end in sight. In order to bolster their own sagging economy, psychologists have used the shortage of psychiatrists, especially in rural areas, as an argument for extending prescription authority. Psychologists are more widely dispersed in remote areas than are psychiatrists, which was enough to persuade New Mexico and Louisiana to grant such authority to psychology in 2002 and 2004, respectively.

Despite opposition from psychiatry, which has enlisted the formidable help of the American Medical Association, psychology will attain prescription authority for three reasons: (1) psychology can solve the shortage of psychiatrists that exists in nonmetropolitan areas; (2) the hyped-up demand for psychotropic drugs will require more dispensers; and (3) society is pushing healthcare downward. Nurses, particularly nurse practitioners and physician assistants, are doing more of the work of primary care physicians, and practical nurses are doing more of the work of registered nurses. In turn, PCPs are doing the first tier of what has heretofore been the domain of specialists. In like fashion, psychologists are doing much of the work once considered the sole province of psychiatry (e.g., hospitalization, court commitment for mental illness, forensic testimony, child custody determination, and much more). It remains to be seen whether psychologists, once they can prescribe, will demonstrate a balance between when to prescribe and when to do psychotherapy. The expediency of the prescription pad over the labor intensiveness of psychotherapy, along with the greater economic reward for rapid dispensing of medication, may prove to be as irresistible for psychology as it has been for psychiatry.

This expansion, however, may be on shaky ground because a backlash against overly prescribing is always a possibility, even if a remote one. There is an impressive body of research indicating that psychotropic medications are not nearly as effective as once thought (Zito, Safer, dosReis, Gardner, Boles, & Lynch 2000; see also W. Glasser, chapter 6 in this volume). In addition, there are research indications that psychotherapy may be as effective as antidepressants, and in some cases, even more effective (Antonuccio, Danton, & DeNelsky, 1999). The problem with getting accurate scientific data lies in the descriptive nature of psychiatry, contaminating experimental and control groups with less than pure cases.

To use an analogy, pretend that pulmonology is still in the descriptive stage in which psychiatry finds itself. This would mean that diagnoses are made from an observation of symptoms only, with laboratory tests nonexistent. Let us say that one hundred of our patients exhibit the symptoms of pneumonia: fever, difficulty in breathing, pulmonary rasping, fluid in the lungs, malaise, and so on, and that the diagnosis of pneumonia is made solely on the basis of these symptoms. Because no objective tests are available, the pulmonologist does not know that forty of these patients have bacterial pneumonia, forty have viral pneumonia, and twenty have inhalation or other types of pneumonia. Among the latter group we can even include SARS, which is often difficult to distinguish from viral pneumonia and requires its own test.

The patients are randomly assigned to two groups, one receiving antibiotics and the other receiving antiviral medication. Our conclusion, without any other evidence, will be that antibiotics are forty percent effective (the number of persons with bacterial pneumonia), and antiviral medication is also forty percent effective (the number of patients with viral pneumonia). In the remaining twenty percent (those with inhalation pneumonia or SARS), neither is very effective. Not knowing that our groups are contaminated with three different types of pneumonia, each requiring a different treatment, the false conclusion is reached that in the treatment of pneumonia, antibiotics and antivirals are equally effective (or noneffective, considering that neither is even fifty percent effective). In actuality, both antibiotics and antivirals are effective with bacterial and viral pneumonias, respectively.

This is the state of descriptive psychiatry today. Research on depressives addresses varying conglomerate groups of depression, probably requiring different types of treatments. We have teased out bipolar depression and lithium as its treatment of choice, but the other depressions are murky and undifferentiated. Why would a reactive depression to a loss require the same medication as a chronic depression (dysthymia) with no demonstrable loss? Would not psychotherapy to heal the loss be more appropriate? Antidepressants that reduce symptoms also curtail the healing aspects of bereavement. In other words, treating grief with antidepressants stops the positive work of mourning. Although the patient might feel better, the underlying grief remains unresolved and returns to haunt the individual years later. Unfortunately, much treatment with antidepressant medication is hit or miss; if something does not work, the physician adds another like medication, then possibly another, and so on. If all else fails, the severely depressed patient is seen as a candidate for electroconvulsive therapy (ECT), a relic that is back in vogue.

The boom in psychopharmacology goes on with varying degrees of effectiveness, and the boldness of its practices (especially off-label applications) can be startling unless one considers that it is adding mightily to the mental health–industrial complex. So named by Duhl, Cummings, and Hynes (1987) and patterned after the military–industrial complex identified by President Eisenhower (1960) and the medical–industrial complex identified by Relman (1980), the mental health–industrial complex involves professionals joining with drug companies to push their psychotropic wares, while cooperating with hospitals to fill psychiatric beds, neither necessarily in the interest of best practices.

THE INVENTIVENESS CONTINUES

Having looked at two entrenched markets (ADD/ADHD and DID) and mental health's enormous medication market (depression), it would be interesting to dabble in two fanciful markets that (if one can stifle laughter) demonstrate the inventiveness of a profession that is allowed to create disorders with no semblance of scientific validation or clinical efficacy and effectiveness, but with a potential for expanding a shrinking economic psychotherapy base. Disorders such as ADD/ADHD, depression, and posttraumatic stress disorder are generally accepted. The objection is that they are stretched to include persons who originally would not have been regarded as being afflicted.

There are a number of so-called syndromes, however, that flourish even though they are far from being generally accepted. They make their appearance, are given a great deal of attention for a short period, then subside, and even vanish. These never attain the rank of listing in the DSMs, but they temporarily create a revenue stream for lawyers, forensic psychologists, new-age therapists, and continuing education offerings. During its heyday, chronic sugar intoxication was blamed for everything from hyperactivity and learning disorders in children to murder by adults. It peaked with the celebrated diminished capacity "Twinkie" defense of a double murder in San Francisco and has all but vanished, other than persisting as a cruel joke. Somnambulism syndrome—violence and even murder committed while sleepwalking—provided incomes for defense lawyers and forensic psychologists for a time and was the subject of several approved continuing education offerings. When juries stopped buying into the notion, it also vanished. These new syndromes make a splash, then disappear after juries and the public reject them.

Far more enduring is the battered woman syndrome (Walker, 1984). Although it has never made the DSM as a disorder, it is based on widely accepted psychological constructs and is generally accepted with some reservations. Although it addresses male power/dominance, it has been pointed out that the syndrome fails to explain the reverse power thrust exhibited by some women. These are women who deliberately provoke their husbands by outrageously flirting with other men, then use the sanctions and approbation imposed against the husband as their own power base. Nonetheless, battered woman syndrome, along with rape trauma syndrome, has enjoyed wide credibility and acceptance over time.

Reverse Seasonal Affective Disorder (Reverse SAD)

In contrast, and hot off the griddle, is a new syndrome that is just beginning its trek through fame to oblivion, it is hoped, the sooner the better. Where millions of Americans reportedly suffer depression during the winter months (called Seasonal Affective Disorder, or SAD), researchers at none other than the National Institute of Mental Health (NIMH) have identified depression that afflicts persons during daylight savings time (Spencer, 2003). Called Summer Seasonal Affective Disorder, or reverse SAD, it strikes in late April and early May. NIMH purports that the nation's suicide rate peak in midsummer may reflect severe cases of reverse SAD. This runs counter to the generally accepted concept in suicide prevention that depressed persons are re-energized after the long winter and are more likely to commit the suicide they have been pondering. Undeterred, NIMH insists that although severe reverse SAD afflicts only about one percent of Americans, compared with the five percent afflicted with severe forms of winter SAD, milder cases of reverse SAD abound and are reflected in warm weather "grouchiness." The reader is implored not to laugh out loud, while this author, as both a psychologist and a taxpayer, worries that NIMH may have run out of things to do.

Compassion Fatigue Syndrome

Compassion fatigue, or "secondary trauma," is said to be the leading cause of burnout in the healthcare industry, costing millions of dollars in sick time and staff turnover annually (Stamm, 2003). Ostensibly, there is a "soul weariness" that comes with caring, characterized by nightmares, strange fears, and generalized helplessness. There are now therapists who conduct psychotherapy with colleagues suffering from compassion fatigue. Retreats for renewal and healing of healthcare workers are being offered all over the country (La Rowe, 2003).

Psychotherapists, who constantly deal with highly charged emotions in their patients, are particularly vulnerable to compassion fatigue syndrome. However, those at risk constitute a large pool of potential patients and encompass all healthcare, mental health, and helping professionals, including: social workers, counselors, psychologists, nurses, paramedics, crisis workers, EMS personnel, nurse practitioners, physician assistants, and drug and alcohol counselors. All settings are included: inpatient, outpatient, emergency room, ambulatory, and home care (PESI Healthcare, 2003, p. 2).

For some strange reason physicians are the only healthcare workers not specifically mentioned as being at risk. Either they are lacking in compassion, or they have discovered a vaccine and are guarding it as a secret. It would not be surprising if the syndrome were expanded to include the children of healthcare workers with compassion fatigue. Certainly a parent so depleted cannot provide the caring a child needs. Besides, extending the risk to children would create a sure-fire market.

WHAT HAPPENED TO PARITY?

A bitter economic lesson was recently dealt to the field of mental health. After practitioners pinned their hopes on a series of rapidly enacted parity laws, mandating a level playing field between physical and mental health funding, it was disclosed that there was less spent on mental health and chemical dependency (MH/CD) treatment in 2001 than before the enactment of the surprisingly large number of parity laws. The federal government enacted a weak parity law in 1996, and despite vigorous attempts to strengthen it, the law was renewed in its same anemic form in 2001, the year of its expiration.

In the meantime, in an effort to go far beyond the Congress, thirty-four states enacted much tougher parity laws. This climaxed an unprecedented level of legislative success on the part of mental health professionals, who had rallied to save their economic base. This success boomeranged, however, because parity laws cannot require the same co-payments and other procedures for medical versus psychiatric bills. For the most part, an equal lifetime benefit for the two was the usual mandate.

Employers, fearing an explosion of costs for MH/CD wherever tough parity laws were enacted, came up with even more draconian managed care. They contracted with vendors that made behavioral care harder to get by assigning mental health claims to a nastier and far more difficult review process than those for medical/surgical care. Mental health spending, as a share of total health spending, not only dropped following the successful drive for parity legislation, it continues to drop (Carnahan, 2002) now that insurers and employers have responded adversely.

This is only one of many examples of unintended consequences resulting from well-meaning, politically driven healthcare initiatives that lack a sound economic base. Only when mental health becomes an integral part of physical health, each indistinguishable from the other, will there be parity (Cummings, 2002). This is inevitable, because psychological stress and distress accompany all disease and are often at the root of physical complaints, whereas most illness is the result of faulty lifestyles.

MANUALIZING THE MADNESS

In the face of a shrinking patient base, mental health has developed some interesting methods for increasing demand for its services, all the while defying sound economics. The following is a manualized summary of the principles underlying current expansion efforts.

First, take a treatment method or technique that is widely known to mental health professionals and invent a new syndrome, or even better, a series of syndromes to which the treatment may be readily applied. This adheres to the Palmer method of healthcare economics: when all one has is a hammer, label all objects as nails.

This first principle (fabrication), however, cannot succeed without corollaries. A number of seemingly successful inventions have backfired: therapists have gone to jail or lost their licenses, and the field has suffered a black eye, at least temporarily, from concepts such as repressed memories of incest abuse, parentally sponsored satanic cults, rebirthing, Twinkie diminished capacity, somnambulism, and abduction and sexual abuse by space aliens, to name a few. There must follow the second, third, and fourth principles, respectively, of durability, viability, and plausibility. Although somewhat interchangeable, these are listed separately for purposes of elucidation.

Durability

To survive the test of time, a new syndrome must rest on treatment methods that are widely taught in graduate schools and accessible to most clinicians, as well as universally accepted by the public. It does not matter if these techniques originally had nothing to do with the fabricated syndrome inasmuch as wide acceptance of the treatment will be interpreted to mean the syndrome itself has credibility, a welcome form of the halo effect.

Unfortunately, even in the face of these precautions, miscalculations will occur and new syndromes will backfire. Do not despair; merely abandon the syndrome and pretend it never existed. Professional societies have considerable experience with this procedure, so it should not be difficult. Journal editors must be especially vigilant, making certain the syndrome never again appears in the scientific and professional literature. The public has a short memory and can be easily distracted by the emergence of the next, even more attractive, syndrome.

Viability

To be economically viable a fabricated syndrome must produce a substantial new revenue stream or greatly increase revenue from an existing syndrome by redefining it to apply to more people. The greater the population potentially covered by the syndrome, the greater the economic viability. Attention deficit disorder is a classic example. It can probably be stretched to apply to fifty percent of boys in any given classroom and further extended to include a vast number of girls and adults. An even more stellar example is depression, which now includes any slight mood changes resulting from daily living and can potentially encompass ninety-nine percent of the population, possibly excluding only unipolar hypomanics. Dissociative identity disorder is useful in that it can be manufactured on the spot with susceptible and rapidly proliferating borderline personality disordered (BPD) patients, a cohort that can easily be increased if one's practice is sagging or reduced if it is prospering. It also has the charm of giving troublesome patients the fun of multiplying their personalities instead of making the psychotherapist's life miserable.

No effort will succeed, however, if insurers, employers, and the government do not accept the existence of the fabricated or overly extended syndrome. Public opinion is critical, because it will pressure all three groups. Pop culture, movies, television, and trial lawyers are all helpful in shaping public opinion. Government is, of course, subject to political pressure and is helpless when its own NIMH comes up with fanciful entities such as reverse seasonal affective disorder (i.e., summer depression).

Corporations that are worker-oriented will choose mental health plans that provide benefits for whatever malady the culture has accepted. The most difficult group to persuade is the managed care companies, but all is not lost. Their previous practice of blanket denial of claims has come under scrutiny, and they must justify rejections. The business interests that control managed care fortunately do not know a real disorder from a fabricated one, and have no idea where to draw the line on greatly overblown syndromes. This bafflement is reflected in their escalating costs. Easiest of all are trial lawyers, who jump at the chance to embrace any syndrome, no matter how flimsy, that might benefit their client's case.

Plausibility

In order for a new or overblown syndrome to be plausible, a number of inviolate rules exist.

1. Determine if the fabrication has the potential to reflect popular societal trends. Relativism (all behavior is normalized so there are no consequences to one's choices in life) should be coupled with victimology (no one is at fault, and everyone in difficulty is a victim). This will result in wide acceptance because it ensures that no one is a nitwit. Narrative and other postmodernist therapies that deconstruct all reality are in keeping with the fabrication of syndromes they can then address.
2. Make certain the fabrication is politically correct and offends no one, especially the nitwits that no longer exist.
3. Imply a neuropsychological connection for the syndrome, but make it vague and discourage any research that would establish or reject a biological basis. ADD/ADHD, as currently formulated, is a model to be emulated.
4. Accuse skeptics of lacking compassion for those who suffer from the ravages of the syndrome whose existence they doubt. This is especially effective if the syndromes in question involve women or children.
5. Publish scientific-appearing books, even if the content is faulty, unproven, or bordering on gibberish. It does not matter if very few people read these books because their mere existence will make the inventor of the syndrome appear erudite. The heavier the volume, the more impressive, especially when lawyers wave it before a jury that is adjudicating the harm that has come to a patient because an insurance company failed to cover the syndrome as a reimbursable benefit. Avoid refereed journals that will likely reject the syndrome or, even worse, publish critiques that will make it appear unscientific. Seek out sympathetic or quasi-scientific journals, but be cognizant that journal articles do not have the gravitas of books.

These simple guidelines should help increase the rate of fabrication of syndromes, enhance their success, and expand the shrinking economic base of mental health. The alternative is to create a sound economic and scientific base, a more enduring outcome but a much more difficult endeavor.

GOING ABOUT IT THE RIGHT WAY

Among the ways of appropriately expanding the economic base of mental health, perhaps the most immediate and potentially rewarding for patients, physicians, and psychologists alike is to expand the role of the psychotherapist to that of a primary care provider (Cummings, 2002). The healthcare system is burdened by the sixty to seventy percent of patients visiting primary care physicians whose symptoms reflect psychological distress rather than disease, or whose physical illness is exacerbated by psychological factors (Cummings et al., 2002). Primary care physicians (PCPs) do not have time in the usual "seven-minute" office visit to address these problems, and the patient continues to somatize psychological problems into physical symptoms that demand an increasingly costly series of office visits, laboratory tests, and medical procedures, all of which bring little or no relief to the patient. Attempts to refer these patients to psychotherapy result in less than ten percent actually visiting a psychologist.

In systems where behavior care providers (BCPs) have co-located with PCPs in the primary care setting, the PCP has only to walk the patient a few steps down the hall to the office of the BCP. The "hallway handoff," as this process is called in integrated behavioral/primary care systems, results in ninety percent of these patients entering psychotherapy, data that is consistent in the integrated programs of Kaiser Permanente, the 167 installations of the U.S. Air Force, the Veterans Administration, community health centers, and many others (see Cummings, O'Donohue, Hayes, & Follette, 2001). By reconceptualizing the role of the psychotherapist as a behavioral primary care provider, the flow of patients into mental health can be expanded by an astounding nine hundred percent. And this is no fabrication. (See Cummings, 2002, for a discussion of and cited writings on mental healthcare economics).

Following carefully thought-out economic principles, backed by solid science, not only will increase psychology's patient base but will go a long way toward restoring the field's fading reputation.

REFERENCES

Acocella, A. (1998, April 6). The politics of hysteria. *New Yorker*, 64–79.

American Psychiatric Association (1994). *Diagnostic and Statistical Manual of Mental Disorders* (4th ed.). Washington, DC: Author.

Antonuccio, D.O., Danton, W.G., & DeNelsky, G.Y. (1999). Raising questions about antidepressants. *Psychotherapy and Psychosomatic Medicine, 68*(1), 3–14.

Bahnson, C.B. & Smith, K. (1975). Autonomic changes in a multiple personality. *Psychosomatic Medicine, 37*, 85–86.

Brende, J.O. (1984). The psychophysiologic manifestations of dissociation: Electro-dermal responses in a multiple personality patient. *Psychiatric Clinics of North America, 7,* 41–50.

Brokaw, T. (2000, May 4). In-depth: Attention deficit/hyperactivity disorder. *NBC Nightly News,* New York.

Brown, L. (1999, December). *Treating Older Adults: A Symposium.* Orlando, FL: Milton H. Erickson Foundation, Annual Meeting.

California Psychological Association (2002, February). *CPA Summit Meeting.* Sacramento, CA.

Carnahan, I. (2002, January 21). Asylum for the insane. *Forbes,* 33–34.

Cormier, J.F. & Thelen, M.H. (1998). Professional skepticism of multiple personality disorder. *Professional Psychology: Research and Practice, 29,* 163–167.

Cummings, N.A. (1990). Collaboration or internecine warfare: The choice is obvious, but elusive. *Journal of Counseling and Development, 68,* 503–504.

Cummings, N.A. (2002). Are healthcare practitioners economic illiterates? *Families, Systems, and Health, 20*(4), 383–393.

Cummings, N.A. & Wiggins, J.G. (2001). A collaborative primary care/behavioral health model for the use of psychotropic medication with children and adolescents: The report of a national retrospective study. *Issues in Interdisciplinary Care, 3*(2), 123–128.

Cummings, N.A., O'Donohue, W.T., & Ferguson, K.E. (Eds.), (2002). *The Impact of Medical Cost Offset on Practice and Research: Making It Work for You.* Foundation for Behavioral Health: Healthcare Utilization and Cost Series, Vol. 5. Reno, NV: Context.

Cummings, N.A., O'Donohue, W.T., Hayes, S.C., & Follette, V. (2001). *Integrated Behavioral Healthcare: Positioning Mental Health Practice with Medical/Surgical Practice.* San Diego, CA: Academic.

Dell, P.E. (1988). Professional skepticism about multiple personality disorder. *Journal of Nervous and Mental Disease, 176,* 528–531.

Duhl, L.J., Cummings, N.A., & Hynes, J.J. (1987). The emergence of the mental health complex (pp. 1–14). In L.J. Duhl and N.A. Cummings (Eds.), *The Future of Mental Health Services: Coping with Crisis.* New York: Springer.

Eisenhower, D. (1960, January). *Presidential Farewell Address.* Washington, DC: The White House.

La Rowe, K.D. (2003, August). Seminar: *The Caregiving Personality and Secondary Traumatic Stress.* Eau Claire, WI: PESI Healthcare.

Lesse, S. (1982). Editorial: The uncertain future of clinical psychiatry. *American Journal of Psychotherapy, 37*(2), 306–312.

Lilienfeld, S.O. & Lynn, S.J. (2003). Dissociative identity disorder: Multiple personalities, multiple controversies, (pp. 109–142). In S.O. Lilienfeld, S.J. Lynn, & J.M. Lohr, (Eds.), *Science and Pseudoscience in Clinical Psychology.* New York: Guilford.

Ludwig, A.M., Brandsma, J.M., Wilbur, C.B., Bendefeldt, F., & Jameson, D.H. (1972). The objective study of a multiple personality: Or, are four heads better than one? *Archives of General Psychiatry, 26,* 298–310.

Marmer, S.S. (1998, December). Should dissociative identity disorder be considered a bona fide psychiatric diagnosis? *Clinical Psychiatry News.*

PESI Healthcare (2003). *How to Transform Compassion Fatigue.* Eau Claire, WI: Author.

Pollock, W. (2000). *Real Boys' Voices.* New York: Random House.

Pope, H.C., Oliva, P.S., Judson, J.L., Bodkin, J.A., & Gruber, A.J. (1999). Attitudes toward DSM-IV dissociative disorders diagnoses among board-certified American psychiatrists. *American Journal of Psychiatry, 156,* 321–323.

Prince, M. (1905). *The Dissociation of a Personality: A Biographical Study in Abnormal Psychology.* New York Longmans, Green.

Rabasca, L. (2000). APA participates in White House meeting that questions psychotropic drug use among preschoolers. *Monitor on Psychology, 31*(5), 10.

Relman, A. (1980). The medical–industrial complex. *New England Journal of Medicine, 303*(17), 996–998.

Schreiber, F.R. (1973). *Sybil.* New York: Warner.

Spanos, N.P. (1996). *Multiple Identities and False Memories.* Washington, DC: American Psychological Association.

Spencer, J. (2003, May 22). When blue skies bring on the blues: Research shows why some despair on sunny days and relish gloom of winter. *Wall Street Journal,* D1-2.

Stamm, B.H. (2003). *Secondary Traumatic Stress: Self-Care Issues for Clinicians, Researchers and Educators.* Eau Claire, WI: PESI Healthcare.

Thigpen, C.H. & Cleckley, H.M. (1957). *The Three Faces of Eve.* New York: McGraw Hill.

Walker, L.E. (1984). *The Battered Woman Syndrome.* New York: Springer.

Willis, D.J. (2003). The drugging of young children: Why is psychology mute? *The Clinical Psychologist, 56*(3), 1–2.

Wright, R.H. & Cummings, N.A. (Eds.), (2001). *The Practice of Psychology: The Battle for Professionalism.* Phoenix, AZ: Zeig, Tucker & Theisen.

Zito, J.M., Safer, D.J., dosReis, S., Gardner, J.F., Boles, M., & Lynch, F. (2000). Trends in prescribing of psychotropic medication to preschoolers. *Journal of the American Medical Association, 283,* 1025–1030.

6

WARNING: PSYCHIATRY CAN BE HAZARDOUS TO YOUR MENTAL HEALTH

William Glasser

This chapter explains my position on the current state of the mental health delivery system. In the forty-five years I've been in psychiatric practice, I have counseled in every area of psychiatry except with small children. Regardless of their symptoms, all who came or were sent to me for counseling had the same basic problem: They were unhappy. Their lives were not going the way they desired them to go, and in almost all instances it was because they were not getting along with the important people in their lives to the extent they wanted. They were not mentally ill. There was no pathology in their brains or brain chemistry. The term mental illness should not be applied to these unhappy people. That diagnosis should be reserved for people who have pathology in their brains, such as people who suffer from Parkinson's or Alzheimer's diseases. These long-established mental illnesses are treated by neurologists, not psychiatrists.

The most accurate way to describe these unhappy people is that although they are not mentally ill, they are not nearly as mentally healthy as they would like to be. Currently, the best way to help them is through counseling. However, I would like to offer an alternative. I believe that unhappy people can be taught to improve their own mental health through Choice Theory, a new form of psychology I created to help people improve their relationships (Glasser, 1998). When they do, they will be both happier and mentally healthier than they are now. Better relationships are the key to mental health and happiness. The Choice Theory approach provides a way for huge numbers of unhappy people to help themselves to better mental health when they can't afford or won't accept counseling. And they can do so at little or no cost to themselves or anyone else.

By the year 1990, mental health—never a strong component of psychiatry—had almost disappeared from the profession. What the vast majority of psychiatrists (whom I refer to as the psychiatric establishment) do today is diagnose unhappy people as mentally ill and prescribe psychiatric drugs to treat them. These psychiatrists call themselves biological psychiatrists. They do little or no counseling. Some who prescribe brain drugs exclusively call themselves psychopharmacologists. For reasons I explain shortly, none of them seems to have any concern for mental health. In all my years in practice, I have counseled unhappy people successfully and never prescribed a psychiatric drug (Glasser, 2000). I counsel without drugs by teaching people in layman's terms to apply Choice Theory to the way we choose to live our lives.

There is no longer a concerted effort from the psychiatric establishment to create a counselor–patient relationship and talk about the problems of those who suffer from psychiatric symptoms, such as those described in detail in the DSM-IV (a compilation of psychological symptoms, many of which are put together as syndromes and called mental illness). The biological psychiatrist will maintain that a patient's symptoms are part of a "mental illness" caused by a brain chemistry imbalance that can only be corrected with drugs. Most of the few psychiatrists who still counsel almost always combine this effort with psychiatric drugs, and many imply that the drugs are the most important component of their treatment.

What the current psychiatric establishment is doing that harms the mental health of those treated extends far beyond the psychiatrist's office. Almost all health professionals seem to be caught in this neurochemical "web" (Black, 2003). Psychiatric drugs that can harm the brain dominate the entire "mental health" landscape. To give an example of the magnitude of this domination, in 2001, 111 million prescriptions were written for just one class of drugs: serotonin reuptake inhibitors (SSRIs) such as Paxil, Prozac, and Zoloft. This represents a fourteen percent increase over the year 2000, and the numbers are still climbing (*Los Angeles Times*, 2002). Recent studies show that this class of drugs may be no more effective than placebos for depression (Kirsch, Moore, Scoboria, & Nicholls, 2002).

General practitioners, as much or more than psychiatrists, have begun diagnosing mental illnesses and prescribing Prozac and other similar brain drugs. Pediatricians are diagnosing attention deficits (ADD or ADHD) in children and prescribing Ritalin, a strong synthetic cocaine that acts on the child's brain in ways that are not yet known and may never be known. Psychologists, social workers, and counselors are diagnosing mental illnesses and teaming with general medical practitioners and psychiatrists to get drug prescriptions for their clients. Often this is done without the prescribing doctor examining in any depth the people for whom they prescribe.

These psychotropic drugs are not harmless. There is a large body of scientifically sound psychiatric research that lays out in detail the harm these drugs can do both to mental health and to the brain itself. At the same time this research points out that these drugs are nowhere near as effective as claimed by the companies that make them (Antonuccio, Danton, & DeNelsky, 1999; Fisher & Greenberg, 1997; Zito, Safer, dos-Resi, Gerdner, Boles, & Lynch, 2000). In February, March, and April of 2004, the FDA issued several warnings directly to physicians regarding serious side effects of antidepressants, including the increased risk of suicide, especially in adolescents. This is the dark side of biological psychiatry that is rarely discussed.

Still, it might be argued that it is worthwhile risking the damage these drugs may do to one's brain if there are no safe effective alternatives to them. But there are. Quick effective counseling without brain drugs has advanced beyond what it was twenty-five years ago. The problem is that most unhappy people who could benefit from counseling cannot afford the costs of talking to a counselor, much less a psychiatrist. Their health insurance will cover brain drugs for years on end, but rarely more than a few counseling sessions will be reimbursed.

Damaging as this practice may be, the real horror of this system is the harm it does to our innate desire to try to take care of ourselves. The message that now comes through loud and clear from biological psychiatry is that *when you are diagnosed with a mental illness there is nothing you can do to help yourself*. The message I am striving to convey is that no matter what "mental illness" a person may be diagnosed with there is no pathology in the brain. The correct diagnosis is *unhappiness*, and there is a great deal that patients can do to help themselves or family members become happier or mentally healthier.

The media went "gaga" when John Forbes Nash, Jr. recovered from schizophrenia, a supposedly incurable mental illness that even with the best psychiatric care separates its sufferers permanently from reality. But as you saw in the movie *A Beautiful Mind* this is not the case at all. Many psychiatrists, including myself, don't believe schizophrenia is a mental illness. Schizophrenia is only one of the hundreds of ways that unhappy people like Nash deal with their unhappiness. One of the first psychiatrists to deny the existence of mental illness was Thomas Szasz (1961), who warned that such diagnosis is a mistake. No psychiatrist did much for John Nash. What he did to recover, he eventually did for himself, together with the help of his loyal wife and the tolerance of the Princeton Math Department, which let him wander its halls for years.

Unfortunately, near the end of the movie, a blatant untruth stated that his unanticipated recovery was greatly furthered by the use of modern brain drugs. Written in Nash's biography (Nasar, 1998), and shown somewhat in the movie, is that he did not take his brain drugs regularly before 1970 and after that year took none at all. I think it is more accurate to say his much later recovery was aided by the happiness of being awarded the 1994 Nobel Prize for economics, which earned him much respect from his colleagues. His wife divorced him but always provided him with the safety and comfort of a home. He may have wandered around Princeton during the day but he was never homeless. His recovery occurred despite his psychiatric care, not because of it.

THE DIFFERENCE BETWEEN PHYSICAL HEALTH AND MENTAL HEALTH

Most people know a lot about physical health but very little about mental health. When health is discussed in the media, the focus is almost always on curing and preventing physical illness, as if our population is either physically ill or physically healthy. This focus is extremely misleading; the vast majority of us are neither physically ill nor physically healthy. Only a very small percentage of people are so physically ill that they carry a medical diagnosis such as cancer, heart disease, or diabetes. Even a smaller percentage is so physically healthy they are fit to run a marathon. This leaves millions of us who are neither physically ill nor in top physical condition. We are somewhere in the middle between illness and good health.

Therefore, the best way to describe the physical health of the whole population is to use a continuum, shown below, with relatively few of us at either end and most of us somewhere in the middle.

Physically Ill ———— Out of Shape ———— Physically Healthy

Physical illness, always based on pathology, is shown at the left, and physical health at the right. The vast majority of us who occupy the middle can best be described as out of shape. In the affluent, indolent, well-nourished society we live in, I still think it is fair to say that most of us in the middle would like to be more physically fit. And almost all of us are well aware of what we need to do to get there: exercise more and eat less. However, from experience, we are also painfully aware that knowing what to do is far easier than doing it. To get encouragement, attention, and instruction we may enroll in a fitness class or employ a personal trainer. But whether we do it alone or with help, we still have to do it. No one or no medication can do it for us.

With that in mind, I'd like to offer a mental health continuum that is analogous to the physical health continuum:

Mentally Ill ———— Unhappy ———— Mentally Healthy

On the left are the relatively few mentally ill people who suffer from brain pathology. Their mental illnesses correspond to physical illnesses such as cancer, heart disease, and diabetes. Examples of these mental illnesses are Alzheimer's disease, Parkinson's disease, epilepsy, brain tumors, or multiple sclerosis. Any neurology text will list these and many more. Pathology in the brain can lead to much unhappiness, but these diseases are not how we express unhappiness. They are diagnosed and treated by neurologists, not psychiatrists.

The "mental illnesses" that establishment psychiatrists diagnose, treat, and list in the DSM-IV should not be labeled illnesses because none of them is associated with any brain pathology (Glasser, 2002). These "illnesses" are the many ways in which unhappy people express their unhappiness. As you can see in the physical and mental health continuums shown above, the mental equivalent of out of shape is unhappy. If those in the middle of each continuum—out of shape or unhappy—know what to do and are willing to do it, they can move toward the healthy end of the continuum.

The difference between the continuums is that those who are out of shape know what to do. They must exercise and lose weight. Information that teaches how to do this is available in hundreds of reliable books. Those who worry that they may be too out of shape to risk exercising can go to a doctor for a physical examination. If there is no pathology, the doctor will suggest a gradual increase in exercise and decrease in food intake.

On the other hand, it is unlikely that those with symptoms of unhappiness such as anxiety or depression know what to do to improve their mental health. They may look for a self-help book, but these are rare. As far as I can ascertain, there was no book that specifically taught how to improve mental health until I wrote *Psychiatry Can Be Hazardous to Your Mental Health* (Glasser, 2003). You were on your own if you wanted to move toward the healthy end of the mental health continuum.

Those persons in the middle of the mental health continuum are in a more hazardous place than those in the middle of the physical health continuum. They not only don't know what to do, but if they seek help from an establishment psychiatrist they may end up worse off than before. Instead of receiving assurances that they are not ill, which a medical doctor provides to those who are out of shape, they will be diagnosed as suffering from a mental illness caused by pathology in their brains or brain chemistry. They will be told that they need brain drugs to treat the "pathology" they do not have. They will also be told that they might benefit from counseling. However, the emphasis will be that psychotropic drugs are the important part of the treatment. Current psychiatric thinking is blind to the fact that if the brain is not diseased, then the problem is that the patient is unhappy and the symptoms are a way of expressing this unhappiness.

As difficult as it is for doctors to accept the concept of a mental health continuum, they easily understand the concept of a physical health continuum. Very likely they use it to improve their own physical health. When they're out of shape, they know they're not ill and have no need for drugs. They will diet and exercise like anyone else.

By diagnosing mental illness that does not exist, psychiatry is a hazard to mental health. Prescribing drugs that interfere with the brain's normal functioning is a further hazard to mental health and to the integrity of the brain itself. But by far the greatest hazard to mental health is being given the message that we can do nothing to help ourselves. I attempt to teach that by learning Choice Theory there is a lot that we can do for ourselves or to help an unhappy family member toward better mental health, at no risk and little cost. When establishment psychiatrists make a diagnosis, especially based on symptoms of anxiety or depression, they tell patients that a neurochemical imbalance in the brain is causing these symptoms. The fact that there is not a shred of valid evidence to support this claim doesn't seem to bother them. An unshaken belief in mental illness has convinced these psychiatrists that it is impossible for anyone to suffer from the symptoms described in the DSM-IV and still have a physically and chemically normal brain.

In making the case for mental illness, the psychiatric establishment has replaced science with "common sense." If a patient has symptoms, something must be wrong with the brain. Because no reputable scientist has ever found anything pathological in the brain structure or chemistry of anxious or depressed patients, biological psychiatrists focus on what is fleeting, rapidly changeable, and can't be seen under a microscope: abnormal brain chemistry. Because brain chemistry changes continually as behavior changes, one does not have the same brain chemistry when happy as when fearful, angry, or depressed. But because brain chemistry changes does not make it abnormal.

To prove what they claim is true about brain chemistry, establishment psychiatrists employ pseudoscience and say abnormal brain chemistry is shown by brain activity. They scan the brain and show that parts are either more or less active when one is depressed, fearful, or angry. They then make a huge leap of intuition and claim that the scanned change in brain activity represents ever-changing brain chemistry. A further leap leads them to conclude that it is the change in brain chemistry that is causing fear, anger, or depression. That conclusion is about as scientific as my taking a patient's heart rate when he is calm, then pointing a gun at him, shooting a few bullets past his ears, taking his heart rate again and telling him that he has heart disease because it is now beating abnormally fast. In this scenario it would be abnormal if it remained the same.

There is another huge difference between being physically ill and mentally ill. If a person has a physical illness such as clogged coronary arteries, the doctor can offer a specific diagnosis and an effective surgical treatment. He may also offer a statin to lower cholesterol. But in no instance will he try to force this treatment on a patient. However, when a psychiatrist diagnoses a patient as mentally ill—most often when the diagnosis is schizophrenic—he is almost certain to tell the patient that pathology in the brain supports his diagnosis and then prescribe drugs to treat it. If the patient disagrees or resists, the psychiatrist may do something no other doctor will do: try to force the patient to take the medication he believes is needed, even if the patient has to be locked up in order to be watched. Siebert (2003) provides a first-hand account of how a patient's freedom is threatened whenever an establishment psychiatrist gives a diagnosis of schizophrenia. To get a patient locked up, the psychiatrist has to declare that the patient is a danger to himself or others in the community. Some people diagnosed with schizophrenia may indeed be dangerous, but in the vast majority of cases these symptoms are not associated with harmful behavior directed at oneself or others.

By far the most dangerous persons in any community are unhappy young men between the ages of eighteen and thirty. They are especially dangerous when they drink, but no one suggests locking them up or even restricting their access to alcohol. Given care, support, and protection or just avoiding psychiatric care, as John Nash managed to do, they can learn to help themselves. Few people—no matter what their "mental illness" diagnosis is—can be accurately assessed as dangerous enough to themselves or others that they have to be forcibly medicated or locked up.

Psychiatrists who tell a patient or the patient's family that these restrictions are necessary are not avoiding the truth as they see it. They are insistent because they believe they are telling the truth: the patient is mentally ill and needs psychiatric drugs, incarceration, or both. If these psychiatrists are shown evidence that supports what I claim about mental illness and medication (Glasser, 2003), they will insist that this research is wrong. They may claim that there is better or more recent brain research to back up their stance. But I advise caution. There is overwhelming evidence to show that the research they cite is funded by the companies that make the drugs they are prescribing. This is about as valid as the research funded for years by the tobacco companies that concluded "scientifically" that cigarettes were neither addicting nor harmful.

If this were just an academic argument about the validity of the diagnosis of mental illness, I would not be writing this. But what's at stake is not academic. It is the mental health of our population and, on a more personal level, the mental health of a family member or a good friend. Still, I do not advise patients to stop taking a drug if they or their families are convinced this drug is helping. Even if they do stop taking it, they should do so slowly because an abrupt withdrawal from these strong brain-altering drugs may also be harmful to the functioning of their brain.

Why Psychiatry Maintains the Fiction of Mental Illness and Disregards Mental Health

When a patient is diagnosed with a mental illness such as depression, schizophrenia, bipolar disease, or obsessive compulsive disorder and treated with a brain drug, he or she becomes one of the millions of geese who lay golden eggs for the multibillion-dollar brain drug industry. This industry masquerades as mental health's best friend, generously funding a variety of groups and activities that promote mental illness and the use of their drugs to treat it. Examples of this funding are lucrative research grants to psychiatrists who come up with supportive research, plush psychiatric conferences, liberal grants to mental health associations that vigorously support mental illness and brain drugs, enticing grants to patient advocacy groups that do the same, and millions of dollars to high-powered public relations and advertising firms to promote the "new drugs" that treat "mental illness" and persuade the media to support the value of brain drugs. The last thing the psychiatric establishment and the drug companies want is for people to get the idea that they can improve their own mental health or help loved ones improve theirs at little or no expense.

MOVING TOWARD MENTAL HEALTH

It may be easier to help oneself move from unhappiness to mental health than it is to move from being out of shape to physically fit. Those persons in the out-of-shape, middle range of the physical health continuum are not in pain. They enjoy eating and sitting around. It feels good to remain in the middle. Most find that making the effort to diet and exercise is difficult and painful. We know we'll feel guilty if we start to diet and exercise, then give it up. So most of us are content to live a sedentary life, top off our bellies, and hope for the best.

In contrast, those in the middle of the mental health continuum are unhappy and often suffer from painful symptoms such as depression and anxiety. Once they accept that they are not mentally ill and that there are easy-to-understand ways to move toward being mentally healthy, they have an incentive to begin improving their lives. This effort is not painful; it feels good. Each step they take in the direction of mental health increases their incentive to go further.

Being mentally healthy means enjoying the company of the people you know, especially family and friends. Mentally healthy people like people in general and are more than willing to help an unhappy family member, friend, or colleague feel better. To a great degree, they lead a tension-free life, laugh a lot, and rarely suffer from the aches and pains that many people accept as an unavoidable part of living. They enjoy life and have no trouble accepting that other people are different from them. They don't criticize or try to change anyone. They are creative in their endeavors and usually fulfill more of their potential than those who are mentally unhealthy. Even in difficult situations when they are unhappy, they know why they are unhappy and will attempt to do something about it. Being physically healthy is not a prerequisite for mental health. A person may be physically handicapped like Christopher Reeve and still fit this criterion.

My mission is to encourage people to be more aggressive in protecting themselves from wrong diagnoses and harmful brain drugs by learning how they can help themselves to be happier and more mentally healthy. Patients and their families should ask any doctor who diagnoses them as mentally ill and advises drugs to explain the basis behind the diagnosis and treatment. Are there alternatives to what is being suggested that don't involve drugs? Remember, there is no pill for unhappiness. Any pill that makes one feel better can be addicting. It would be most helpful for patients to sit down and read a few of the books that seek to help people move toward being mentally healthy. Personally, I strongly recommend *Beyond Prozac: Healing Mental Health Suffering Without Drugs* by Terry Lynch, M.D. (2001). If I ever get seriously unhappy, I plan to camp on his doorstep.

Preparing Patients to Help Themselves

In the last twenty-five years, the psychiatric establishment has almost completely reversed direction. It no longer supports the belief, commonly held for centuries and as sensible today as ever, that a person who is unhappy and capable of carrying on a conversation should seek counseling. I take this belief a step further. If a person is capable of reading and talking about what they've read, there is a good chance they can learn to help themselves by reading books that offer step-by-step support and talking to others about how they can implement the ideas they glean. There are millions of unhappy people who will never seek counseling but could easily and pleasurably join a low-cost or cost-free Choice Theory Focus Group and learn to help themselves.

The current psychiatric belief is that even those who are in contact with reality and could be counseled are still mentally ill and better treated with psychiatric drugs. Some of the establishment psychiatrists that patients are almost sure to see if they belong to an HMO may be interested in counseling but rarely are given permission to provide it. After doing little more than compiling a brief checklist of symptoms, they will tell the patient and/or the patient's family that he or she is mentally ill or suffers from a mental disorder.

This now-dominant psychiatric practice, supported by a multimillion-dollar media blitz paid for by the drug industry, has been so successful that it has been accepted not only by most psychiatrists but by almost all medical doctors, many psychologists, social workers, and counselors. It is the way that the current mental health system makes money from unhappiness and is embraced by a general public that has no easy access to the truth.

We have learned to go for the quick fix. Our society has become accustomed to the concept of medicating discomfort with over-the-counter pills, syrups, and potions. The public likes the simplicity of the argument: a person with psychological problems is ill, and all that's necessary to make life better is to take a pill. The public has no awareness that the price of this pill is to blind patients to the concept that they can pursue happiness and mental health on their own. There is a further price to be paid, however, by taking strong brain drugs. Many of them harm the brain and, in so doing, cause the symptoms that are at the far left of the mental health continuum.

This harm may be called side effects by physicians, but once these chemicals are in your brain there is nothing "side" about them. In his book, *Prozac Backlash*, Joseph Glenmullen, M.D. (2000) points out many of these side effects and also explains that some of them start when the drug is discontinued. Thus, even getting off the drug is not always safe. The worst side effect he discusses is called tardive dyskinesia, which causes a person to lose control over many muscles, including facial muscles, resulting in uncontrollable writhing and grimacing. In many cases, it appears incurable. It is very hard to predict who will get this disease and what drug dose is safe.

At this time no one knows specifically what causes the symptoms described as illnesses in the DSM-IV. There are a lot of inferences such as lowered serotonin, a brain chemical found to be lower than normal in stressed rats who "appear" to the researchers to be depressed. They use rats because the only accurate way to determine serotonin levels is to grind up the brain and assay the ground-up material. But even if the inference in the comparison of rats to humans is correct, no one yet knows whether the depression lowered the serotonin or the lowered serotonin caused the depression. Psychiatrists who use brain scans to diagnose depression are guessing it's the latter and trying to persuade physicians and their patients to go along with this guess.

I'd like to offer a plausible explanation for the cause of many of the hard-to-understand psychological symptoms such as hallucinations, delusions, and mania. I believe they stem from a person's creativity, much as dreams do. A better understanding of this creativity may help us deal more effectively with its unwanted aspects.

When medical doctors tell patients that their symptoms are caused by a disease, disorder, or an illness such as heart disease, they have explicit pathological proof for their diagnosis from one or more of the following: physical pathology found on examination; pathology found from x-ray, Cat-Scan, or MRI procedures; microscopic pathology seen on slides; and/or chemical pathology derived from testing blood or other body fluids. When psychiatrists say that symptoms are caused by a mental illness, they haven't a shred of similar evidence. To label a person mentally ill, which now translates in almost everyone's mind as some sort of brain pathology, is to stigmatize millions of people who should not be subjected to the rejection, ostracism, harmful drugs, and brutal electric shocks to the brain that can and often do accompany this erroneous label.

Unusual, crazy, or frightening as these symptoms may be, they are no more caused by mental illness than was Timothy McVeigh's act of blowing up the federal building in Oklahoma City in 1995. He turned out to be the most dangerous American who ever walked the streets of our country but no one called him mentally ill. What unhappy people have in common is their unpredictable behavior. People who knew McVeigh before and after he committed the crime were well aware that McVeigh was unhappy. What they didn't know was what he was planning to do. There is no limit to the illogical destructiveness of unhappy people, just as there is no limit to the kindness, caring, and self-sacrifice of mentally healthy people. In both cases, their brains are normal; it is how they choose to use them, and the reasoning behind this choice, that differentiates mental health from mental illness (Glasser, 2003). For example, when your computer fails to work the way you want it to, it is a thousand times more likely that the trouble will be in the way you are using it or in the software than in the computer itself. You need to use it more accurately or find better software. You don't need to fix the computer any more than you need to "fix" a normal brain with drugs or electric shocks.

Dealing with Depression

In the treatment of depression, the placebo effect of sugar pills is strong evidence that unhappiness, not mental illness, is the cause of the symptoms. If depression were caused by a chemical imbalance in the brain, then it should not be relieved by a sugar pill. Yet evidence is mounting that given with care, conviction, and time with the doctor who gives it, the sugar pill works better than antidepressant drugs such as Prozac, Paxil, and Zoloft (Vedantam, 2002). It is also interesting that brain activity scans are used to confirm the "positive effect" of these drugs on the brain. The PET scans of people on sugar pills show equal or even greater brain activity in the same areas than those of people on the real drugs. Placebos also can be more effective because they do not have the adverse side effects of real medication.

For example, patients who are depressed because they are unhappy with a relationship might go to their doctor, who prescribes a medication that she says with some conviction (because she believes she is telling you the truth) is the latest medication for depression. "It has helped many of my patients. I think it has a good chance of helping you. It takes a while to work but please call me in a week and tell me how you are doing." With this much attention, patients, most of whom want to please an attentive doctor, will report improvement. What is interesting is that after Vedantam's 2002 research was finished, some of the patients who reported strong positive placebo effects were told that they, indeed, had received a sugar pill. They relapsed immediately. The placebo effect had been shattered by this revelation.

Studies such as this on the effectiveness of placebos have been going on for centuries and nearly always turn out the same. What is vastly different with psychtropic drugs is the huge media support for their effectiveness, almost all of it financed by drug companies, with the complete cooperation of the psychiatric establishment. There are billions to be made with these drugs. On the other hand, there are no corporate profits in counseling or programs to improve mental health.

Like a psychiatric cancer, the false belief in mental illness that only a drug can cure has invaded our entire society, reducing the use of counseling, and standing directly between a patient and mental health by convincing the patient he is mentally ill. What is so ironic is that the HMOs, who mostly control access to psychiatric care, have climbed on the mental illness/brain drug bandwagon because they see counseling as more expensive than drugs, although the drugs are not cheap. To put a patient on Paxil for a year, 365 pills at $3.00 each, costs more than a thousand dollars and carries little certainty that the patient's "disease" will be improved to where he has no need for further drugs. On the contrary, once the drugs are started, their use tends to escalate, especially because many of them are addictive. The Choice Theory Focus Groups I advocate (Glasser, 2003) teach patients how to live their lives more effectively and cost them little or nothing. Because they can continue using what they have learned, the results can be much longer lasting than those from drugs. This would appear to be a win–win opportunity for both patients and HMOs.

HMOs interested in the mental health program I suggest—that is, offering unhappy symptomatic people the option of enrolling in a Choice Theory Focus Group—could easily have one or two of the psychiatrists who work for them devote a few hours a week to setting up and supporting this program. Considering how many HMOs there are, the impact could be astounding. This is an interesting challenge for HMOs that would cost them next to nothing to put into place.

A further benefit to the HMO's mental health program is that it would provide medical doctors with another option for the many unhappy patients they see every day who complain of pain or discomfort for which no physical cause can be found. Even after the expensive MRIs and CAT scans are done and a lot of doctor time invested, patients suffering chronic pain from fibromyalgia and other problems keep returning to their doctors. I recognize that these patients will be highly skeptical of any mental health program, protesting that what they need is more physical care and better medication and that their mental health is fine.

Yet for the nine years that I was the psychiatrist for the Los Angeles Orthopedic Hospital, I worked with more than fifty patients with chronic pain. No cause for their pain had been established, and I found them remarkably open to the idea that the pain might not be medically treatable. I spent time with them and created a relationship with them. The results in many cases were very good. The Choice Theory Focus Group program was not in place then. But I can see now that a program giving these patients usable mental health information plus time and attention could have been quite effective. Such group programs should be active and incorporate a great deal of give and take, not just lecturing and listening. A friendly, we'd-like-to-see-you-again approach would encourage attendance. There would be none of the long waiting times followed by the hurried encounters patients run into now when they finally see a doctor.

Encouraging Mental Health Associations to Get Involved

The natural place to begin reforming the mental health field is in the many mental health associations that span our country. Mental health associations could begin doing what their name implies: improve the mental health of the community by offering access to ongoing Choice Theory Focus Groups at no cost to participants. These are not therapy groups. Anyone who has read my book (Glasser, 2003), in which I describe such a group in action, and who has some teaching skills, can get a group started. (There is also a demonstration video available, showing a Choice Theory Focus Group in progress. Information on this tape can be found on the Internet at www.wglasser.com.) Once initiated, these groups can continue on their own without leaders. This is what Alcoholics Anonymous has been doing since the 1920s with staff members and trained volunteers.

Unsatisfying Relationships Are the Main Cause of Unhappiness

Unhappiness is best described as a time and place when our life is not the way we'd like it to be. We can be in this unhappy place for a moment or many years, but as soon as we realize we are in it, we want to do whatever we can to get out of it. However, most of the time we don't know what to do. If our unhappiness continues for weeks, symptoms such as depression, anxiety, mania, panic, headaches, chronic pain, and even symptoms associated with what is called schizophrenia can appear. Because we are creative, there is always the possibility that a new symptom will present itself. This is one of the reasons that the DSM-IV volume has grown so large.

Assuming that we are physically healthy and have sufficient food and shelter, we experience more unhappiness in unsatisfying relationships than in any other situation, with marriage leading the list. The initial symptoms are commonly anger and depression. The depression will persist if we don't do anything to improve our mental health. If it continues, additional symptoms such as fatigue, headache, listlessness, difficulty sleeping, and loss or gain of appetite may add to or replace depression. It is virtually impossible to be unhappy for longer than a few months and remain symptom free.

It is safe to say that no one can avoid unhappiness. All we can do is try to understand what is wrong and from this understanding try to figure out how to get along better than we do now with the important people in our lives. If we can improve our relationships, we will improve our mental health and our symptoms will disappear. The idea behind the Choice Theory Group program is to help people who don't need psychiatric care or psychiatric drugs—the vast majority of us—learn coping and awareness skills that will help them improve their relationships and carry over their new-found contentment into every aspect of their lives.

This is my vision for the future of the mental health field.

REFERENCES

Antonuccio, D.O., Danton, W.G., & DeNelseky, G.Y. (1999). Raising questions about antidepressants. *Psychotherapy and Psychosomatic Medicine, 68*(1), 3–14.

Black, A. (2003). Prescription for scandal. In William Glasser (author and Ed.), *Psychiatry Can Be Hazardous to Your Mental Health,* Chapter 13. New York: HarperCollins.

Fisher, S. & Greenberg, R.P. (1997). *From Placebo to Panacea: Putting Psychiatric Drugs to the Test.* New York: John Wiley.

Glasser, W. (1998). *Choice Theory.* New York: HarperCollins.

Glasser, W. (2000). *Counseling with Choice Theory: The New Reality Therapy.* New York: HarperCollins.

Glasser, W. (2002). *Unhappy Teenagers, How Parents and Teachers and Can Reach Them.* New York: HarperCollins.

Glasser, W. (2003). *Psychiatry Can Be Hazardous to Your Mental Health,* New York: Harper-Collins.

Glenmullin, J. (2000). *Prozac Backlash.* New York: Simon & Shuster.

Los Angeles Times. (1 July 2002). Health Section.

Kirsch, I., Moore, T., Scoboria, A., & Nicholls, S. (2002), The emperor's new drugs. *Prevention and Treatment* (5), 22–37.

Lynch, T. (2001). *Beyond Prozac: Healing Mental Health Suffering without Drugs.* New York: Simon & Schuster.

Nasar, S. (1998). *A Beautiful Mind.* New York: Simon & Schuster.

Siebert, A. (2003). In W. Glasser, *Psychiatry Can Be Hazardous to Your Mental Health,* Chapter 13. New York: HarperCollins.

Szasz, T. (1961) *The Myth of Mental Illness.* New York: Paul Hoeber.

Vedantam, S. (2002). Sugar pills fight depression, *Washington Post,* May 7.

Zito, J.M., Safer, D.J., dosResi, S., Gerdner, J.F., Boles, M., & Lynch, F. (2000). Trends in prescribing of psychtropic medications to preschoolers. *Journal of the American Medical Association, 283,* 1025–1030.

OTHER BOOKS ON CHOICE THEORY

Glasser, W. (2002). *Unhappy Teenagers, How Parents and Teachers and Can Reach Them.* New York: HarperCollins.

Glasser, W. (2000). *Counseling with Choice Theory, The New Reality Therapy.* New York: HarperCollins.

Glasser, W. (2000). *Getting Together and Staying Together.* New York: HarperCollins.

Glasser, W. (1999). *The Language of Choice Theory.* New York: HarperCollins.

7

ATTENTION DEFICIT HYPERACTIVITY DISORDER: WHAT IT IS AND WHAT IT IS NOT

Rogers H. Wright

It is almost axiomatic in the mental health field that fads will occur in the "diagnosis" and treatment of various types of behavioral aberrations, some of which border on being mere discomforts. Although the same faddism exists to some degree in physical medicine, its appearance is not nearly as blatant, perhaps in part because physical medicine is more soundly grounded in the physical sciences than are diagnoses in the mental health field. These fads spill over into the general culture, where direct marketing often takes place. One has to spend only a brief period in front of a television set during prime time to discover ADHD (Attention Deficit Hyperactivity Disorder), SAD (Social Anxiety Disorder), or IBS (Irritable Bowl Syndrome). Even when purporting to be informational, these are more or less disguised commercials, inasmuch as they posit a cure that varies with the drug manufacturer sponsoring the television ad.

The other certainty is that these "diagnoses" will fall from usage as other fads emerge, as was the case a decade or so ago with the disappearance of a once-common designation for what is now sometimes called ADHD. That passing fad was known as minimal brain syndrome (MBS) and/or food disorder (ostensibly from red dye or other food additives). From this author's perspective, these fad "diagnoses" don't really exist. Other writers in this volume (e.g., Cummings, Rosemond, and Wright) have commented on the slipperiness of these "diagnoses"—that is, the elevation of a symptom and/or its description to the level of a disorder or syndrome— and the concomitant tendency to overmedicate for these nonexistent maladies.

CHILDREN AND ADHD

Certainly, there are deficiencies of attention and hyperactivity, but such behavioral aberrancies are most often indicative of a transitory state or condition within the organism. They are not in and of themselves indicative of a "disorder." Every parent has noticed, particularly with younger children, that toward the end of an especially exciting and fatiguing day children are literally "ricocheting off the walls." Although this behavior may in the broadest sense be classifiable as hyperactivity, it is generally pathognomonic of nothing more than excessive fatigue, for which the treatment of choice is a good night's sleep. Distractibility (attention deficit) is a frequent concomitant of excessive fatigue, particularly with children under five years of age, and can even be seen in adults if fatigue levels are extreme or if stress is prolonged. However, such "symptoms" in these contexts do not rise to the level of a treatable disorder.

Conversely, when distractibility and/or hyperactivity characterize the child's everyday behavior (especially if accompanied by factors such as delayed development, learning difficulties, impaired motor skills, and impaired judgment), they may be indicative of either a neurological disorder or of developing emotional difficulties. However, after nearly fifty years of diagnosing and treating several thousand such problems, it is my considered judgment that the distractibility and hyperactivity seen in such children is not the same as the distractibility and hyperactivity in children currently diagnosed as having ADHD. Furthermore, the hyperactivity/distractibility seen in the non-ADHD children described above is qualitatively and quantitatively different, depending on whether it is caused by incipient emotional maldevelopment (functional; i.e., nonorganic) or whether it is due to neurological involvement.

It is also notable that most children whose distractibility and/or hyperactivity is occasioned by emotional distress do not show either the kind or degree of learning disability, delayed genetic development, poor judgment, and impaired motor skills that are seen in children whose "distractibility/hyperactivity" is occasioned by neurological involvement. Only in children with the severest forms of emotional disturbance does one see the kind of developmental delays and impaired behavioral controls that are more reflective of neurological involvement (or what was known as MBS until the ADHD fad took hold). Differentiating the child with actual neurological involvement from the child that has emotionally based distractibility is neither simple nor easy to do, especially if the behavioral (as opposed to neurological) involvement is severe.

A major and profound disservice occasioned by the current fad of elevating nonspecific symptoms such as anxiety and hyperactivity to the level of a syndrome or disorder and then diagnosing ADD/ADHD is that we lump together individuals with very different needs and very different problems. We then attempt to treat the problem(s) with a single entity, resulting in a one-pill-fits-all response. It is also unfortunately the case that many mental health providers (e.g., child psychiatrists, child psychologists, child social workers), as well as many general care practitioners (e.g., pediatricians and internists), are not competent to make such discriminations alone. Therefore, it follows that such practitioners are not trained and equipped to provide ongoing care, even when an appropriate diagnosis has been made.

To add to an already complicated situation, the symptom picture in children tends to change with time and maturation. Children with neurological involvement typically tend to improve spontaneously over time, so that the symptoms of distractibility and hyperactivity often represent diminished components in the clinical picture. Conversely, children whose distractibility and hyperactivity are emotionally determined typically have symptoms that tend to intensify or be accompanied/replaced by even more dramatic indices of emotional distress.

Management of Children Exhibiting "ADHD" According to Etiology

It is apparent that somewhat superficially similar presenting complaints (i.e., distractibility and hyperactivity) may reflect two very different causative factors, and that the successful treatment and management of the complaint should vary according to the underlying causation. Neurological damage can stem from a number of causative factors during pregnancy or the birth process, and a successful remedial program may require the combined knowledge of the child's pediatrician, a neuropsychologist specializing in the diagnosis and treatment of children, and a child neurologist. In these cases appropriate medication for the child is often very helpful.

Psychotherapy for the child (particularly younger children) is, in this writer's experience, largely a waste of time. On the other hand, remedial training in visual perception, motor activities, visual–motor integration, spatial relations, numerical skills, and reading and writing may be crucial in alleviating or at least diminishing the impact of symptoms. Deficits in these skills can be major contributors to the hyperactivity and distractibility so frequently identified with such children. Counseling and psychotherapeutic work with the parents is very important and should always be a part of an integrated therapeutic program. Such children need to be followed by an attending pediatrician, a child neurologist, a child neuropsychologist, and an educational therapist, bearing in mind that treatment needs change throughout the span of remediation. For example, medication levels and regimens may need to be adjusted, and training programs will constantly need to be revised or elaborated.

It is also noteworthy that so-called tranquilizing medication with these children typically produces an adverse effect. This writer remembers a situation that occurred early in his practice, a case he has used repeatedly to alert fledgling clinicians to the importance of a comprehensive initial evaluation and ongoing supervision in the development of neurologically involved children.

John, a two-and-a-half-year-old boy, was referred by his pediatrician for evaluation of extreme hyperactivity, distractibility, and mild developmental delay. The psychological evaluation elicited evidence of visual perceptual impairment in a context of impaired visual motor integration, a finding suggestive of an irritative focus in the parietal-occipital areas of the brain. This finding was later corroborated by a child neurologist, and John was placed on dilantin and phenobarbital. A developmental training program was instituted, and the parents began participation in a group specifically designed for the parents of brain-injured children. Over the next couple of years, the patient's progress was excellent, and his development and learning difficulties were singularly diminished. The parents were comfortable with John's progress and with their ability to manage it, so they decided to have a long-wanted additional child. In the meantime, the father's work necessitated moving to another location, leading to a change of obstetrician and pediatrician.

The second pregnancy proceeded uneventfully and eventuated in the birth of a second boy. Shortly after the mother returned home with the new infant, John began to regress, exhibiting a number of prior symptoms such as hyperactivity and distractibility, as well as problems in behavioral control. The new pediatrician referred the family to a child psychiatrist, who promptly placed John on a tranquilizer. Shortly thereafter, John's academic performance began to deteriorate dramatically, and his school counseled the parents about the possibility that he had been promoted too rapidly and "could not handle work at this grade level."

At this point, the parents again contacted this writer, primarily out of concern for John's diminished academic performance. Because it had been more than two years since John had been formally evaluated, I advised the parents that another comprehensive evaluation was indicated. The parents agreed, and a full diagnostic battery was administered to John, the results of which were then compared to his prior performance. It immediately became apparent that he was not functioning at grade level, and that the overall level of his functioning had deteriorated dramatically.

In his initial evaluation, John's functional level had been in the Bright Normal range (i.e., overall IQ of 110 to 119), whereas his current functioning placed him at the Borderline Mentally Retarded level (IQ below 60). The history revealed nothing of significance other than the behavioral regression after the birth of the sibling and the introduction of the new medication. I advised the parents that I thought the child was being erroneously medicated, with consequent diminution of his intellectual efficiency, and that the supposition could be tested by asking the attending child psychiatrist to diminish John's medication to see if the child's performance improved.

The attending child psychiatrist was quite upset by the recommendations and the implications thereof and threatened to sue me for "practicing medicine without a license." I informed the physician that I was not practicing medicine but rather neuropsychology, along with deductive reasoning known as "common sense," which we could test by appropriately reducing John's dosage level for a month and then retesting him. Faced with the alternative of a legal action for slander or libel for having accused this neuropsychologist of a felony, the child psychiatrist agreed.

Upon retesting a month later, the child's performance level had returned to Bright Normal, and his academic performance and behavior in school had improved dramatically. By this time approximately six to eight months had elapsed since the birth of the sibling, and John had become accustomed to his new brother. All concerned agreed that the medication had not been helpful and that the child should continue for another three to six months without medication. Subsequent contact with the parents some six months later indicated that John was doing well at school. The parents were quite comfortable with the behavioral management skills they had learned, which enabled them to handle a child with an underlying neurological handicap.

As noted earlier, the marked distractibility and/or hyperactivity in children with neurological involvement tends to diminish through adolescence, especially after puberty, as do many of the other symptoms. As a consequence, these children present a very different clinical picture in adolescence and adulthood. Typically, they are characterized by impulsivity, at times poor judgment, and excessive fatigability. It is generally only under the circumstances of extreme fatigue (or other stress) that one will see fairly dramatic degrees of distractibility and hyperactivity. Thus, an appropriate diagnosis leading to productive intervention is difficult to make.

Conversely, children who exhibit the symptoms of distractibility and hyperactivity on an emotional basis typically do not show the diminution of symptomatology with increasing age. In fact, the symptoms may intensify and/or be replaced by even more dramatic symptoms, especially during puberty and adolescence (Myklebust, 1973). It should also be emphasized that the kind of distractibility and hyperactivity exhibited by the emotionally disturbed youngster is very different in quality and quantity from that of a youngster whose hyperactivity and distractibility has a neurological basis (Myklebust, 1973; Ochroch, 1979). Unfortunately, it is also frequently the case that a youngster with a neurological handicap may have significant emotional problems overlaying the basic neurological problems, making diagnosis even more complicated (Small, 1980). But the overriding problem confronting parents today is the misdiagnosis of emotionally-based symptoms that brings the recommendation of unwarranted medication.

In the largest study of its kind, Cummings and Wiggins (2001) retrospectively examined the records of 168,113 children and adolescents who had been referred and treated over a four-year period in a national behavioral health provider operating in thirty-nine states. Before beginning treatment, sixty-one percent of the males and twenty-three percent of the females were taking psychotropic medication for ADD/ADHD by a psychiatrist, a pediatrician, or a primary care physician. Most of them lived in a single-parent home, and lacked an effective father figure or were subjected to negative and frequently abusive male role models. Behavioral interventions included a compassionate but firm male therapist and the introduction of positive male role models (e.g., fathers, Big Brothers, coaches, Sunday school teachers, etc.) into the child's life. Counseling focused on helping parents understand what constitutes the behavior of a normal boy.

After an average of nearly eleven treatments with the parent and approximately six with the child, the percentage of boys on medication was reduced from sixty-one percent to eleven percent, and the percentage of girls on medication went from twenty-three percent to two percent. These dramatic results occurred despite very strict requirements for discontinuing the medication, which seems to point to an alarming overdiagnosis and overmedication of ADD/ADHD and greater efficacy of behavioral interventions than is generally believed to be the case by the mental health community.

ADULT ADHD

The wholesale invasion of ADHD in childhood and adolescence is accompanied by a concurrent explosion of such diagnoses into adulthood. One cannot watch television without being bombarded by the direct marketing that asks: "Do you find it difficult to finish a task at work? Do you frequently find yourself daydreaming or distracted? You may be suffering from ADD. Consult your physician or WebMD." Of course, adult ADD exists; children with real ADD will grow into adulthood. But the symptoms described in this aggressive TV marketing are more reflective of boredom, the mid-day blahs, job dissatisfaction, or stress than a syndrome or disorder requiring treatment.

Unfortunately, treatment interventions focused primarily on medication and based on such ethereal and universal symptoms promise an instant "cure" for the patient who now does not have to confront possible unhappiness or stress. Such simple solutions also find great favor with the insurers and HMOs that look for the cheapest treatment. Persons exhibiting "symptoms" are more likely to benefit from a variety of behavioral interventions ranging from vocational counseling for job dissatisfaction and marital counseling for an unhappy marriage, to psychotherapy for underlying emotional stress, anxiety, or depression. Such interventions tend to be time-consuming and costly, with the consequence that the patients may inadvertently ally themselves with managed care companies devoted to the principle that the least expensive treatment is the treatment of choice.

Distractibility and hyperactivity of the type that we have called the "real ADHD" does exist in adults. However, in general, symptoms are much more subtle and, in many if not most cases, overshadowed by other symptoms. Thus, if mentioned at all, distractibility and hyperactivity are rarely significant presenting complaints. Such things as poor judgment, behavioral difficulties, forgetting, difficulties in reading/calculating, and getting lost are typically pre-eminent in the adult patient's presenting complaints. These usually become apparent in adulthood after an accident, strokes (CVA), infections of the brain, and other such events. The very drama of the causative factor typically makes the diagnosis apparent, and treatment providers are "tuned in" to anticipate sequellae secondary to neurological damage: intellectual and/or judgmental deficits, behavioral change, impulsivity, and motor impairment.

It should be emphasized that hyperactivity and distractibility, although present, are less dramatic symptoms that are understandably of less concern to the patient. Furthermore, they often diminish rapidly in the first eighteen months following the neurological event. Even then, the major constellation of symptoms may not be sufficiently dramatic to alert attending medical personnel as to the primary cause of the patient's complaints. This is particularly true of contrecoup lesions occurring most frequently in auto accidents.

Although circumstances resulting in contrecoup damage are frequent and often missed, there are also other, even more significant, types of neurological involvement that may also pass unnoticed. These include early-onset Alzheimer's disease beginning at age fifty and cerebral toxicity resulting from inappropriate medication in the elderly, which is usually misdiagnosed as incipient Alzheimer's. Expectation can unfortunately contribute not only to a misdiagnosis, but also failure to order tests that might elicit the underlying condition. In addition, the converse may infrequently occur: Neurological involvement may be anticipated but is not demonstrable and does not exist. Three illustrative cases follow.

Case 1

Bill, a young construction worker, received notice of his imminent induction into the armed services. Right after lunch on a Friday afternoon, a large section of 2 × 4 lumber dropped from the second story of a work site, striking him butt-first in the right anterior temporal region of the head. He was unconscious for a short period of time, quickly recovered consciousness, and showed no apparent ill effects from the blow. He refused hospitalization, and was taken by his employer to his home.

On the following Monday, Bill phoned his employer saying that he was still "not feeling too good," and given the imminence of his induction into the Army, he "was just going to goof off" until he was "called up." The employer had no further contact with Bill, who was inducted into the Army, where he almost immediately began to have difficulty, primarily of a behavioral type. Throughout his basic training, he tended to be impulsive and to use poor judgment, and he was constantly getting into fights with his companions. He barely made it through training and was shipped overseas where he was assigned to a unit whose primary duty was guard duty.

Throughout his training and his subsequent duty assignment, Bill was a frequent attendee at sick call with consistent complaints of headache, earning him the reputation of "goof-off." His military career was terminated shortly after an apparently unprovoked attack on the officer in charge of the guard detail to which Bill was assigned. After a short detention in the stockade, he was discharged from the Army. His headaches and impulsivity continued into civilian life and prompted Bill to seek medical assistance through the Veterans Administration. The VA clinic's case study included neurological screening tests that were strongly suggestive of brain involvement. Consequently, he was given a full psychological work-up, which revealed intellectual impairment attendant to temporal lobe damage.

Subsequent neurological and encephalographic studies were consistent with the neuropsychological conclusions, and indicated a major focus in the anterior temporal area of the brain. A careful and detailed history was taken, and the incident of the blow to the head was elicited. This case suggests that even though Bill refused hospitalization, because of the severity of the blow it would have been prudent for the employer to insist on a thorough evaluation.

Case 2

James, a man in his late forties, was the son of a Southern sharecropper. Upon graduation from high school, he attended the Tuskegee Institute for a short period before he was drafted into the armed forces. James had a productive military career and upon his discharge moved to California, got married, and proceeded to raise his family. He had trained himself as a finish carpenter and cabinetmaker. His work was highly regarded, and his annual income was well above the average for his field. One of his three children was a college graduate, a second was well along in college, and the third was graduating from high school. James owned his own home and enjoyed a fine reputation as a contributing citizen of his community.

While at work installing a complicated newel post and banister, James became disoriented and tumbled from a stair landing, falling some five feet and landing primarily on his head and shoulders but experiencing no apparent loss of consciousness. He was taken to a hospital for evaluation but was released with no significant findings. Almost immediately thereafter, he began to have difficulty at work. He would become disoriented, could not tell left from right, and made frequent mistakes in measuring, sawing, and fitting even simple elements. Before the accident he seldom if ever missed work, but now he became a frequent absentee. The quality of his work deteriorated and his income plummeted. He sought medical advice and was given a small stipend under the Workers Compensation program.

Over several weeks, he demonstrated no progress, and the attending neurologist and neurosurgeon referred him for neuropsychodiagnostic evaluation as a possible malingerer. The neuropsychologist noted that James' current status was completely at odds with his prior history, and not at all consistent with malingering. For example, the evaluation revealed that this highly skilled cabinetmaker, to his embarrassment, could no longer answer the question, "How many inches are there in two and a half feet?" The neuropsychological finding of pervasive occipital-parietal involvement was subsequently corroborated by electroencephalographic study.

Case 3

An airline captain driving along Wilshire Boulevard in Los Angeles lost consciousness when he experienced a spontaneous cerebral hemorrhage. He was immediately taken to a nearby major hospital where he received immediate and continuing care. Subsequently, a subdural hematoma developed, requiring surgical intervention. The captain recovered and showed no clinically significant signs of neurological involvement. An immediate post-recovery issue was the possibility of being returned to flight status. The attending neurosurgeon referred the patient for a comprehensive neuropsychological evaluation that found no indication of residual neurological deficit. Consequently, the neuropsychologist and the attending neurosurgeon recommended return to flight status.

In summary, in none of the foregoing situations was attention deficit or hyperactivity a significant presenting complaint, although the presence of both was clinically demonstrable at various times in the post-traumatic period. Yet the failure to recognize their presence would not have had a negative impact on treatment planning and or management in any of the three cases. Conversely, if excessive focus on the possible "attention deficits and/or hyperactivity disorder" dictated the nature of the therapeutic intervention, a significant disservice to each of these patients would have resulted.

Traditionally when distractibility and/or hyperactivity are prominent parts of the presenting complaint, the mental health provider directs diagnostic energies toward ascertaining the underlying source of these dysphoric experiences. The distractibility and hyperactivity would have been viewed as secondary symptoms to be tolerated, if possible, until the resolution of the underlying problem resulted in their alleviation. In situations where the symptoms were so extreme as to be significantly debilitating, the mental health provider might reluctantly attempt to provide some symptom relief. However, in such cases this was done with the certain knowledge that it was an expedient, and was not addressing causation.

Times have changed dramatically, reflecting the interaction of a number of factors such as competition and cost controls. With the emergence of a plethora of mental health service providers, psychiatry opted to "remedicalize," essentially abandoning what it refers to as "talk therapy" in favor of medicating questionable syndromes and disorders. Psychology, pushed by its academic wing, could never decide what level of training was sufficient for independent mental health service delivery (i.e., master's versus doctoral degrees), and graduate-level training programs began to turn out hordes of master's-level providers in counseling, social work, education, and school psychology.

Meanwhile, the inclusion of mental health benefits in pre-paid health programs broadened consumption and brought about managed care as a means of reducing consumption of all kinds of health services, including behavioral health services. When the American public's impatience with time-consuming processes is added to managed care's limiting of services in the context of a glut of mental health providers the scene is set for considerable mischief. Add to this brew the fact that psychiatry holds a virtual medication-prescribing monopoly in mental health and that drug manufacturers are constantly developing and marketing new magic pills, it all adds up to an environment that encourages the "discovery" of yet another syndrome or disorder for which treatment is necessary.

SUMMARY

When hyperactivity and/or distractibility is truly one of the presenting symptoms, it is indicative of a complex situation that warrants extensive and thoughtful evaluation, and, more often than not, complex and comprehensive treatment planning from the perspective of a variety of specialists. In situations where the attention deficit and/or hyperactivity reflects problems in parenting, chemotherapeutic intervention for the child is likely to be, at best, no more than palliative and, at worse, may succeed in considerably complicating the situation. In this writer's experience, chemotherapeutic intervention for emotionally disturbed children is a last resort and of minimal value in addressing the overall problem. Psychotherapeutic intervention with the parents, which may or may not include the child, is more often than not the treatment of choice. This is a judgment that is best made only after exhaustive study by pediatrics, psychology, neurology, and perhaps, last of all, psychiatry, which so often seems all too eager to overmedicate (see chapter 6).

Where the presenting complaints of hyperactivity and distractibility are in a context of delayed development, excessive fatigability, learning deficits, and other such signs, the complexity of the diagnostic problem is substantially increased. In such circumstances, it is absolutely not in the child's best interest to limit the diagnostic evaluation to a single specialty. With the increasing evidence that neurological involvement can follow any number of prenatal and postnatal exposures, wise and caring parents will insist on a comprehensive evaluation by specialists in pediatrics, child neurology, and child neuropsychology. More often than not, if medication is indicated, it will be of a type quite different than what is used in the management of so-called ADHD.

Furthermore, treatment intervention and case management will likely involve skilled educational training of the specialized type developed for use with the brain-injured child (see Myklebust, 1973, 1978; Ochroch, 1979; Small, 1980, 1982; Strauss & Kephart, 1955). In the case of a friendly pediatrician, a concerned psychologist, or a caring child psychiatrist, any or all attempting unilaterally to diagnose and/or manage the treatment regimen, the concerned and caring parent is well advised to promptly seek additional opinions. For a comprehensive description of the type of evaluation that is most productive in the management of children of this kind, see Small (1982).

REFERENCES

Cummings, N.A. & Wiggins, J.G. (2001). A collaborative primary care/behavioral health model for the use of psychotropic medication with children and adolescents: The report of a national retrospective study. *Issues in Interdisciplinary Care, 3*(2), 121–128.

Myklebust, H.R. (1973). Identification and diagnosis of children with learning disabilities: An interdisciplinary study of criteria. *Seminars in Psychiatry, 5*(1), 74–93.

Myklebust, H.R. (Ed.) (1978). *Progress in Learning Disabilities*. New York: Grune & Stratton.

Ochroch, R.A. (1979). A review of the minimal brain dysfunction syndrome. In R. Ochroch (Ed.), *The Diagnosis and Treatment of Minimal Brain Dysfunction in Children: A Clinical Approach.* New York: Human Sciences.

Small, L. (1980). *Neuropsychodiagnosis in Psychotherapy,* (rev. ed.). New York: Brunner/ Mazel.

Small, L. (1982). *The Minimal Brain Syndrome: Diagnosis and Treatment.* New York: Free Press.

Strauss, A. & Kephart, N. (1955). *The Psychotherapy and Education of the Brain Injured Child,* Vol. 2. New York: Grune & Stratton.

8

THE MYTH OF CONTINUING EDUCATION: A LOOK AT SOME INTENDED AND (MAYBE) UNINTENDED CONSEQUENCES

Rogers H. Wright

The last part of the twentieth century witnessed the rise of consumerism, a development that in short order pervaded the entire culture. The manifestations of this infatuation were widespread throughout society, as protectors of the public welfare passed a variety of legislation designed to ensure the quality and quantity of all sorts of goods and services. To be sure, the public got better safer automobiles (sometimes) and improved air quality and environment, if one ignored the dangers posed by Methyl Tertiary-Butyl Ether (MTBE) contaminating our water supply or the outrageous additional costs of the corn product ethanol lacing our gasoline. Certainly one of the intended, although unstated, consequences of the ethanol outrage is that the corn producers of the Middle Western states are happy with the broadened markets for their crop, and their senators and congresspersons are pleased by the increased probability of their reelection.

Another of the stellar jewels of this "let's protect the public" fervor is the well-meaning intent to improve professional services and procedures, especially those of health services, through the medium of continuing education (CE), which also appears to have unstated but

143

intended consequences The long-existing myth in healthcare was that once the "doctor" passed his state licensing examination, he was never involved with another book until someone "read over him," part of the process of noting his "passing." In amazingly short order, the idea of lifelong education for the health service provider magically spread to every form of professional service delivery. An immediate concern was, "How do we motivate all these practitioners to participate?" The solution was soon forthcoming in the form of mandating participation in CE as a condition for renewing/maintaining one's professional credentials.

Certain other problems became quickly apparent, such as who would administer the CE programs and who would be responsible for their content. This was readily settled by giving professional societies and associations responsibility for the "quality" of the CE programs by setting standards for providers of CE services, at best a specious proposal for ensuring the quality and relevance of the CE product. An apparently intended consequence is that by approving providers both the professional association and the credentialing agency avoid liability and/or responsibility (legal and otherwise) for the content of the CE offerings. The unintended consequence is that the content of current CE offerings ranges from very good to awful. Concomitantly, the relevant state regulatory agency is charged with administering the program, thereby ensuring provider compliance. It is not shocking that another immediate "intended/unintended consequence" was that both the professional associations and the governmental agencies needed additional staff and compensation to implement and maintain such important services devoted to and expended in the public interest.

These proposals found great favor, and in short order virtually every professional service provider was faced with the necessity of participating in continuing education. This chapter views the implications of these developments from the perspective of the profession of psychology. However, personal communications with colleagues in law, medicine, accounting, nursing, dentistry, real estate, and so on indicate that the difficulties touched on in this chapter have universality for all service providers.

THE WORKINGS OF THE CONTINUING EDUCATION SYSTEM

From an economic standpoint, and perhaps from other perspectives as well, CE is comparable to Al Capone's handling of prohibition. However, because consuming alcoholic beverages is a voluntary activity, whereas the maintenance of one's professional credentials (dependent on meeting CE requirements) is economically life sustaining, the CE industry has the advantage of a captive consumer pool never enjoyed by Capone. Initially, CE requirements were modest in that the number of CE hours required for renewing one's credentials was minimal.

Even so, and almost from the outset, some practices were problematic. For example, regulatory boards almost immediately began requiring that CE hours encompass certain subject matter. California's credentialing board, the Psychology Examining Committee (PEC), required every psychologist to complete a course in "human sexuality," later adding participation in courses in "child abuse," and so on. As an aside, this writer shared with many others the perception that: (1) the content of the "sexuality" course was little more than pornography, whereas the child abuse content was superficial, and in several instances misguided; and (2) politically appointed regulatory boards and/or politically elected directors of professional associations make politically motivated (and frequently wrong-headed) decisions about the content of training and/or professional practice.

Despite these and other complaints, the PEC continued the requirements; moreover, with time—and the need for more revenue, personnel, and the like—it increased CE requirements substantially. Currently, CE requirements vary from state to state, ranging from twenty to forty hours per credential period. For example, California requires thirty-six hours of CE credit across the two-year life of one's credentials; this averages eighteen units per calendar year, the equivalent of a college semester of work each year. The cost of fulfilling these CE requirements is quite substantial. The approximately $25 per course-hour average cost is further inflated by "processing" charges imposed by each entity (i.e., the credentialing board, national and/or state association, etc.) even remotely involved. An additional and substantial cost is travel and per diem expenses for CE meetings, which are typically held in larger cities.

The consumer of professional services might well ask, "Why does this concern me?" The answer, of course, is that the service provider will not subsidize the additional several thousand dollar overhead cost of this program, so the cost is passed on to the consumer in the form of additional charges for professional services rendered. Thus, it behooves the consumer to know whether CE programs are delivering as promised. Sadly, it must be reported that there is virtually no objective, credible data addressing this issue. Furthermore, the governmental agencies, professional associations, and continuing education vendors are not at all forthcoming about the gross or net incomes derived from these activities. Thus, to date the consuming public lacks definitive, objective, reliable data on which to base an appraisal of CE.

It has become apparent that CE is a stupendously big business with enormous cash flows. The advertisements for these programs list an average cost well above $100 per participant/per event, the price paid by the vendors to the national and state professional associations to certify the educational offerings. Add vendors' profit margins and processing costs charged by governmental credentialing agencies, and the aggregate receipts reflect a very substantial ongoing business with a guaranteed consumer base. Who can beat that?

What is wrong with professional societies and/or regulatory agencies making money? The answer, of course, is nothing at all, presuming that their doing so is not at the expense of the public or the professionals they ostensibly serve. Unfortunately, the monies are all too frequently consumed by enlarging the bureaucracies of the organizations overseeing the CE programs. Because the cost of CE programs increases the cost of professional services, the justification for their continued existence must be based on more than bland assurances of efficacy promulgated by the participating agencies.

ARE CE PROGRAMS REALLY NECESSARY?

Those with vested interests in CE programs would answer with a resounding affirmative. But do the offerings themselves actually result in increased quality and more effective services? An observation of the offerings by those not directly involved raises serious questions as to the merit and efficacy of many, if not most, CE programs.

Given today's litigious climate, it is doubtful that the cliché of graduating and never opening another book would be a frequently encountered phenomenon. Every health practitioner has a dubious and unwelcome companion in the legions of trial lawyers who are ready to pounce on the unwary. Thus, if only for reasons of enlightened self-interest, most service providers feel a compulsion to keep themselves informed of developments in their field.

Keeping in mind that the avowed purpose of continuing education is to ensure the public welfare, one next must look at the means that affect the realization of this goal. First, professional societies in particular make little, if any, effort to evaluate the content quality of CE programs. The American Psychological Association (APA) specifically disclaims such efforts, stating instead that its responsibilities end with the certification of a provider or organization as meeting the APA's standards of competence. This "institutional cover" thus enables virtually anyone to operate with apparent association approval. It is a sad fact that in the organization's current Web site listings, CE programs are being offered by individuals whose stated training neither qualifies them for APA membership nor for practice as a psychologist in the state of California.

In addition to the national professional organizations operating CE programs, nearly every state has an organization of psychology professionals, and most state associations also operate CE programs similar to those offered by the APA. In California alone there are thousands of mental health providers (psychologists, psychiatrists, social workers, counselors, etc.), virtually all of whom are mandated to participate in the CE enterprise. Consequently, and bluntly stated, CE is one hell of a big business with a great many vested interests (state regulatory agencies, national and state professional societies, and continuing education vendors including colleges and universities). These entities rake in really big bucks, adding staggering and incalculable costs to the price of delivered professional services.

Thus, from the standpoint of justifying the increased cost of service delivery alone, it is reasonable to expect that CE programs would long ago have provided significant demonstrable and credible evidence of CE's contributions to increasing the quality of delivered professional services. However, this writer has seen no definitive evidence to show that all this fuss and fury is, in fact, worthwhile or that it meets legitimate public and professional needs. In their comprehensive and thoughtful review of the continuing education process, Jacobs et al. (in press) suggest that there have been no significant efforts by psychology to evaluate CE's impact on service delivery from the standpoint of either the consumer or the provider. They add that the interests involved in the CE enterprise are so complex that doing away with the system is unlikely.

Another dimension by which the reader can derive some sense of the value of CE programs to the public and the mental health profession is by examining the kinds of material and activities that are categorized as continuing education. This should evoke some serious questions among even the most enthusiastic CE advocates. For example, the APA's CE Web page for the month of January 2004 (APA, 2004) contained upwards of 200 offerings. One of the approved providers—Alliant International University, with campuses throughout California—detailed their ambitious Spring 2004 CE offerings, which included such topics as: Buddhist Meditation for Psychotherapists; Buddhist Psychology for Psychotherapists; The Good Divorce: Long Term Applications for Children and Family; Facilitating and Leading Change in Complex Organizations; Human Sexuality: A Basic Training for Those Who Work with the Sexuality of Others; Sexual Orientation: Current Theory and Trends in Working with Lesbians, Gays, and Bisexual Patients; Animal Abuse: Assessment and Treatment of Adults and Children. All courses run six to eight hours or more, and not one costs less than $100.

In this same timeframe, the mail produced a brochure offering CE courses in California sponsored by the New England Educational Institute of Pittsburgh, Maine, an organization that also is approved by the APA to offer CE. California and the warmer states are favored spots for winter-time CE offerings under the rubric of the "First Annual California Symposium," this group offered Introduction and Overview of Buddhist Schools of Mindfulness; Meditation, Breath Control, Concentration, and Absorption Training; Deepening Insight: Cultivating the Witnessing Mind; Mindfulness and Practices from the Nondual; Working with Client's Pain, Suffering and Hopelessness; Dropping the Need for Happy Endings, Acknowledgements and Possibilities; and Practical Methods of Spiritually Based Therapy. Without any knowledge of the efficacy of the foregoing courses, this writer was relieved to note others entitled "Overview of the Anxiety Disorders" and "Cognitive Behavioral Conceptualization of Anxiety Disorders." At least the latter might have a more clearly defined relationship to improving competence and/or quality in the delivery of psychological services.

This potpourri of CE offerings is further broadened by offerings of credit for reading an edition of a national psychological newspaper, *The National Psychologist,* and taking a thirteen-question multiple choice quiz on the contents of one's reading. In the test accompanying the January–February 2004 edition of *The National Psychologist,* one of the questions concerns an interview with the newly designated chief executive officer of the APA. The multiple choice question asks the reader to identify a statement of the CEO on the purposes of the APA: that is, creating an organization of diverse membership and recruiting racial minorities to add to the diversity. Really, how many organizations these days would not declare that as their intent? One also gets continuing education credits for attending professional meetings (e.g., conventions, etc.), where at least providers might be exposed to new developments in their fields. It is arguable that any of the foregoing subjects might in some way have a positive impact on the consumer of psychotherapeutic services, although for many, if not most, of the offerings, the direct positive benefit to a consumer is difficult to ascertain.

One of the inherent problems in the enterprise of continuing education—an enterprise rapidly approaching the proportions of a scam—is the differentiation between that which is psychotherapeutic and psychotherapy itself. For example, the coeditor of this volume relates that when he was operating one of the world's major mental health service provider organizations, he received a claim from a practitioner who billed for additional services that apparently consisted of holding a mineral rock during the psychotherapeutic session. When his billing for psychological services was denied, the provider insisted that he learned about the therapeutic properties of mineral rocks in a CE course.

Many activities have a psychotherapeutic value: for example, talking with a bored bartender while imbibing one's favorite alcoholic concoction. Although this may be very therapeutic for the consumer, it is not psychotherapy. Nor can the bored bartender charge an additional fee as a psychotherapist, although many of them probably wish they could. Although holding a mineral rock, petting animals, and focusing on "emotions" may have some psychotherapeutic value, most practitioners would agree that these activities are not even definable, let alone billable, as psychotherapy.

Another major area of difficulty and perhaps an unintended consequence of continuing education has to do with the power that has accrued to regulatory boards and/or professional associations. This power has carried with it an aura of omniscience and omnipotence frequently exercised in a charged political and politicized context. Thus, we continue to see efforts to mandate CE courses ranging from political correctness, an esoteric subject matter needed by only a few highly specialized providers, to topics that all mental health professionals already know, and sometimes to topics that are unproven and even nonexistent. For example, several years ago a California regulatory board attempted to mandate that all providers under their jurisdiction complete a course in Ebonics, the alleged "street language" of one of the state's minority groups. Fortunately, a storm of protest forced the board to rescind that order.

Other questionable mandated courses in such subjects as human sexuality abound, as if the psychologist has not already received such training. The hidden motive in the latter is the intent to assure that the latest in political correctness has been imparted to the ignorant practitioner. Another example: the California Board of Psychology and the California Board of Behavioral Science (BBS) require a one-time CE course aimed at providing training and education in long-term care for the elderly. Having worked at length with the elderly, I am assured that most psychologists in a lifetime of practice will probably never see a patient who qualifies under those terms. Geriatric Psychopharmacology is another course offered to fulfill four hours of required CE credit, even though psychologists and social workers cannot prescribe in California.

Behavioral healthcare providers, as a group, have a long tradition of social concern, and the professional Dudley DoGooders among us frequently feel compelled to try to force their value systems on their errant colleagues and the world at large. Unfortunately and regrettably the "Dudleys" are all too frequently joined in their arrogance and social engineering efforts by regulatory boards and professional associations because of political correctness or perceived political pressures. This volume abounds with examples of such well-intentioned but often destructive efforts. However, we are not alone in these shenanigans. The television evening news chronicled a situation wherein a bar association was being sued by one of its own members challenging the bar's CE requirement for training in "ethnic sensitivity."

A final area of concern is the rush to provide and mandate participation in courses formulated to attract so-called subgroups within the field. In the introduction to this volume, I commented on the economic interests that drive representatives of "minority groups" to make claims about the necessity of exposure to the heritage and culture of such groups as a qualification for providing psychotherapeutic benefits to them. After fifty years of delivering psychodiagnostic and psychotherapy services to a exceedingly wide range of human beings, and as an educator, researcher, and participant/leader in the development of professional psychology, it is my considered judgment that all too frequently joining the patient's efforts to focus on cultural idiosyncracies, minority group identification, rage attacks, sexuality, injustices, victimization, and the like is to become complicit in the consumers' preoccupation with symptoms rather than the causation of their problem. It also does serious disservice to the maxim that it is not what the therapist understands, it is what the patient (consumer) comes to understand that is compellingly critical to a successful psychotherapeutic experience.

Over the years I've had to undergo four root canals, each done by personal friends and each of which ended up disastrously, ultimately causing the loss of the affected tooth. A few months ago, I had a fifth dental flare-up, but this time I called a friend who practices oral surgery and asked for a referral. He recommended and I subsequently consulted an endodontist and had my first successful root canal experience. To this day, I neither know nor care whether the endodontist has ever taken a CE course, but I do know that he doesn't do anything but root canals. The general dentists I had consulted previously were sincere and well-meaning; the problem was that they don't do many root canals.

In my practice when I am, for whatever reason, referring someone for psychological services, I really do not bother to review a list of their CE experiences. I look for someone who has a long history of success in a particular field and is experienced in providing the type of psychological services I believe are needed. No amount of CE "weekend training" will compare with that. In fact, in my experience, an all too frequent consequence of CE training is that it encourages the impulsive and headstrong provider to venture into new areas best left to others. To ensure that the consumer receives quality service, the provider should be an originally well-trained, knowledgeable, and experienced professional operating within the limits of personal competence. Odd, isn't it that psychology's code of ethics— established long before anyone even thought about continuing education—says exactly the same thing?

REFERENCES

American Psychological Association. (2004). Continuing education for January. Office of Continuing Education. www.apa.org/continuingeducation.

Jacobs, W.J., McKnight, P., McKnight, K., & Sechrest, L. (in press). Why legislatures, courts, attorneys, the media, and consumers of psychological services ought to get worked up about continuing professional education: A return to the roots. *Journal of Consulting and Clinical Psychology.*

Section C
Political Influence on Science and Practice

9

SUPPRESSING INTELLIGENCE RESEARCH: HURTING THOSE WE INTEND TO HELP

Linda S. Gottfredson

Research on intelligence is a tale of good and evil, or so the media would have us think. We are presented as mean-spirited pseudoscientists who are greasing the slippery slope to oppression and genocide with their elitist racist ideologies about human differences. On the other side are the earnest souls who would save us from those horrors by exposing the unscientific and immoral basis of the so-called "science" of intelligence differences. Even when the science is conceded to be accurate, it is often labeled dangerous and irresponsible (Block & Dworkin, 1974). If not life-imperiling, it at least threatens the foundations of American democracy. In short, the world must be made safe from intelligence research.

Perhaps ironically, institutional psychology has been busy doing just that for over thirty years. The media can keep repainting its libelous portrait of intelligence research only with the complicity of intelligence's mother field, psychology. Although intelligence tests are frequently cited as psychology's biggest success, psychology often treats researchers who study the origins and consequences of individual and group differences in general intelligence as its biggest embarrassment, the troublesome child or mad uncle whom a socially ambitious family would lock up or have disappear. In doing so, it has undermined the integrity of psychological science, encouraged fiction-driven social policies that continue to disappoint and ratchet up blame, and blinded us to the daily risks and challenges faced by the less able among us.

A CASE STUDY IN SUPPRESSION: ARTHUR JENSEN AND THE SILENCED MAJORITY

Psychology is not a monolith, of course, but a semi-organized social system governed by regard and reputation, often dispensed (as well as coveted) by official representatives such as journal editors, awards committees, and association officers. It therefore seems emblematic that the American Psychological Association (APA) has never given an award to Arthur R. Jensen, the greatest contemporary scholar of intelligence and one of the fifty most "eminent psychologists of the twentieth century" (Detterman, 1998; Dittman, 2002, p. 29). Neither has the newer but more scientifically oriented American Psychological Society (APS).

Fair, Formidable, Fearless—and Correct After All

Jensen personifies the dedicated empiricist who seeks scientific truths, not popular acclaim. He would rather be right than seem right, which is personally costly when the truth is unpopular. He incurred steep costs by publishing and defending his 1969 *Harvard Educational Review* article, "How Much Can We Boost IQ and Scholastic Achievement?" (Jensen, 1969), and he continues to incur costs with his subsequent work. Recognizing that Jensen "will not receive the honors his work merits from organizations like the American Psychological Association," editor Douglas Detterman (1998) dedicated a special issue of the journal *Intelligence* ("A King Among Men") to honoring Jensen.

Peers wrote with the highest praise for the scientist and the man, and with outrage at the abuse Jensen has suffered for maintaining his scientific integrity. Despite repeatedly being abused by "thugs with pens" and threatened physically, Jensen has "[f]or more than 40 years … unflinchingly strived to make psychology an honest science" (Scarr, 1998, pp. 227, 231). "Indeed, few people now alive have had more impact on the field" of human intelligence (Sternberg, 1998, p. 213). As a scholar, Jensen is "formidable" (Deary & Crawford, 1998, p. 274), "exceptional," "innovative," "prolific" (Nettlebeck, 1998, pp. 233, 239), "inspirational" (Rushton, 1998, p. 218), and "the quintessential scientist" (Kaufman, 1998, p. 253). He has "an ingenious ability to develop quantitative analyses that address fundamental issues in highly original ways that advance our knowledge of critical issues in the field" (Brody, 1998, p. 246); he does research of "exceptional thoroughness and scientific rigor" (Vernon, 1998, p. 267) that is "intensive, detailed, exhaustive, fair-minded, temperate, and courageous" (Bouchard, 1998, p. 283); and he "has continued to blaze trails where others would not lead but many would later follow" (Gottfredson, 1998, p. 291). One commentator became "so thoroughly impressed by Jensen's empiricism, wisdom, and sense of fairness" after reading Jensen's "brilliant, data-based, meticulous critique" of the commentator's own work, one that had made him "sweat" to see Jensen "so familiar with my work and … start his attack with smoking guns" (Kaufman, 1998, p. 250).

Detterman (1998, p. 177) emphasized an "unusual" trait of Jensen's "that [may be] impossible for Jensen's critics to understand" but which has allowed him to prevail scientifically. It is not the "thick skin" that many peers mentioned, but Jensen's "healthy agnosticism about everything."

> For years, his critics have called him every name in the book and have accused him of all kinds of biases and prejudices. In fact, I have never known anybody with fewer prejudices. The biggest prejudices scientists usually have are those in favor of their own ideas…. However, Jensen has no loyalty whatsoever to any theory or hypothesis even if they come from his own ideas. He would gladly know the truth even if it proved him wrong. In fact, he would be excited to know the truth.

Even into the late 1980s, Jensen assumed that only a small minority of experts shared his conclusions about intelligence. A handful had agreed publicly with the suddenly "notorious" Dr. Jensen, the inveterate Hans J. Eysenck (e.g., Eysenck, 1971) being the most vocal among them. More expressed their agreement only privately to him. Among the "closet Jensenists" in psychology were luminaries who could have provided Jensen's conclusions with strong and credible public support but instead asked him not to reveal their views. Beyond these small minorities, Jensen generally heard only resounding silence or condemnation from fellow psychologists.

The results of a 1984 survey (Snyderman & Rothman, 1988) of experts on intelligence and mental testing therefore surprised even Jensen. The experts' modal response on every question that involved the "heretical" conclusions from Jensen's 1969 article was the same as his (Jensen, 1998, p. 198). The experts' mean response overestimated test bias, however, because there is none against blacks or lower social class individuals (Jensen, 1980; Neisser et al.1996; Snyderman & Rothman, 1988, p. 134; Wigdor & Garner, 1982). Here, in abbreviated form, are the survey's major questions and the 600 experts' responses.

> Q: What are the important elements of intelligence?
> A: "Near unanimity" (96 to 99 percent) for abstract thinking or reasoning, problem-solving ability, and capacity to acquire knowledge (p. 56).
> Q: Is intelligence best described as a single general factor with subsidiaries or as separate faculties?
> A: A general factor (58 percent, or 67 percent of those responding; p. 71).
> Q: What heritability would you estimate for IQ differences within the white population?
> A: Average estimate of 57 percent (p. 95).
> Q: What heritability would you estimate for IQ differences within the black population?
> A: Average estimate of 57 percent (p. 95).
> Q: Are intelligence tests biased against blacks?
> A: On a scale of 1 (not at all or insignificantly) to 4 (extremely), mean response of 2 (p. 117).
> Q: Are intelligence tests biased against lower social class individuals?
> A: On a scale of 1 (not at all or insignificantly) to 4 (extremely), mean response of 2 (p. 118).
> Q: What is the source of average social class differences in IQ?
> A: Both genetic and environmental (55 percent, or 65 percent of those responding; p. 126).
> Q: What is the source of the average black–white difference in IQ?
> A: Both genetic and environmental (45 percent, or 52 percent of those responding; p. 128).

Supposedly a fringe scientist, Jensen was actually in the mainstream because the mainstream had silently come to him (Gottfredson, 1997a). Meanwhile, public opinion was still being pushed in the opposite direction, creating an ever-greater gulf between societal perception and scientifically informed thought.

The Silent Majority

It is no mystery why so many experts in intelligence-related fields moved intellectually in Jensen's direction. New research, often conducted by researchers eager to prove him mistaken (e.g., Brody, 1992, p. ix), kept supporting his conclusions. But why was the migration seemingly so secretive? And why did Jensen's colleagues keep silent while the media promulgated clear falsehoods as scientific truths, especially when, as Snyderman and Rothman (1988) demonstrated, the media portrayed expert opinion on intelligence as the opposite of what it really was? Worst of all, why did Jensen's peers turn away, or even throw a few stones themselves, while a brethren scholar with whom they agreed was viciously attacked?

Self-Serving Self Censorship

The ferocity of attacks on Jensen after publication of his 1969 article signaled what could happen to anyone who violated the new taboo against discussing the relation between intelligence and genes or race. If any reminder were needed, it was soon provided when Harvard psychologist Richard Herrnstein (1971) published an article in *The Atlantic Monthly* arguing that social class inequalities are rooted partly in genetic differences in IQ, a speculation since confirmed (Rowe, Vesterdal, & Rodgers, 1998). Herrnstein did not mention race, but was immediately denounced as racist (Herrnstein, 1973).

In fact, one need not mention either genes or race but merely take intelligence differences seriously to be accused of racism. Early in my career I reported that bright boys who had attended a school for dyslexics did not enter the usual high-level jobs (medicine, law, science, and college teaching). They had nevertheless succeeded at a high level by entering prestigious or remunerative occupations that required above-average intelligence but relatively little reading or writing: specifically, top management and sales positions. A colleague accused me of saying that "blacks can't make it because they are dumb." She taught me that the taboo's boundaries are broad but uncertain and that enforcement begins on its far outskirts.

It is understandable that many people keep far away from those amorphous but stinging boundaries. Moreover, the farther one goes into forbidden territory, the more numerous and more severe the sanctions become: first the looks of disapproval and occasional accusations of racism, then greater difficulty getting promotions, funding, or papers published, and eventually being shunned, persecuted, or fired. Experiencing the first mild sanction is enough to cause many to envision the worst and reverse course. As one chaired professor told me, just seeing how Jensen was mistreated was enough to convince her, like others, to cease studying cognitive differences and switch fields in the early 1970s.

Because individual and group differences in phenotypic intelligence have substantial effects on so many social phenomena (e.g., Gordon, 1997; Lubinski & Humphreys, 1997), intelligence is relevant to many fields of psychological inquiry, among them education, child development, parenting, health behavior, vocational development, career counseling, and personnel selection. Avoiding the phenomenon, therefore, requires actively walling it off in a great variety of fields. Common forms of self-censorship include intentionally omitting relevant facts or findings from one's publications, ignoring them in others', failing to draw obvious connections between phenomena, neglecting to dispute clear but convenient falsehoods and to perform analyses that might produce the politically wrong answer, committing a deliberate act of omission, to which one leading social scientist later confessed (Coleman, 1990–1991). Researchers may also refuse to share relevant data with other scholars who are willing to perform the politically sensitive analyses that they are not, such as estimating the contribution of genetic differences to the mean black–white IQ difference (Rowe, 1997).

Cordoning off data, analyses, and conclusions according to the strictures of political correctness creates a safe distance between oneself and controversial research and researchers, but it simultaneously isolates those individuals and renders their research less credible to the scientifically uninformed. As they become the untouchables, "prudence" compels some of the discipline's informed members to distance themselves from them or their ideas by casting aspersions, lest potential critics think that they, too, harbor the proscribed thoughts. The best informed, who are often called upon for expert comment, cannot endorse clear falsehoods without jeopardizing their own standing within the discipline, but they sometimes dispute minor issues in a manner that the uninformed mistake for wholesale repudiation (Gottfredson, 1994a; Page, 1972).

Scientific societies also engage in various forms of self-censorship, presumably to avoid tainting themselves by giving credence to the disapproved person or idea. Although Jensen received honors before his 1969 publication (Guggenheim Fellowship, fellowship at Stanford's Center for Advanced Study in the Behavioral Sciences), he has received none since then from American psychology for his remarkable scientific contributions. His only award in more than thirty years came on the eve of his eightieth birthday in 2003: the Award for Distinguished

Contributions in Individual Differences from the International Society for the Study of Individual Differences, a small international society of academic psychologists.

American psychological societies have even withdrawn lifetime achievement awards from intelligence researchers, as did the APA in 1997 from the 92-year-old internationally eminent Raymond B. Cattell, whom detractors accused of scientific racism (Laurance, 1997) on the eve of the award ceremony. In like manner, various scientific and professional societies have invited Jensen to address their members, only to rescind their invitations when some critic objected. While APA president in 1975, Donald Campbell urged participants at the annual convention's membership meeting to do "plenty of hissing and booing" at Jensen's invited address on test bias (Jensen, 1983, p. 308), APA's Board of Directors later forced Campbell to apologize to Jensen, but then expunged the apology from its official minutes.

In fact, psychologists and their organizations often led the charge against Jensen. One of APA's larger divisions (Division 9, Society for the Psychological Study of Social Issues, SPSSI) immediately orchestrated a media campaign to discredit many of the main points in Jensen's 1969 article (Jensen, 1972, pp. 31–37). Psychologists at various regional meetings that year also organized calls to censure Jensen and expel him from the APA (Jensen, 1972, p. 39). SPSSI's president at the time, Martin Deutsch, soon announced that he had found fifty-three errors in Jensen's article, "all unidirectional and all anti-black," and that there must be "some other motive, not scientific," behind them. He finally provided the list two years later after APA's Committee on Ethical Standards intervened, but there were no errors among the fifty-three items (Jensen, 1983, p. 307). Psychologist Jerry Hirsch (Hunt, 1999, pp. 73–74) captured the tenor of the time when he repeatedly wrote and spoke about Jensen having "avowed goals" that were "as heinously barbaric as were Hitler's and the anti-abolitionists." With psychologists themselves loudly attempting to extrude the "heinous" Dr. Jensen from the discipline, it is no wonder that most others watched in silent fear.

This may also help explain why professional associations have, with a few exceptions (Jensen, 1983, p. 307), seemed deaf to requests for assistance from members targeted for harassment for their research. These requests surged in the 1980s when some universities acceded to demands that particular faculty's intelligence research be suppressed by banning requisite funding, blocking promotions and merit pay, requiring that lectures be given by videotape, instigating investigations for hate crimes, threatening dismissal, and the like (Gottfredson, 1996c; Hunt, 1999; Kors & Silverglate, 1998; Lynn, 2001; Rushton, 1994). Although individual officers sometimes provide generous personal support (ex-APA president Robert Perloff being one, in my case), timely institutional action to protect the targeted members' academic rights has been rare because it requires, at minimum, getting a majority vote in one or more committees to take action that critics are likely to block or protest.

Censorship for the Public Good

There are inter- and intradisciplinary squabbles throughout the sciences, and academe is no less immune to petty politics and backbiting than any other realm. But the social processes that suppress unpopular intelligence research are extreme. They involve repeatedly violating the most fundamental norms of science, and often common decency as well. The daily personal slights can be humorous in hindsight, as when colleagues stumble over themselves to avoid being physically near the shunned colleague. However, having former friends violate the norms of civility and science to destroy one's career is not. Otherwise decent people who behave indecently toward fellow scholars usually justify it as a moral necessity. They are fighting evil, and proudly so.

Book and journal editors sometimes explicitly cite moral necessity to legitimate their holding "controversial" intelligence research to more numerous and onerous standards before judging it worthy of publication or dissemination. For example, in explaining why he was rejecting a paper I submitted to *The Public Interest* in 1986, editor Nathan Glazer stated that, although finding it scientifically sound, there were social "considerations" that "overweigh the claims of social science." (The manuscript described the employment inequalities that black–white differences in general intelligence typically create under race-blind hiring.) He would later write in *The New Republic* (Glazer, 1994, p. 16), in response to publication of *The Bell Curve* (Herrnstein & Murray, 1994), that:

> Our society, our polity, our elites, according to Herrnstein and Murray, live with an untruth: that there is no good reason for this [racial] inequality, and therefore society is at fault and we must try harder. I ask myself whether the untruth is not better for American society than the truth .... For this kind of truth, ... what good will come of it?

Perhaps more common than editors explicitly rejecting manuscripts on solely unscientific grounds is their (and their reviewers') enforcing much stiffer scientific standards for politically incorrect intelligence research. When acknowledging their double standards, they usually justify the practice as ethically required to prevent the research in question from causing harm, although what that harm might be is never clear. Jensen's files are full of such reviews.

Consider, for example, the reason that Charles Kiesler, then editor of the *American Psychologist* (and APA's chief executive officer for many years), gave Jensen for rejecting a paper he had submitted to that journal. After acknowledging that the manuscript had "taken an inappropriate length of time to make it through the review process," Kiesler stated that "My own feeling as Editor is that since this area is so controversial and important to our society, I should not accept any manuscript that is less than absolutely impeccable." One problem, he suggested, was that "In this paper there is a hanging implication that any differences that are demonstrated to exist are genetic" (January 17, 1980, letter from Kiesler to Jensen). The paper had tested "Spearman's Hypothesis," that mean black–white differences in mental test scores are larger on more *g*-loaded tests, suggesting that the racial difference lies principally in *g*, the general intelligence factor.

The claim of protecting the nation and its citizens from harm is sometimes merely a self-serving pretext, but it might often be sincere. The media and strident critics of intelligence research have for decades demonized researchers like Jensen and have forecast the most despicable crimes against humanity should their conclusions prevail. The implication of ABC's November 22, 1994, national newscast was surely not lost on viewers when, while exposing the supposedly unsavory history of intelligence research behind *The Bell Curve*, news anchor Peter Jennings followed photographs of Jensen and other supposed race scientists with footage of Nazi soldiers and what appeared to be death camp doctors and prisoners. His broadcast illustrates how taboos exercise control by triggering revulsion, not thought. To question the accuracy of the reportage or argue the merits of academic freedom would be tantamount to indicting oneself for sheltering the evil that others would have us crush by any means possible.

Indeed, many people have treated Jensen as vile and dangerous. For a long time Jensen received death threats, needed bodyguards while on his campus or others, had his home and office phones routed through the police station, received his mail only after a bomb squad examined it, was physically threatened or assaulted dozens of times by protesters who disrupted his talks in the United States and abroad, regularly found messages like "Jensen Must Perish" and "Kill Jensen" scrawled across his office door, and much more (Jensen, 1972, 1983, 1998). Psychologists Richard Herrnstein and Hans Eysenck also had such experiences during the 1970s for defying right thinking about intelligence. Eysenck, for example, was physically assaulted by protesters during a public lecture at the London School of Economics (Herrnstein, 1973; Rushton, 1994).

Critics have associated a belief in the hereditary basis of intelligence with evil intent so frequently and for so long that merely mentioning "IQ" is enough to trigger in many minds the words "pseudoscience," "racism," and "genocide." Even recent APA president Robert Sternberg keeps this malicious association alive by regularly ridiculing and belittling empirically minded intelligence researchers—for example, comparing Jensen, in a book meant to honor him, to a child who would not grow up (Sternberg, 2003)—referring to their work as "quasi-science" (Science and pseudoscience, 1999, p. 27) that has "recreated a kind of night of the living dead" (Sternberg, 1997, p. 55). In addition, he sprinkles his descriptions with mentions of racism, slavery, and even Soviet tyranny (e.g., Sternberg, 2003; see also Sternberg, 2000; Sternberg & Wagner, 1993).

Critics have yet to explain why we should assume that a belief in the heritability of many human differences is dangerous and that a belief in man's infinite malleability is not. Why is the former belief always yoked to Hitler, but the latter never to Stalin, who outlawed both intelligence tests and genetic thinking? Stalin killed at least as many as did Hitler in his effort to reshape the Soviet citizenry (Courtois, 1999). Why does it accord humans less dignity to acknowledge and accommodate their biological differences than to deny them or try to stamp them out? Most important, why should we wager our collective future on assuming it safer to deny than to face the implacable empirical realities affecting our lives? Moral panics preclude such reflection.

THREE FICTIONS AND THEIR CASCADING DAMAGE TO PSYCHOLOGY AND SOCIETY

Critics have moved the study of intelligence out of the scientific realm into a moral one where they set the rules (Nyborg, 2003). Scientists who flout their moral strictures are judged scientifically misguided or corrupt and thus stripped simultaneously of both scientific and moral authority. Those who flaunt allegiance to these rules are held up as good scientists, in both senses of the term. Most social scientists now take for granted the new etiquette on what they must say and seem to believe.

Fiction-Driven Science and Failed Social Policy

Fear thinned the ranks of empirically minded intelligence researchers when Jensen came under attack in 1969. Since then, graduate students and young academics in related fields have been systematically socialized by both mentors and media to avoid "sensitive" issues in intelligence research. The new tacit knowledge, or street smarts, for career advancement in academe includes all forms of self-censorship described earlier. The walls that authors erect to seal off unwanted facts and inferences about intelligence, genes, and race are so prevalent in scholarly publications today that one tends to notice them only by their absence. An author's "connecting the dots" stands out, either as a breath-catching breach of etiquette or as a breath of fresh air, depending on one's perspective.

The unwanted facts are also kept at bay—"discredited"—by fictions about the nature and origins of human differences. Three fictions have been especially important; all are resolutely held (or at least professed) by most social scientists and policy makers; all require them to defy rather than work with empirical realities. One is the "egalitarian dogma" (Rushton, 1994) or "egalitarian fiction" (Gottfredson, 1994a). The other two are "family effects theory" and "passive learning theory" (Rowe, 1997; cf. Scarr, 1997, on socialization theory). All were once plausible hypotheses, but that was long ago. I describe them briefly in order to illustrate later the cascading harm they cause.

Fiction 1: Egalitarian Dogma

The egalitarian fiction is that demographic groups do not differ meaningfully, on average, in important abilities and aptitudes: that is, whatever their current levels of performance, all groups are equipotential, both now and in the future. Critics argue it would be demeaning and demoralizing to claim otherwise. The American black–white IQ difference is this fiction's key target. Data from large national samples shows that the black–white IQ gap is essentially the same at age three as later in life, and at the end of the twentieth century as at the beginning: about 1.1 standard deviations (Gottfredson, 2003b). The gap has been impervious to social change, affirmative action, secular rises in IQ (the so-called Flynn effect), and endless educational interventions (which was one point of Jensen's 1969 article). The lower average black IQ has yet no definitive explanation, genetic or environmental, but it is clearly exceedingly stubborn. It is not a chimera of test bias (Neisser et al., 1996).

Tightly held and ferociously protected, the presumption of equipotentiality directs all explanation of social inequalities toward mistreatment or inequalities in the social environment. The fiction also guides much social policy. For example, a foundational assumption of much employment discrimination law and policy is that there would be no racial differences in hiring and promotion but for illegal racial discrimination by employers (Sharf, 1988). Unequal outcomes now trigger the presumption of guilt, which employers must then disprove. As we show, this leads to much mischief in personnel psychology by fueling impossible demands. One man's benevolent lie becomes another man's impossible burden.

Fiction 2: Family Effects Theory This false theory holds that differences in cognitive competence and educational performance can be traced to differences in family advantage. Most efforts to equalize educational achievement, therefore, attempt to provide all students with resources comparable to those of middle-class families, ranging from type of instruction, advanced placement courses, and educational funding to meals, role models, and aspirations. Like the egalitarian fiction, family effects theory locks our attention onto external influences, apparently presuming that most people are just passive, hapless lumps of clay to be molded by circumstance. This is key in propping up the egalitarian fiction, because it "explains" the group differences in test scores.

Differences in cognitive ability can, in fact, be traced partly to differences in environments, but not to those in family effects theory. Behavior geneticists distinguish between two types of environmental influence: shared and nonshared (also called *between*-family and *within*-family effects). Shared influences are those that make siblings more alike. Possible shared influences include parental income, education, childrearing style, and the like, because they impinge on all siblings in a household. Nonshared influences are those that affect individuals and therefore make siblings less alike. Little is yet known about them, but they might include illness, accidents, nongenetic influences on fetal development, and the concatenation of unique experiences.

To the great surprise of even behavior geneticists, shared environmental effects on intelligence (within the broad range of typical environments) wash away by late adolescence. IQ differences can be traced to both genes (40 percent) and shared environments (25 percent) in early childhood, but genetic effects increase in importance with age (to 80 percent in adulthood) whereas shared effects dissipate (Plomin, DeFries, McClearn, & McGuffin, 2001). For example, adoptive siblings end up no more alike in IQ or personality by adolescence than do random strangers, and instead become similar to the biological relatives they have never met.

Scholastic achievement depends primarily on cognitive ability so it, too, is moderately highly heritable, with its heritability overlapping that for IQ. Like IQ, academic performance increases in heritability with age, but unlike IQ it continues to be shaped somewhat by shared influences (Plomin et al., 2001, pp. 199–201). Equalizing shared environments may be a legitimate goal in and of itself, but given the importance of intelligence to learning it can do little to narrow differences in educational achievement or any of education's downstream correlates such as occupation and income level.

In fact, despite reform, race and class differences in educational achievement remain large and not much different today than they were decades ago. Still guided by its fictions, however, right thinking continues to accuse schools of failing their disadvantaged students and to demand that they eradicate the achievement gaps forthwith. Under the new No Child Left Behind Act, schools will be punished if they do not.

Currently one of the biggest puzzles for family effects theory is that academic achievement gaps do not narrow even in settings where all the supposedly important environmental resources are present (Banchero & Little, 2002). For example, its adherents are now arguing among themselves (Lee, 2002) about the proper cultural explanation for the large black–white achievement gaps that persist in the most socioeconomically advantaged, integrated, liberal, suburban school districts in the United States such as Shaker Heights, Ohio (Ogbu, 2003) and Berkeley, California (Noguera, 2001). Moreover, black–white test score gaps (IQ, SAT, etc.) tend to be larger at higher socioeconomic levels. This finding contradicts the predictions of family effects theory. It is consistent with g-based theory, however, because the latter predicts that black and white children of high-IQ parents will regress part way from their parents' mean toward different population means: IQ 100 for whites and IQ 85 for blacks.

Fiction 3: Passive Learning Theory This false presumption is that intellectual ability is the sum total of exposures to opportunities to learn: that is, the greater one's exposure to relevant information and good instruction, the more one will know and the smarter one will be. It is a species of environmental determinism and required, in turn, to prop up the other fictions. This theory purports that equalizing students' opportunities to learn will equalize their learning.

The passive learning theory is false because some people "pick up ideas" or "catch on" much quicker than others (they extract more from each opportunity), and "fast" or "slow" learners usually remain so throughout their educational careers and adult lives. When students are free to learn at their own pace, the brightest students often learn at least five times faster than the slowest. To a large extent, that is what higher intelligence means. The theory is also false because people are not merely passive learners, but seek out information and select different opportunities to learn when given a choice.

The great spread of intelligence levels among high school students predicts—and we actually observe—that many students perform at least two to four grade levels above or below their grade in any given core subject, whatever the instructional regime. The National Assessment of Educational Progress (NAEP) vividly illustrates the very different learning curves among students. For example, the ninetieth percentile of nine-year-olds (~IQ 120) performs in reading, math, and science at the level of the twenty-fifth percentile of seventeen-year-olds (~IQ 90) (National Center for Education Statistics, 2000). Between-race differences are not as large as within-race differences, of course, but they are still substantial. For instance, black twelfth graders average four to five grade levels behind whites on NAEP tests of reading, math, and science (Gottfredson, 2003b).

It is educational malpractice to assume that all students benefit equally from the same instruction. One-size-fits-all instruction impedes learning among those for whom the cognitive fit is poor. The instructional style that most helps slow students (highly structured, concrete, step-by-step instruction that leaves no gaps for students to fill in) impedes the learning of bright students, who profit most from more abstract, incomplete instruction that allows them to restructure information in unique ways (Snow, 1996). Targeting instruction to students' individual cognitive needs would likely improve achievement among all, but it would not cause the slow learners to catch up with the fast. The fast learners would improve more than the slow ones, further widening the learning gap between them and seeming to make the "rich richer." This is currently politically unacceptable.

The Devolution of Fiction-Driven Science

Fiction-driven policies have fallen far short of expectation in all arenas of life where intelligence affects performance. They will continue to do so. Rather than question the fictions, however, social scientists have been revising their theories and reallocating blame among external forces for stifling talent in some demographic groups. For example, at the time Jensen wrote his 1969 article, policy analysts still presumed that equalizing educational access and resources would equalize learning and life chances for the disadvantaged. When that policy and subsequent ones failed, theories of inequality evolved from shifting the presumed material causes of social inequality to its psychic ones. Thus, the proffered cures now include providing equal regard as well as equal funding. Neither public policy nor public science may yet consider the well-documented role of intelligence. Clinging to its fictions, ideologically correct social science increasingly resembles the decaying Ptolemaic theory of the heavens (Gottfredson, 2003d).

Psychology's Ptolemaists seize every new straw of hope for explaining group differences in success without recourse to ability differences, no matter how improbable in light of the relevant evidence (e.g., stereotype threat; Gottfredson, 2002b). So, too, do they lunge for every new environmental nostrum for those presumably nonexistent ability differences, no matter how elusive or contrary to established evidence the purported cure may be (e.g., the still-mysterious cause of the secular increases in IQ, or "Flynn effect").

At the same time they devoutly keep intelligence a "neglected aspect" in their work (Lubinski & Humphreys, 1997). *A Common Destiny* (Jaynes & Williams, 1989) provides a highly visible example. It was the work of a National Research Council (NRC) panel charged with cataloguing the nature and sources of black–white differences in success and well-being. As Humphreys (1991) describes, however, it failed even to mention IQ or ability differences or refer to work that did. Other high-profile task force reports have mentioned intelligence research only to summarily dismiss it as noxious (College Board, 1999).

The fictions about intelligence essentially deny that it exists, which virtually no one believes. Many people just want a more "democratic" view of it. Not surprising, psychology's supply rose to meet public demand, and the new egalitarian perspectives on human intelligence were instantly blessed by opinion makers. Chief among them are the "multiple intelligence" theories by psychologists Howard Gardner (1983, 1998) and Robert Sternberg (1997). The eager acceptance of their theories by educators, psychologists, and others occurred despite the lack of credible evidence that their proposed intelligences actually exist, that is, as independent abilities of comparable generality and practical importance to g. Gardner has rejected even measuring his eight intelligences, let alone demonstrating that they predict anything (Hunt, 2001; Lubinski & Benbow, 1995). Study-by-study dissections of Sternberg's multiple-intelligence research program reveal no such evidence (Brody, 2003a,b; Gottfredson, 2003a,c). If anything, they confirm that all three of his proposed intelligences are just different flavors of g itself, as probably are most of Gardner's (Carroll, 1993, p. 641).

Their empirically vacuous (Kline, 1991; Messick, 1992) "modern understandings" of intelligence are now widely cited, however, as additional scientific proof that the empirically minded scientists of intelligence are hopelessly, stubbornly mistaken, especially if they pay scant attention to the new theories. Like the media, both Gardner and Sternberg frequently ridicule the 100-year-old tradition of intelligence research and pepper their discussions with allusions to its supposedly unsavory adherents and undemocratic values (e.g., Gardner, 1998, p. 23; Sternberg, 2003). The new theories thus advance on their political appeal, not on any scientific merits. The popularity of the multiple-intelligence theories among psychology's consumers may enhance institutional psychology's political standing in the short term, but its pursuit of political acceptability cultivates wish over wisdom and cheap moralizing over hard work. It handicaps honest, intensive, exhaustive, fair-minded, temperate, and courageous science while giving an advantage to academic opportunism.

POLITICIZED SCIENCE, USURPED RIGHTS

In claiming to protect the public from dangerous questions and answers, journal editors and reviewers imply that their fellow citizens are apt to misuse the information (become oppressors) or be psychologically crippled by it (be victimized). They imply that democracy is best served by keeping its citizenry ignorant of matters that they deem themselves more fit to decide. Researchers likewise usurp the rights belonging to others when they skew their own work to fit political pressures or predilections. Such usurpation may involve acts of omission, as with self-censorship, or acts of commission, as when empiricists misuse science to actively promote a particular political view. Wolf (1972) describes how common the latter was during the 1960s on matters of race.

Two fairly recent examples from selection psychology show how even the most senior leaders in psychology have sometimes practiced politics in the guise of science. Both reflect the pressure that the egalitarian fiction puts on employment practice. The presumption in employment law today is that employment inequality results from illegal discrimination until employers prove otherwise. This puts enormous pressure on employers to do whatever it takes to achieve racial balance in selection despite the typically large average racial differences among applicants in requisite skills, abilities, and, eventually, job performance.

Race Norming Test Scores

The first example of politics in scientific garb is a National Research Council's recommendation (Hartigan & Wigdor, 1989) that the U.S. Department of Labor (DOL) race norm its employment tests. Race norming guarantees racial balance—quota hiring—because it involves ranking all applicants separately by race and then selecting the same percentage of top scorers within each race. The NRC panel confirmed that the DOL's test battery was unbiased and valid for predicting job performance; however, it provided a convoluted statistical argument that race norming was nonetheless justified on scientific grounds. It is not, and psychologists on the panel later admitted that. Specifically, it represents a particular definition of fairness (not bias), and thus is a "values" call, not a technical matter (Sackett & Wilk, 1994, pp. 931–936).

One might want for political reasons to grant bonus points for race on tests that are psychometrically sound, as was the DOL's aptitude test battery, but race norming cannot be justified on technical grounds because it always introduces racial bias (favoring the lower-scoring races) and reduces predictive validity (Blits & Gottfredson, 1990a; Gottfredson, 1994b). Psychometrician Lloyd Humphreys (1989, p. 14), always a straight talker, wrote in a letter to *Science* that the NRC's high-profile recommendation was a value judgment "camouflaged by rhetoric [and] statistical legerdemain."

In this case, the attempted usurpation of rights was foiled when it was exposed as a covert move for quota hiring (Blits & Gottfredson, 1990a,b; Gottfredson, 1990). In 1991, the U.S. Congress voted overwhelmingly to outlaw race norming in employment after it learned that the Labor Department had been race norming its employment tests for a decade and that the U.S. Equal Employment Opportunity

Commission (EEOC) had started threatening private employers if they did not adopt the "scientifically justified" practice.

The racial preferences that race norming entails are hardly trivial. What the NRC report did not say was that blacks scoring at the fifteenth percentile in skill level on DOL's test would have been judged equal to whites and Asians scoring at the fiftieth percentile, and blacks at the fiftieth percentile would be rated comparably skilled as whites and Asians at the eighty-four percentile (Blits and Gottfredson, 1990a). Seldom apprised of such facts, most people greatly underestimate how discrepant the pools of qualified applicants are from which racial balance is supposed to emerge.

Another illustration, pertinent to the next example, is that approximately seventy-five percent of whites versus only twenty-eight percent of blacks exceed the minimum IQ level (~IQ 91)—a ratio of three to one—usually required for minimally satisfactory performance in the skilled trades, fire and police work, and mid-level clerical jobs such as bank teller (Gottfredson, 1986, pp. 400–401). The potential pools become increasingly racially lopsided for more cognitively demanding jobs. Workers in professional jobs such as engineer, lawyer, and physician typically need an IQ of at least 114 to perform satisfactorily. About twenty-three percent of whites but only one percent of blacks exceeds this minimum.

Racially Gerrymandering Test Content

Employers can hardly ignore differences in mental competence because the general mental ability factor g is the best single predictor of performance in jobs and school, especially in the higher ranks of both (Schmidt & Hunter, 1998). When used in a race-blind manner, valid and unbiased selection procedures, therefore, virtually guarantee substantial disparate impact in most circumstances, with the imbalance becoming more extreme in the higher levels of education and work (Gottfredson, 1986; Sackett, Schmitt, Ellingson, & Kabin, 2001; Schmidt & Hunter, 1998). Developing tests that measure cognitive skills more effectively tends only to worsen the proscribed disparate impact. Adding relevant noncognitive predictors to the mix does little to reduce the racial imbalance (Schmitt, Rogers, Chan, Sheppard, & Jennings, 1997).

The egalitarian fiction requires psychologists to defy this reality in order to perform the impossible ("psychomagic"), or at least seem to. Many selection professionals preferred race norming because it harms productivity less than other methods of filling racial quotas.

After the practice was banned, a movement developed among selection psychologists to "improve" selection procedures by, in effect, making them less reliable and less valid (Gottfredson, 1994b, 2002b). Proponents of the new techniques (e.g., test score banding) created the aura of improvement with adventitious labeling, for example, modern, innovative, sophisticated, nontraditional, broader, and more equitable; not giving undue weight to small differences; assessing the whole person; and having higher authenticity or "fidelity" (face validity).

The police selection test developed in 1994 for Nassau County, New York, represents one such "technical advance." The ten members of a joint Nassau County–U.S. Department of Justice (DOJ) team set out to develop a police selection test with less disparate impact (more racially balanced results). Since 1977, the county had been unable to satisfy the DOJ's employment discrimination unit under its various consent decrees. (Recall the three to one ratio given above for the proportion of whites vs. blacks exceeding the ability level below which performance in police work tends to be unsatisfactory.) Seven of the team's eight psychologists constituted a Who's Who of APA's large Division 14 (Industrial and Organizational Psychology), four of whom had previously served as its president.

Several years and millions of dollars later, this high-powered team claimed to have succeeded in developing a test that virtually eliminated disparate impact while simultaneously improving selection validity. Water could run uphill, after all. Once again, leading psychologists found a seemingly scientific solution to an intractable political–legal dilemma. DOJ immediately began pressing other police jurisdictions nationwide to replace their more "discriminatory" tests with the new selection battery.

A close look at the several-volume technical report for the Nassau test battery revealed that the team had succeeded in reducing disparate impact by gerrymandering the test to assess only traits on which the races differed little or not at all (Gottfredson, 1996a,b). The joint Nassau–DOJ team had administered its nearly day-long, 25-part experimental battery to all 25,000 applicants, but settled on the battery's final composition only after examining the scores it yielded for different races. The experimental battery was then apparently stripped of virtually all parts demanding cognitive ability. The only parts actually used to rank applicants were eight noncognitive personality scales (all commercial products owned by members of the team) and the ability to read above the first percentile of currently employed police officers (near illiteracy). Selection for cognitive competence had been reduced to little more than the toss of a coin, despite the team's own careful job analysis showing that "reasoning, judgment, and inferential thinking" were the most critical skills for good police work.

The new police test was made to appear more valid than the county's previous ones by, among other things, omitting key results required by legal and professional guidelines, transforming the data in ways that artificially reduced the apparent validity of the cognitive subtests relative to the noncognitive ones, and making a series of statistical errors that more than doubled the final battery's apparent predictive validity (from .14 to .35). When exposed, the test created a scandal in Division 14 ("The Great Debate of 1997" in Hakel, 1997, p. 116), partly because other leading selection psychologists expected its use would produce less effective policing and degrade public safety (Schmidt, 1996).

Nassau County was stuck with the cognitively denuded test, and its training academy soon felt the predictable effects. Although the Justice Department eventually stopped promoting the test after the scandal became public, other test developers were already sitting on DOJ's doorstep ready to provide it with others of the same type. It can be very lucrative for a test developer to please the nation's enforcer of "nondiscriminatory" employment testing, which for decades has brooked no opposition among test developers and users to its aggressive enforcement of the politically correct view on ability differences.

CAUSTIC SCIENCE: CONSTRUCTING AND CURING THE INCORRIGIBLY RACIST SOCIETY

The would-be censors of "sensitive" intelligence research assert that the nation will be healthier by remaining ignorant of selected realities. They suggest that the truth, especially on racial differences in cognitive ability (genetic or not), can only do harm and that their untruths only good. Again, why should we think so? Intelligence researchers are willing to agree that disseminating information more widely may hold some risks, which is why they discuss how to minimize them (Loehlin, 1992). In contrast, the censors have yet to consider whether the collective fraud they nurture might also do harm. We have just seen one example where it could threaten public safety. And it may wreak more insidious, self-perpetuating damage to the body politic.

All populations exhibit a wide and enduring dispersion in general intelligence. All develop social institutions that adjust to this dispersion in some manner. The ways a society organizes and reorganizes itself to accommodate its substrate of human talents are among the "third-order" effects of *g* that Gordon (1997) enumerates and the "cascading effects" that Lubinski and Humphreys (1997) describe. Fictions about intelligence likewise have societal-level effects when they require us to deny and defy empirical realities that persistently intrude themselves into a nation's life.

The dogma of equipotentiality dictates that explanations of racial inequalities lie in mistreatment and disadvantage. No explanation may "blame the victim" or challenge the fictions currently undergirding ideologically correct thinking. But failure begets blame, and blame seeks a target. Because overt discrimination is rare today, the persistent, pervasive, and seemingly inexplicable failure of fiction-driven policies for achieving racial parity in all life outcomes is taken to reflect the presence of an even worse culprit, one that not only creates inequality everywhere, despite all countermeasures, but also remains invisible. The evil on which right thinkers have settled is covert racism. Psychologists and others now tell us that racial animus is unconscious and has become "institutionalized" throughout American life. That we cannot directly see the racism and may even deny it only shows how deeply woven it is into the fabric of our minds and institutions. No self-defense, no exoneration is possible in the face of social inequality. Only group parity, we are told, can tell us when the hidden evil has been exorcised.

We have already seen one of the earliest policies for rooting out invisible racism: making racial imbalance in employment prima facie evidence of illegal discrimination. However, curative enthusiasms have moved far beyond that. Even the most objective, most carefully vetted procedures for identifying talent are instantly pronounced guilty of bias or "exclusion" when they yield disparate impact in hiring, college admissions, placement in gifted education, and the like. Indeed, the very notions of objectivity and merit are now under attack by influential intellectual elites (Farber & Sherry, 1997).

When faithful and fair application of the law yields disparate impact in arrest or incarceration rates, American jurisprudence must be considered inherently racist (see arguments in Crenshaw, Gotanda, Peller, & Thomas, 1995). When earnest, socially liberal teachers fail to narrow the stubborn achievement gaps between races and classes, they must be unconsciously discriminatory and require diversity training. Because American institutions still routinely fail to yield the desired racial balance, those who created and supposedly control those institutions—majority Americans—must be deeply, unconsciously, inveterately racist and creators of a society where appearances to the contrary are just a smokescreen to hide their built-in privileges. Under the equipotentiality fiction, there can be no other legitimate explanation, and any attempt at one serves only to evade responsibility.

The major culprit is actually the *g*-loadedness of modern life. Intelligence is not just an academic ability; virtually all of life's arenas require continual learning, reasoning, and problem solving of some sort. The advantages of higher *g* sometimes differ greatly from one arena to another, but they increase whenever situations and tasks are unfamiliar, ambiguous, unpredictable, changing, unscripted, unsupervised, untutored, multifaceted, or otherwise complex, that is, when they call for learning and judgment. Moreover, the practical advantages of higher *g*, both large and small, are pervasive and compound over time and life spheres (see reviews in Gottfredson, 1997b, 2002a).

The current war against social and economic inequality is therefore substantially a futile and fratricidal war against the manifestations of *g* itself. If such signs are interpreted as evidence of the oppression of some by others, then we shall never lack for fresh evidence. Moreover, the seeming oppression will be greater wherever *g* has greater functional value, such as in the higher levels of education and work. Groups that succeed at higher levels will, by virtue of that success, be presumed guilty of practicing, condoning, or benefiting from oppression. The guilty will be all the more contemptible should they refuse to confess and atone for their transgressions. In order to protect lower-scoring minorities and less able individuals from being victimized by the truth, we now must convict all others of grievous sins. The nation must cure itself by turning its institutions inside out, and its principles upside down.

Harming the Less Intelligent: Living Daily with Reality

Fewer, but still many, social scientists hold to a fourth false credo, that intelligence has little or no functional utility, at least outside schools. Moreover, they often add that the advantages and disadvantages of high or low IQ are mostly "socially constructed" to serve the interests of the privileged. This view was articulated in an influential article published soon after Jensen's 1969 article by economists Samuel Bowles and Herbert Gintis (1972/1973). They argued that higher IQ does not have any functional utility, even within schools, and that IQ tests are simply a tool created by the upper classes to maintain and justify their privileges. They dismissed talk of "objectivity" and "merit" as just smoke blown to obscure this fact. Psychologist Robert Sternberg implies much the same when he suggests that the *g* factor dimension of intellectual differences is an artifact of Western schooling (Sternberg et al., 2000, p. 9) and that using cognitive tests such as the SAT to sort people is akin to the way slavery and religious prejudice were once used to keep disfavored groups down (Sternberg, 2003).

However, when critics argue that IQ differences have little or no functional meaning beyond that which cultures or their elites arbitrarily attach to them for selfish purposes, they simultaneously turn attention away from the very real problems that lower intelligence creates for less able persons. As Herrnstein and Murray (1994) note, the critics generally have little contact with the downtrodden they would protect. These bright opinion makers may be living comfortably with their fictions and benevolent lies, but lower IQ individuals must live daily with the consequences of their weaker learning and reasoning skills. Their distant protectors would seem to be the limousine liberals of intelligence. They do not realize that everyday tasks that higher IQ individuals consider so simple might create obstacles to the well-being of others less cognitively blessed.

Functional Literacy and Daily Self-Maintenance

Citizens of literate societies take for granted that they are routinely called upon to read instructions, fill out forms, determine best buys, decipher bus schedules, and otherwise read and write to cope with the myriad details of everyday life. But such tasks are difficult for many people. The problem is seldom that they cannot read or write the words, but usually that they are unable to carry out the mental operations the task calls for to compare two items, grasp an abstract concept, provide comprehensible and accurate information about themselves, follow a set of instructions, and so on. This is what it means to have poor "functional literacy."

Functional literacy has been a major public policy concern, as illustrated by the U.S. Department of Education's various efforts to gauge its level in different segments of the American population. Tests of functional literacy essentially mimic individually administered intelligence tests, except that all their items come from everyday life, such as calculating a tip (see extended discussion in Gottfredson, 1997b). As on intelligence tests, differences in difficulty rest on the items' cognitive complexity (their abstractness, amount of distracting irrelevant information, and degree of inference required), not on their readability per se or the level of education test takers have completed. Literacy researchers have concluded, with some surprise, that functional literacy represents a general capacity to learn, reason, and solve problems, a veritable description of g.

The National Adult Literacy Survey (Kirsch, Jungeblut, Jenkins, & Kolstad, 1993) groups literacy scores into five levels. Individuals scoring on Level 1 have an eight percent chance of successfully performing tasks similar in difficulty to locating an expiration date on a driver's license and totaling a bank deposit slip. They are not routinely able to perform Level 2 tasks, such as determining the price difference between two show tickets or filling in background information on an application for a social security card. Level 3 difficulty includes writing a brief letter explaining an error in a credit card bill and using a flight schedule to plan travel. Among Level 4 tasks are restating an argument made in a lengthy news article and calculating the money needed to raise a child, based on information in a news article. Only at Level 5 are individuals routinely able to perform mental tasks as complex as summarizing two ways that lawyers challenge prospective jurors (based on a passage discussing such practices) and, with a calculator, determining the total cost of carpet to cover a room.

Although these tasks might seem to represent only the inconsequential minutiae of everyday life, they sample the large universe of mostly untutored tasks that modern life demands of adults. Consistently failing them is not just a daily inconvenience, but a compounding problem. Likening functional literacy to money—it always helps to have more—literacy researchers point out that rates of socioeconomic distress and pathology (unemployment, adult poverty, etc.) rise steadily at successively lower levels of functional literacy, which mirrors the pattern for IQ (Gottfredson, 2002a).

Weaker learning, reasoning, and problem-solving ability translates into poorer life chances. The cumulative disadvantage can be large, because individuals at literacy Levels 1 or 2 "are not likely to be able to perform the range of complex literacy tasks that the National Education Goals Panel considers important for competing successfully in a global economy and exercising fully the rights and responsibilities of citizenship" (Baldwin, Kirsch, Rock, & Yamamoto, 1995, p. 16). Such disadvantage is common, because forty percent of the adult white population and eighty percent of the adult black population cannot routinely perform above Level 2. Fully fourteen percent and forty percent, respectively, cannot routinely perform even above Level 1 (Kirsch et al., 1993, pp. 119–121). To claim that lower ability citizens will only be victimized by the public knowing that differences in intelligence are real, stubborn, and important is to ignore the practical hurdles they face.

Health Literacy, IQ, and Health Self-Care

The challenges in self-care for lower-IQ individuals are especially striking in health matters, where the consequences of poor performance are tallied in excess morbidity and mortality. Health psychologists have ignored the role of competence in health behavior, focusing instead on volition. Patient "noncompliance" is indeed a huge problem in medicine, but health literacy researchers, unlike health psychologists, have concluded that it is more a matter of patients not understanding what is required of them than being unwilling to implement these requirements (reviews in Gottfredson, 2002a; 2004).

Health literacy is functional literacy in health-related tasks, such as determining from a prescription label how many pills to take. Health scientists have concluded that it, too, represents a general ability to learn, reason, and solve problems (for extended discussion and citations see Gottfredson, 2002a; 2004). Accordingly, as in other domains of literacy, comprehension is not improved by providing health information in oral rather than written form. Also comparable is that distressing proportions of the population are unable to perform the simple health-related tasks that usually require little or no instruction.

For example, twenty-six percent of outpatients in several large urban hospitals could not determine from an appointment slip when the next visit was scheduled, and forty-two percent could not understand instructions for taking medicine on an empty stomach. Among those with "inadequate" literacy, the failure rates on these two tasks were forty percent and sixty-five percent, respectively. Substantial percentages of this low-literacy group were unable to report, when given prescription labels containing the necessary information, how to take the medication (twenty-four percent), how many times the prescription could be refilled (forty-two percent), or how many pills of the prescription should be taken (seventy percent). Taking medications improperly can be as harmful as not taking them at all, and the pharmacy profession has estimated that about half of all prescriptions are taken incorrectly.

As in other performance domains, training and motivation do not erase the disadvantages of lower comprehension abilities. For instance, many patients who are under treatment for insulin-dependent diabetes do not understand the most elemental facts for maintaining daily control of their disease. In one study, about half of those with "inadequate" literacy did not know the signs of very low or very high blood sugar, both of which require expeditious correction, and sixty percent did not know the corrective actions to take. Like hypertension and many other chronic illnesses, diabetes requires continual self-monitoring and frequent judgments by patients to keep their physiological processes within safe limits during the day. Persistently high blood sugar levels can lead to blindness, heart disease, limb amputation, and much more. Low functional literacy has been linked to the number and severity of illnesses, worse self-rated health, far higher medical costs, and (prospectively) more frequent hospitalization. These relations are not eliminated by controlling for education, socioeconomic resources, access to healthcare, demographic characteristics, and other such variables.

Because health literacy is a rough surrogate for g, it produces results consistent with research on IQ and health. To take several examples, intelligence at time of diagnosis correlates .36 with diabetes knowledge measured one year later (Taylor, Frier, Gold, & Deary, 2004). IQ measured at age eleven predicts longevity, incidence of cancer, and functional independence in old age, and these relations remain robust after controlling for deprived living conditions (Deary, Whitemann, Starr, Whalley, & Fox, 2004). Another prospective epidemiological study found that the motor vehicle death rate for men of IQ 80 to 85 was triple and for men of IQ 85 to 100 it was double the rate for men of IQ 100 to 115 (O'Toole, 1990). Youthful IQ was the best predictor of all-cause mortality by age forty in this large national sample of Australian Army veterans. Furthermore, IQ's predictive value remained significant after controlling for all fifty-six demographic, health, and other attributes measured (O'Toole & Stankov, 1992).

As in education, equal resources do not produce equal outcomes in health. Like educational inequalities, health inequalities increase when health resources become equally available to all, such as happened to the British government's dismay after it instituted free national healthcare. Although health improves overall, it improves least for less-educated and lower-income persons. They seek more, but not necessarily appropriate care when cost is no barrier; adhere less often to treatment regimens; learn and understand less about how to protect their health; seek less preventive care, even when free; and less often practice the healthy behaviors so important for preventing or slowing the progression of chronic diseases, the major killers and disablers in developed nations.

Good health depends as much today on preventing as on ameliorating illness, injury, and disability. Preventing chronic disease is arguably no less cognitive a process than preventing accidents, the fourth leading cause of death in the United States behind cancer, heart disease, and stroke. As described elsewhere (Gottfredson, 2004), preventing both illness and accidents requires anticipating the unexpected and "driving defensively," in a well-informed way, through life.

> Their cognitive demands are comparable—remain vigilant for hazards and recognize them when present; remove or evade them in a timely manner; contain incidents to prevent damage or limit it if begun; and modify behavior and environments to prevent reoccurrence. Health workers can diagnose and treat incubating problems, such as high blood pressure or diabetes, but only when people seek preventive screening and follow treatment regimens. Many do not. Perhaps a third of all prescriptions are taken in a manner that jeopardizes the patient's health. Non-adherence to prescribed treatment regimens doubles the relative risk of death among heart patients. For better or worse, we are largely our own primary healthcare providers.

> *Gottfredson & Deary (2004)*

Family effects theory and passive learning theory work no better in health matters than in education. Just as equal access to healthcare tends to increase class differences in health, greater access to health information results in larger knowledge gaps between groups. Infusing more knowledge into the public sphere about health risks (smoking) and new diagnostic options (Pap smears) results in already informed persons learning the most and more often acting on the new information. This may explain why an SES-mortality gradient favoring educated women was developed for cervical cancer after Pap smears became available.

Lower-IQ individuals extract less benefit from the same resources than do brighter individuals. Providing them with equal resources does not change that. Hospitals are now making an effort to render information more cognitively accessible to patients, if only to avoid lawsuits from aggrieved patients who did not understand that to which they were consenting. Both curative and preventive care might be more effective if healthcare providers recognized and more effectively accommodated the great diversity in cognitive competence among patients. There is much of practical value they could learn from the vast nomological network of knowledge about *g*.

Unfortunately, the health sciences and medicine are also in the grip of right thinking about human diversity. After it became clear that health inequalities could not be explained by inequalities in material resources and access to healthcare, it became fashionable in health epidemiology to blame class and race differences in health on the psychic damage done by social inequality. We are now to believe that social inequality per se is literally a killer (Wilkinson, 1996). Physicians, like teachers, are increasingly being accused of racism and given sensitivity training when they fail to produce racial parity in outcomes (Satel, 2000). Mindful of ideologically correct thought, health literacy researchers who mention intelligence do so only to reject out of hand the notion that literacy might reflect intelligence, because any such notion would be racist and demeaning.

In the meantime, inadequate learning and reasoning abilities put many people at risk for taking medications in health-damaging ways, failing to grasp the merits of preventive precautions against chronic disease and accidents, and failing to properly implement potentially more effective but complex new treatment regimens for heart disease, hypertension, and other killers. To intentionally ignore differences in mental competence is unconscionable. It is social science malpractice against the very people whom the "untruth" is supposedly meant to protect.

REFERENCES

Baldwin, J., Kirsch, I.S., Rock, D., & Yamamoto, K. (1995). *The Literacy Proficiencies of GED Examinees: Results from the GED-NALS Comparison Study*. Washington, DC: American Council on Education and Educational Testing.

Banchero, S. & Little, D. (2002, November 13). "Minorities score poorly even at high scoring schools." *Chicago Tribune.*

Blits, J.H. & Gottfredson, L.S. (1990a). Employment testing and job performance. *The Public Interest*, Winter, No. 98, 18–25.

Blits, J.H. & Gottfredson, L.S. (1990b). Equality or lasting inequality? *Society, 27*(3), 4–11.

Block, N.H. & Dworkin, G. (1974). IQ, heritability, and inequality. *Philosophy and Public Affairs, 4*, 40–99.

Bouchard, T.J., Jr. (1998). Intensive, detailed, exhaustive. *Intelligence, 26*(3), 283–290.

Bowles, S. & Gintis, H. (1972/1973). IQ in the U.S. class structure. *Social Policy, 3*(4 & 5), 65–96.

Brody, N. (1992). *Intelligence* (2d ed.). San Diego, CA: Academic.

Brody, N. (1998). Jensen and intelligence. *Intelligence, 26*(3), 243–247.

Brody, N. (2003a). Construct validation of the Sternberg Triarchic Abilities Test (STAT): Comment and reanalysis. *Intelligence, 31*, 319–329.

Brody, N. (2003b). What Sternberg should have concluded. *Intelligence, 31*, 339–342.

Carroll, J.B. (1993). *Human Cognitive Abilities: A Survey of Factor-Analytic Studies*. New York: Cambridge University Press.

Coleman, J.S. (1990–1991). The Sidney Hook Memorial Award Address: On the self-suppression of academic freedom. *Academic Questions, 4*, 17–22.

College Board (1999). *Reaching the Top: A Report of the National Task Force on Minority High Achievement*. New York: College Board Publications.

Courtois, S. (1999). Introduction: The crimes of Communism. In S. Courtois, N. Werth, J-L. Panné, A. Paczkowski, K. Bartošek, J-L. Margolin, & M. Malia (Eds.), *The Black Book of Communism: Crimes, Terror, Repression* (pp. 1–31). Cambridge, MA: Harvard University Press.

Crenshaw, K., Gotanda, N., Peller, G., & Thomas, K. (1995). *Critical Race Theory: The Key Writings That Formed the Movement.* New York: New Press.

Deary, I.J. & Crawford, J.R. (1998). A triarchic theory of Jensenism: Persistent, conservative reductionism. *Intelligence, 26*(3), 273–282.

Deary, I.J., Whiteman, M.C., Starr, J.M., Whalley, L.J., & Fox, H.C. (2004). The impact of childhood intelligence on later life: Following up the Scottish Mental Surveys of 1932 and 1947. *Journal of Personality and Social Psychology, 44*, 217–231.

Detterman, D.K. (1998). Kings of men: Introduction to a special issue. *Intelligence, 26*(3), 175–180.

Dittman, M. (2002, July/August). Study ranks the top 20th century psychologists. *APA Monitor*, 28–29.

Eysenck, HJ. (1971). *Race, Intelligence, and Education.* London: Maurice Temple Smith [American title *The IQ Argument*. New York: Library Press].

Farber, D.A. & Sherry, S. (1997). *Beyond All Reason: The Radical Assault on Truth in American Law.* New York: Oxford.

Gardner, H. (1983). *Frames of Mind: The Theory of Multiple Intelligences.* New York: Basic.

Gardner, H. (1998). A multiplicity of intelligences. *Scientific American Presents, 9*(4), 18–23.

Glazer, N. (1994). The lying game. *The New Republic*, October 31, 15–16.

Gordon, R.A. (1997). Everyday life as an intelligence test: Effects of intelligence and intelligence context. *Intelligence, 24*(1), 203–320.

Gottfredson, L.S. (1986). Societal consequences of the g factor in employment. *Journal of Vocational Behavior, 29*, 379–410.

Gottfredson, L.S. (1990, December 6). When job-testing "fairness" is nothing but a quota. *Wall Street Journal*, p. A18.

Gottfredson, L.S. (1994a). Egalitarian fiction and collective fraud. *Society, 31*(3), 53–59.

Gottfredson, L.S. (1994b). The science and politics of race-norming. *American Psychologist, 49*(11), 955–963.

Gottfredson, L.S. (1996a, October 24). Racially gerrymandered police tests. *Wall Street Journal*, p. A16.

Gottfredson, L.S. (1996b). Racially gerrymandering the content of police tests to satisfy the U.S. Justice Department: A case study. *Psychology, Public Policy, and Law, 2*(3/4), 418–446.

Gottfredson, L.S. (1996c). The new challenge to academic freedom. *Journal of Homelessness and Social Distress, 5*, 205–212.

Gottfredson, L.S. (1997a). Mainstream science on intelligence: An editorial with 52 signatories, history, and bibliography. *Intelligence, 24*(1), 13–23.

Gottfredson, L.S. (1997b). Why g matters: The complexity of everyday life. *Intelligence, 24*(1), 79–132.

Gottfredson, L.S. (1998). Jensen, Jensenism, and the sociology of intelligence. *Intelligence, 26*(3), 291–299.

Gottfredson, L.S. (2002a). g: Highly general and highly practical. In R.J. Sternberg & E.L. Grigorenko (Eds.), *The General Factor of Intelligence: How General Is It?* (pp. 331–380). Mahwah, NJ: Erlbaum.

Gottfredson, L.S. (2002b). Where and why g matters: Not a mystery. *Human Performance, 15*(1/2), 25–46.

Gottfredson, L.S. (2003a). Dissecting practical intelligence theory: Its claims and evidence. *Intelligence, 31*, 343–397.

Gottfredson, L.S. (2003b). Implications of cognitive differences for schooling within diverse societies. Manuscript submitted for review.

Gottfredson, L.S. (2003c). On Sternberg's "Reply to Gottfredson." *Intelligence, 31,* 415–423.

Gottfredson, L.S. (2003d). What if the hereditarian hypothesis is true? University of Delaware, manuscript submitted for review. Intelligence, 32, 225–232.

Gottfredson, L.S. (2004). Intelligence: Is it the epidemiologists' elusive "fundamental cause" of social class inequalities in health? *Journal of Personality and Social Psychology, 44,* 615–629.

Gottfredson, L.S. & Deary, I.J. (2004). Intelligence predicts health and longevity, but why? *Current Directions in Psychological Science, 14,* 117–129.

Hakel, M.D. (1997). Highlights of SIOP's twelfth annual conference. *TIP: The Industrial Organizational Psychologist, 35*(1), 114–118.

Hartigan, J.A. & Wigdor, A.K. (Eds.) (1989). *Fairness in Employment Testing: Validity Generalization, Minority Issues, and the General Aptitude Test Battery.* Washington, DC: National Academy Press.

Herrnstein, R.J. (1971, September). I.Q. *The Atlantic Monthly,* pp. 43–64.

Herrnstein, R.J. (1973). *I.Q. in the Meritocracy.* New York: Little, Brown.

Herrnstein, R.J. & Murray, C. (1994) *The Bell Curve: Intelligence and Class Structure in American Life.* New York: Free Press.

Humphreys, L.G. (1989, July 7). "Fairness in employment testing" [Letter to the editor]. *Science,* p. 14.

Humphreys, L.G. (1991). Limited vision in the social sciences. *American Journal of Psychology, 104*(3), 333–353.

Hunt, E. (2001). Multiple views of multiple intelligence *[review of Intelligence reframed: Multiple intelligence in the 21st century], Contemporary Psychology, 46*(1), 5–7.

Hunt, M. (1999). *The New Know-Nothings: The Political Foes of the Scientific Study of Human Nature.* New Brunswick, NJ: Transaction.

Jaynes, G.D. & Williams, R.J., Jr. (Eds.) (1989). *A Common Destiny: Blacks and American Society.* Washington, DC: National Academy Press.

Jensen, A.R. (1969). How much can we boost I.Q. and scholastic achievement? *Harvard Educational Review, 39,* 1–123.

Jensen, A.R. (1972). *Genetics and Education.* New York: Harper & Row.

Jensen, A.R. (1980). *Bias in Mental Testing.* New York: Free Press.

Jensen, A.R. (1983). Taboo, constraint, and responsibility in educational research. *Journal of Social, Political, and Economic Studies, 8,* 301–311.

Jensen, A.R. (1998). *The g Factor: The Science of Mental Ability.* Westport, CT: Praeger.

Kaufman, A.S. (1998). A new twist on Jensenism. *Intelligence, 26*(3), 249–253.

Kirsch, I.S., Jungeblut, A., Jenkins, L., & Kolstad, A. (1993). *Adult Literacy in America: A First Look at the Results of the National Adult Literacy Survey.* Washington, DC: National Center for Education Statistics.

Kline, P. (1991). Sternberg's components: Non-contingent concepts. *Personality and Individual Differences, 12*(9), 873–876.

Kors, A.C. & Silverglate, H.A. (1998). *The Shadow University: The Betrayal of Liberty on America's Campuses.* New York: Free Press.

Laurance, J. (1997, August 16). Award withheld for psychologist accused of racism. *The Independent (London),* International Section, p. 11.

Lee, F.R. (2002, November 30). Why are black students lagging? *New York Times.*

Loehlin, J.C. (1992). Should we do research on race differences in intelligence? *Intelligence, 16*(1), 1–4.

Lubinski, D. & Benbow, C.P. (1995). An opportunity for empiricism: Review of Howard Gardner's *Multiple Intelligences: The Theory in Practice. Contemporary Psychology, 40,* 935–938.

Lubinski, D. & Humphreys, L.G. (1997). Incorporating general intelligence into epidemiology and the social sciences. *Intelligence, 24*(1), 159–201.

Lynn, R. (2001). *The Science of Human Diversity: A History of the Pioneer Fund.* New York: University Press of America.

Messick, S. (1992). Multiple intelligences or multilevel intelligence? Selective emphasis on distinctive properties of hierarchy: On Gardner's *Frames of Mind* and Sternberg's *Beyond IQ* in the context of theory and research on the structure of human abilities. *Psychological Inquiry, 3*, 365–384.

National Center for Education Statistics (2000, August). Results over time—NAEP 1999 long-term trend summary data tables. <http://nces.ed.gov/nationsreportcard/tables/Ltt1999/> (accessed July 6, 2003).

Neisser, U., Boodoo, G., Bouchard, T.J., Jr., Boykin, A.W., Brody, N., Ceci, S.J., Halpern, D.F., Loehlin, J.C., Perloff, R., Sternberg, R.J., & Urbina, S. (1996). Intelligence: Knowns and unknowns. *American Psychologist, 51*, 77–101.

Nettlebeck, T. (1998). Jensen's chronometric research: Neither simple nor sufficient but a good place to start. *Intelligence, 26*(3), 233–241.

Noguera, P. (2001). Racial politics and the elusive quest for excellence and equity in education. *In Motion Magazine.* http://www.inmotionmagazine.com/er/pnrp1.html.

Nyborg, H. (2003). The sociology of psychometric and bio-behavioral sciences: A case study of destructive social reductionism and collective fraud in 20th century academia. In H. Nyborg (Ed.), *The Scientific Study of General Intelligence: Tribute to Arthur R. Jensen* (pp. 77–79). New York: Pergamon.

Ogbu, J.U. (2003). *Black American Students in an Affluent Suburb.* Mahwah, NJ: Erlbaum.

O'Toole, B.J. (1990). Intelligence and behavior and motor vehicle accident mortality. *Accident Analysis and Prevention, 22*, 211–221.

O'Toole, B.I. & Stankov, L. (1992). Ultimate validity of psychological tests. *Personality and Individual Differences, 13*, 699–716.

Page, E.B. (1972). Behavior and heredity. *American Psychologist*, pp. 660–661.

Plomin, R., DeFries, J.C., McClearn, G.E, & McGuffin, P. (2001). *Behavioral Genetics* (4th ed.). New York: Worth and W.H. Freeman.

Rowe, D.C. (1997). A place at the policy table? Behavior genetics and estimates of family environmental effects on IQ. *Intelligence, 24*(1), 53–77.

Rowe, D.C., Vesterdal, W.J., & Rodgers, J. L. (1998). Herrnstein's syllogism: Genetic and shared environmental influences on IQ, education, and income. *Intelligence, 26*, 405–423.

Rushton, J.P. (1994). The egalitarian dogma revisited. *Intelligence, 19*(3), 263–280.

Rushton, J.P. (1998). The "Jensen Effect" and the "Spearman–Jensen Hypothesis" of black–white IQ differences. *Intelligence, 26*(3), 217–225.

Sackett, P.R., Schmitt, N., Ellingson, J.E., & Kabin, M.B. (2001). High-stakes testing in employment, credentialing, and higher education: Prospects in a post-affirmative-action world. *American Psychologist, 56*(4), 302–318.

Sackett, P.R. & Wilk, S.L. (1994). Within-group norming and other forms of score adjustment in preemployment testing. *American Psychologist, 49*(11), 929–954.

Satel, S. (2000). *PC, M.D.: How Political Correctness Is Corrupting Medicine.* New York: Basic.

Scarr, S. (1997). Behavior-genetic and socialization theories of intelligence: Truce and reconciliation. In R.J. Sternberg & E.L. Grigorenko (Eds.), *Intelligence, Heredity, and Environment* (pp. 3–41). New York: Cambridge University Press.

Scarr, S. (1998). On Arthur Jensen's integrity. *Intelligence, 26*(3), 227–232.

Schmidt, F.L. (1996, December 10). "New police test will be a disaster" [Letter to the editor]. *The Wall Street Journal*, p. A23.

Schmidt, F.L. & Hunter, J.E. (1998). The validity and utility of selection methods in personnel psychology: Practical and theoretical implications of 85 years of research findings. *Psychological Bulletin, 124*(2), 262–274.

Schmitt, N., Rogers, W., Chan, D. Sheppard, L., & Jennings, D. (1997). Adverse impact and predictive efficiency of various predictor combinations. *Journal of Applied Psychology, 82*, 719–730.

Science and pseudoscience. (1999, July/August). *APS Observer*, p. 27.

Sharf, J.C. (1988). Litigating personnel measurement policy. *Journal of Vocational Behavior, 33*, 235–271.

Snow, R.E. (1996). Aptitude development and education. *Psychology, Public Policy, and Law, 2*(3/4), 536–560.

Snyderman, M. & Rothman, S. (1988). *The IQ Controversy, the Media and Public Policy*. New Brunswick, NJ: Transaction.

Sternberg, R.J. (1997). *Successful Intelligence: How Practical and Creative Intelligence Determines Success in Life*. New York: Plume.

Sternberg, R.J. (1998). Costs and benefits of defying the crowd in science. *Intelligence, 26*(3), 209–215.

Sternberg, R.J. (2000). Human intelligence: A case study of how more and more research can lead us to know less and less about a psychological phenomenon, until finally we know much less than we did before we started doing research. In E. Tulving (Ed.), *Memory, Consciousness, and the Brain: The Tallinn Conference* (pp. 363–373). Philadelphia: Taylor & Francis, Psychology Group.

Sternberg, R.J. (2003). "My house is a very very very fine house"—but it is not the only house. In H. Nyborg (Ed.), *The Scientific Study of General Intelligence: Tribute to Arthur R. Jensen* (pp. 77–79). New York: Pergamon.

Sternberg, R.J. & Wagner, R.K. (1993). The g-ocentric view of intelligence and job performance is wrong. *Current Directions in Psychological Science, 2*(1), 1–5.

Sternberg, R.J., Forsythe, G.B., Hedlund, J., Horvath, J.A., Wagner, R.K., Williams, W.M., Snook, S.A., & Grigorenko, A.L. (2000). *Practical Intelligence in Everyday Life*. New York: Cambridge University Press.

Taylor, M.D., Frier, B.M., Gold, A.E., & Deary, I.J. (2004). Psychosocial factors and diabetes-related outcomes following diagnosis of Type 1 diabetes. *Diabetic Medicine, 20*, 135–146.

Vernon, P.A. (1998). From the cognitive to the biological: A sketch of Arthur Jensen's contributions to the study of g. *Intelligence, 26*(3), 267–271.

Wigdor, A.K. & Garner, W.R. (Eds.) (1982). *Ability Testing: Uses, Consequences, and Controversies. Part I: Report of the Committee*. Washington, DC: National Academy Press.

Wilkinson, R. (1996). *Unhealthy Societies: The Afflictions of Inequality*. London: Routledge.

Wolf, E.P. (1972). Civil rights and social science data. *Race, 14*(2), 155–182.

10

PSEUDOSCIENCE, NONSCIENCE, AND NONSENSE IN CLINICAL PSYCHOLOGY: DANGERS AND REMEDIES

Scott O. Lilienfeld, Katherine A. Fowler, Jeffrey M. Lohr, and Steven Jay Lynn

Mental health practices can be bad for your mental health. As counter-intuitive as this conclusion may appear, it has been borne out by a substantial body of research over the past two decades. Although meta-analyses have demonstrated that psychotherapy tends on balance to be helpful (Smith, Glass, & Miller, 1980; Wampold, Mondin, Moody, Stich, Benson, & Ahn, 1997), there is persuasive evidence that certain forms of psychotherapy can be harmful. Moreover, the literature on "deterioration effects" suggests that perhaps three to six percent of clients tend to become worse in response to psychotherapy (Strupp, Hadley, Gomez, & Schwartz, 1978).

Our central thesis is that the field of clinical psychology has for too long neglected a problem that now has come home to roost: the burgeoning industry of pseudoscientific and unscientific psychotherapies (Eisner, 2000; Singer & Lalich, 1996). As a consequence, clinical psychology has placed those who rely on the mental health field at needless risk. As psychologist Richard Gist reminds us, the noble imperative to do something is not a license to do anything. The "almost-anything-goes" attitude, increasingly prevalent in large pockets of the clinical community, must come to an end.

THE ALLURE OF PSEUDOSCIENTIFIC AND UNSCIENTIFIC CLAIMS

Pseudoscientific and unscientific claims hold an understandable allure for practitioners and the general public. Many fringe therapeutic techniques promise quick fixes or overnight cures for longstanding psychological conditions. For example, the developer of Thought Field Therapy, a technique that purportedly cures anxiety disorders by manipulating clients' "energy fields" (which have never been shown to exist), claims to be able to treat phobias in as little as five minutes (Callahan, 1995, 2001). Needless to say, there is no research evidence for this extraordinary assertion.

Many of these techniques also feature numerous bells and whistles that provide them with the superficial veneer of science. For example, the proponents of Eye Movement Desensitization and Reprocessing (EMDR), another technique that has been marketed widely as a "break-through" treatment for anxiety disorders (Shapiro, 1995; Shapiro & Forrest, 1997), claim that lateral eye movements facilitate processing of traumatic memories. Yet meta-analyses suggest that the eye movements play no role in the efficacy of EMDR, which appears to be no more effective than standard treatments that rely on exposing clients to anxiety-provoking imagery (Davidson & Parker, 2001; Lohr, Tolin, & Lilienfield, 1998).

Adding to the allure of these techniques is that they are marketed by highly persuasive, energetic, and even charismatic leaders, some of whom have attained "guru" status among their followers. The preeminent status of these leaders may render their acolytes unlikely to question their confident proclamations, which offer the promise of virtually certain cures. In contrast, the scientific method is inherently uncertain, with its tentative conclusions open to revision. Some practitioners and mental health consumers may therefore turn to fringe therapies in the hope of obtaining definitive answers for intractable psychological conditions.

What is pseudoscience and how does it differ from science? Although a precise definition of pseudoscience is virtually impossible, pseudoscientific claims tend to share a set of loosely correlated features. Although none of these features is necessary or sufficient to qualify a claim as pseudoscientific, the greater their number the more suspect a claim becomes (Herbert et al., 2000; Lilienfeld, 1998). In aggregate, these features constitute helpful "warning signs" to practitioners and the general public.

Among the principal features of pseudoscientific claims are: (a) overuse of ad hoc hypotheses (escape hatches or loopholes) to immunize assertions from falsification; (b) absence of self-correction; (c) evasion of peer review; (d) emphasis on confirmation at the expense of refutation; (e) reversed burden of proof, that is, placing the burden of proof on skeptics rather than on proponents of assertions; (f) absence of "connectivity," that is, failure to build on extant scientific knowledge; (g) overreliance on testimonial and anecdotal evidence; (h) use of obscure or seemingly scientific language to provide claims with the superficial trappings of science, and (i) absence of boundary conditions, that is, a failure to delimit situations under which the claim does not hold (see Bunge, 1984; Lilienfeld, 1998; Lilienfeld, Lynn, & Lohr, 2003; Ruscio, 2001; Stanovich, 2001, for further discussions).

Pseudoscientific claims fulfill most or all of the aforementioned criteria. Unscientific claims, although lacking most of the aforementioned criteria, are largely devoid of research support. Both claims are hazardous, however, pseudoscientific claims are typically more problematic because they possess the superficial trappings of science.

Importance of Open-Minded Skepticism

Before discussing the hazards posed by pseudoscientific and unscientific claims, it is crucial to emphasize that untested clinical interventions may eventually be demonstrated to be efficacious. It would be a serious error to dismiss newly developed procedures out of hand or prior to scientific investigation. Such closed-mindedness has sometimes characterized debates concerning the efficacy of novel psychotherapies (Beutler & Harwood, 2001). Nevertheless, a key tenet of science is that the burden of proof always falls squarely on the claimant, not on the skeptic (Shermer, 1997). A reversed burden of proof, in which the skeptic must show why the claim has little or no merit, has often characterized the proponents of pseudoscientific research programs (Lilienfeld et al., 2003).

Scientific inquiry necessitates a unique blend of open-mindedness and penetrating skepticism (Sagan, 1995; Shermer, 2001). Clinical psychology training programs should inculcate this attitude of open-minded skepticism in their students. Good clinical scientists must constantly walk an epistemic tightrope. They must remain open to novel and untested claims regardless of how implausible they may appear. At the same time, they must subject such claims to incisive scrutiny by designing and conducting rigorous scientific tests. Space engineer James Oberg offered the sage advice, which we term "Oberg's dictum," that keeping an open mind is a virtue, but one's mind should not be so open that one's brains fall out (see Sagan, 1995). Although high standards apply to all domains of scientific inquiry, they are especially crucial in applied areas such as clinical psychology, psychiatry, and social work, in which untested therapeutic practices have the potential to produce harm.

Dangers Posed by Unsubstantiated Mental Health Practices

Some clinical psychologists assume that virtually all mental health practices are helpful, or at worst innocuous. This is not the case. There are several ways in which unsubstantiated mental health practices can cause harm (Beyerstein, 2001; Lilienfeld, 2002b). Some therapies are by themselves iatrogenic. These interventions violate the first canon of the helping professions: *primum non nocere* (first do no harm), often regarded as the gist of the Hippocratic Oath. Although inherently harmful therapies are a major focus of this chapter, we would be remiss not to mention at least three ways in which unvalidated therapies can cause indirect harm.

First, even innocuous practices can produce harm indirectly by depriving individuals of scarce time, financial resources, or both. Economists refer to this side effect as "opportunity cost." Opportunity cost may leave individuals who would otherwise use their time and money to seek out demonstrably efficacious treatments with precious little of either, rendering them less likely to obtain clinical services that could prove beneficial.

Second, the promulgation of dubious assessment and treatment services can undermine the public's faith in the profession of clinical psychology. This can lead the public to place less trust in the assertions of practitioners and clinical researchers, making them less likely to turn to clinical psychologists for needed help and advice.

Third, and perhaps least tangible, is that the promotion and application of unsubstantiated clinical services eat away at the scientific foundations of clinical psychology (Lilienfeld, 1998; McFall, 1991). This erosion of the underpinnings of clinical science may have dire long-term consequences for the profession. As Lilienfeld (2002a) observed:

> Once we abdicate our responsibility to uphold scientific standards in administering treatments, our scientific credibility and

influence are badly damaged. Moreover, by continuing to ignore the imminent dangers posed by questionable mental health techniques, we send an implicit message to our students that we are not deeply committed to anchoring our discipline in scientific evidence or to combating potentially unscientific practices. Our students will most likely follow in our footsteps and continue to turn a blind eye to the widening gap between scientist and practitioner, and between research evidence and clinical work (p. 9).

THE SCIENTIST–PRACTITIONER GAP

The past several decades have witnessed a virtual sea of change in the relation of scientific psychology to professional practice. A disturbingly large number of clinicians base their treatment and assessment practices primarily on clinical experience and intuition rather than on research evidence. As a consequence, an increasing number of critics have argued that the scientist–practitioner gap (e.g., Fox, 1996) poses a grave threat to the scientific foundations of clinical psychology (Dawes, 1994; Kalal, 1999; McFall, 1991; Tavris, 2003a,b).

Admittedly, the problem of unsubstantiated services has dogged clinical psychology virtually since its inception (see Dolnick, 1998). Nevertheless, there is reason to believe that this problem is becoming increasingly acute. Until relatively recently, unvalidated psychotherapies remained safely on the fringes, with little risk of their entering the scientific mainstream. However, recently edited volumes (Shannon, 2002; Corsini, 2001) feature largely or entirely unsubstantiated psychological techniques, including music therapy, aromatherapy, homeopathy, breath work, therapeutic touch, medical intuition, acupuncture, and body-centered psychotherapies. In most chapters these techniques receive minimal critical scrutiny.

There are troubling indications that the problem of unscientific treatments has intensified. For example, a survey by Goisman, Warshaw, and Keller (1999) revealed that the proportion of patients with anxiety disorders who received either behavioral or cognitive-behavioral therapies—interventions found to be efficacious for such conditions—actually declined slightly from 1991 to 1996. This decline is ironic in view of the increasing evidence for the efficacy of these therapies during that time period. Goisman and colleagues further found that anxiety-disordered clients most frequently received psychodynamic therapies, which have not been shown to be effective in the treatment of anxiety disorders.

Two other published surveys (Polusny & Folette, 1996; Poole, Lindsay, Memon, & Bull, 1995) indicate that approximately twenty-five percent of American and Canadian doctoral-level psychotherapists made regular use of suggestive methods such as hypnosis, guided imagery, dream interpretation, free association to childhood memories, journaling, interpretation of ambiguous symptoms, and body work (i.e., a focus on physical sensations), to recover purported memories of child sexual abuse. Nevertheless, research strongly suggests that these and other suggestive techniques that include "truth serum" (a barbiturate that is not in fact a truth serum; Piper, 1993) and "trance writing" (penning reports of abuse while in an apparent trance state) place clients at considerably elevated risk for false memories of abuse (see Lynn, Lock, et al., 2003).

Published surveys also reveal that upwards of one-third of mental health professionals who assess children suspected of having been sexually abused use anatomically detailed dolls (ADDs) to detect such abuse (Davey & Hill, 1999; see Hunsley, Lee, & Wood, 2003, for a review). Yet controlled studies suggest that ADDs are of doubtful validity for detecting child sexual abuse. Even those who believe that ADDs do have some validity agree that they have high false-positive rates, especially among African-American children (Hunsley et al., 2003; Koocher et al., 1995; Wolfner, Faust, & Dawes, 1993). Moreover, ADDs suffer from serious psychometric shortcomings, including inadequate standardization of administration and a virtual absence of norms (Hunsley et al., 2003).

In addition, surveys show that approximately forty percent of doctoral-level clinical psychologists frequently or always administer the Rorschach Inkblot Test and human figure drawings in their assessment batteries, whereas approximately twice that number administer these methods at least occasionally (e.g., Watkins, Campbell, Nieberding, & Hallmark, 1995). Yet these methods have repeatedly been found to be of questionable validity for the substantial majority of clinical uses to which they are put (Hunsley, et al., 2003; Lilienfeld, Wood, & Garb, 2000; Wood, Nezworski, Lilienfeld, & Garb, 2003; see Hibbard, 2003, for a dissenting view).

A variety of influences have conspired to sustain and perhaps widen the already substantial gulf between researchers and practitioners. We focus on two: the substantial proportion of clinical training programs that do not sufficiently emphasize scientific training (Beyerstein, 2001; Lilienfeld, 2002a) and the increasing infusion of postmodern thinking into clinical psychology.

Scientific Training

The problems posed by the paucity of scientific training in numerous clinical Ph.D. and Psy.D. programs have been discussed elsewhere (e.g., Dawes, 1994; Grove, 2000; Lilienfeld et al., 2003; Wright & Cummings, 2000) and are not reiterated in detail here. Suffice it to say that large numbers of students who graduate from these programs appear to lack adequate training in the fundamentals of clinical psychology (e.g., psychometrics, clinical judgment and prediction, methods for disentangling genetic from environmental influences on behavior, applied behavior analysis, personality trait psychology, philosophy of science), although good quantitative data on this topic is sparse.

The authors of this chapter have encountered a Ph.D. clinical psychologist who confessed to being entirely unfamiliar with the classic work of Chapman and Chapman (1967) on illusory correlation despite using projective techniques regularly in his clinical practice, as well as a recent graduate of a Canadian Ph.D. clinical program who had never heard of Paul Meehl, probably the foremost clinical psychologist of the latter half of the twentieth century. Then again, having heard of Meehl provides no guarantee of understanding him. One advanced graduate student in an APA-accredited clinical program asserted confidently that Meehl had settled the clinical–actuarial debate in the 1950s by demonstrating that clinical prediction was almost always superior to actuarial prediction (see Meehl, 1954, and Grove, Zald, et al., 2000, for evidence that actuarial prediction is almost always equal or superior to clinical prediction).

Unfamiliarity with the clinical–actuarial issue is not unusual. In a survey of members of APA's Division 12 (Clinical Psychology), Grove and Lloyd (in preparation) found that thirteen percent of respondents indicated that they had only heard of actuarial prediction methods but were not even moderately acquainted with them. More remarkable, three percent had never heard of actuarial decision-making methods, and a disturbing twenty-two percent believed that actuarial prediction methods tended to be inferior to clinical prediction methods.

Although this lack of knowledge surely has multiple sources, at least some of the blame must be laid on clinical training programs. We ruefully concur with Grove and Meehl (1996), who maintained that:

> In the majority of clinical training programs in clinical psychology… no great value is placed on the cultivation of skeptical, scientific habits of thought; the role models—even in the academy, but more so in the clinical settings—are often

people who do not put a high value on scientific thinking, are not themselves engaged in scientific research, and take it for granted that clinical experience is sufficient to prove whatever they want to believe. There are probably not more than two dozen American psychology departments whose clinical training programs strongly emphasize the need for scientific proof, either as experiments or statistical study of file data, as the only firm foundation for knowledge (p. 318).

Postmodernism

Recent decades have witnessed the increasing influence of an alternative model of clinical knowledge (Kvale, 1992; Tsoi-Hoshmand & Polkinghorne, 1992) based not on scientific research but on postmodern knowledge and theoretical deconstructionism. Indeed, the *American Psychologist*, the flagship journal of the APA, has featured numerous articles on postmodernism over the past fifteen years.

The central tenets of postmodernism include the propositions that (a) all knowledge is contextual and therefore relative, and (b) science represents only one "mode of discourse" among many, and scientific claims to knowledge are no more privileged than alternative claims (e.g., assertions based on intuition or personal experience). Thus, postmodern thought lends itself in many cases to a willingness to accept claims on the basis of subjective convictions rather than scientific research (see Gross & Levitt, 1994). Some postmodern thinkers have even suggested that psychotherapeutic procedures should be based as much on "validation through practice" (Kvale, 1992)—a tacit learning of what works by means of experience—as on research findings derived from controlled outcome studies (see also Schon, 1983). For example, Tsoi-Hoshmand and Polkinghorne (1992) argued that clinical reflection and intuition should be on a par with scientific knowledge in the training of psychotherapists.

Such discussions contain virtually no mention of the factors (e.g., absence of immediate and consistent feedback) that often prevent psychotherapists from learning from experience, or of the numerous social cognitive errors (e.g., selective recall, availability bias, confirmation bias, hindsight bias, illusory correlation) that tend to create an illusion of such learning in its absence (Dawes, 1994; Dawes, Faust, & Meehl, 1989; Garb, 1998). If the history of science has taught us anything, it is that intuition, although often immensely useful in the "context of discovery" (i.e., hypothesis generation), tends to be ill-suited in the "context of justification" (i.e., hypothesis testing; Reichenbach, 1938; see also Myers, 2002, for a superb discussion of the strengths and weaknesses of clinical intuition).

The history of medicine provides a case in point. Most medical historians agree that prior to 1890 virtually widespread medical treatments such as bleeding, purging, and blistering—all derived from a mixture of intuition and informal clinical experience—were either useless or harmful (Grove & Meehl, 1996). Similarly, for several decades of the twentieth century, prefrontal lobotomy was accepted by many mental health professionals as an efficacious procedure primarily on the basis of subjective observation and clinical judgment. One physician who performed lobotomies stated, "I am a sensitive observer, and my conclusion is that a vast majority of my patients get better as opposed to worse after my treatment" (Dawes, 1994, p. 48). This quotation reminds us that informal clinical observations, although potentially helpful in generating fruitful hypotheses, should rarely, if ever, be the final arbiter of treatment efficacy.

SELF-HELP OR SELF-HARM?

In addition to the scientist–practitioner gap, a second major threat to the scientific foundations of clinical psychology—and the mental health of the public—stems from the thriving self-help industry, which produces hundreds of new books, manuals, and audiotapes each year (Rosen, Glasgow, & Moore, 2003). In most major bookstores, the psychology sections are either dwarfed by the size of the self-help and recovery sections (Lilienfeld, 1998) or actually consist almost entirely of self-help books. Rosen (1987) estimated the number of self-help books per year at 2000.

Many self-help books promise rapid or simplistic solutions to complex life problems. Although meta-analyses demonstrate that some self-help materials, particularly those based on sound scientific principles, are efficacious (Gould & Clum, 1993), the overwhelming majority of such material has not been subjected to empirical scrutiny. Indeed, Norcross et al. (2000) estimate that ninety-five percent of such books have no basis in research. This is deeply troubling given that many self-help books have been immense commercial successes. For example, *The Courage to Heal* (Bass & Davis, 1988), a self-help book intended to assist women recovering from the trauma of early abuse, has sold more than 700,000 copies. Incidentally, in its first edition, this book informed readers that "If you think you were abused and your life shows the symptoms, then you probably were" (p. 22).

There is evidence that certain self-help programs are less beneficial than comparable therapist-directed programs, and that some may even be harmful. For example, Matson and Ollendick (1977) found that one in five mothers who used a self-help manual (Azrin & Foxx, 1974) toilet-trained their children successfully. In contrast, four of five mothers in a therapist-led condition did so. Moreover, in the former condition, unsuccessful toilet training was associated with increases in childhood behavior problems and negative mother–child interactions (see Rosen et al., 2003). Zeiss (1978) similarly reported that none of six couples enrolled in a self-help program designed to treat premature ejaculation completed this program.

The self-help industry is not limited to the print media. The past two decades have witnessed a growing cadre of self-help "experts" on talk shows ("psychotainment;" Marano, 1997). It's fair to say that these "experts" are a mixed bag. A few provide reasonably sound wisdom concerning everyday life problems, but many others offer advice of questionable scientific validity (Heaton & Wilson, 1995; Wilson, 2003). For example, the enormously popular self-help guru Tony Robbins informs listeners that he can "cure any psychological problem in a session" and "make someone fall in love with you in 5 minutes" (Griffin & Goldsmith, 1985, p. 41). He has also claimed to revive brain-dead people and allow women to experience orgasms without being touched (Wilson, 2003). As of this writing, these claims still await scientific confirmation.

Potentially Harmful Treatments

There is increasing evidence that some psychological treatments are in themselves harmful. To our knowledge, however, no published source has attempted to compile a list of treatments that have been found to be potentially harmful either to clients or their family members, a void we now attempt to fill.

Attachment Therapies Rebirthing, a controversial treatment for child behavior problems, found its way into the national news under tragic circumstances. In 2000, Candace Newmaker, a ten-year-old girl undergoing treatment at the behest of her adoptive mother, was asphyxiated during a rebirthing session. Rebirthing is one treatment in a class of therapies employed by self-proclaimed "attachment therapists," a group that operates on the principle that children whose behavior does not meet the expectations of their new caretakers have not formed proper attachments. Many, if not most, attachment therapists are not licensed psychologists, and some do not even have advanced degrees in a related discipline.

Rebirthing involves wrapping the child tightly in a blanket in an effort to simulate the birth canal. Adult therapists exert pressure on the tightly wrapped child to simulate the experience of labor contractions, while the child attempts to squeeze her way out. The rationale rests on the dubious idea of recapitulation, that is, that a sequence of events that has gone wrong can be corrected with a different outcome. In this case, the child is "reborn" to the adoptive parent, remedying the negative experience with her birth parents.

Candace never made her way out of the flannel blanket in which she was bound. The four adults present during her rebirthing session ignored her cries for over an hour, as she begged for air, vomited, and pleaded for her life. Although Candace's case was the most well publicized, other children have died as a result of attachment techniques, including four-year-old Krystal Tibbets, who suffocated during a treatment administered by her father at the request of her therapist.

The techniques used by attachment therapists to ostensibly remediate children's problem behavior are invasive and aggressive, often involving restraint, shouting, and humiliation. Some of the major attachment therapy techniques include "holding therapy," in which therapists restrain children for minutes to hours at a time and shout threats and taunts at them; "therapeutic foster care," in which children stay full time with an attachment therapist who enforces military-style ritualized discipline; and discipline techniques involving intense physical labor and deprivation of food, sleep, and education.

The rationale underlying attachment therapy is that separation from a biological parent produces long-lasting ill effects in children, including bottled-up rage that is exhibited as disruptive behavior in the adoptive home. Attachment therapy treats children as vicious, manipulative, and evil, and in some cases even potential serial killers (Mercer, Sarner, & Rosa, 2003). The goal of attachment therapy is to produce a polite, compliant, and affectionate child for the adoptive guardian by coaxing the child into releasing pent-up rage.

Both this philosophy and its desired end-product are based on flawed assumptions. Legitimate researchers conclude that most people develop attachments in their first six to twenty-four months, and that a complete failure to form attachments is very unusual. If it did occur, it would most likely produce a person who had not formed the trust necessary to maintain long-term relationships rather than an aggressive and manipulative psychopath. Additionally, developmental research shows that children adopted early in life typically exhibit no more behavioral or emotional troubles than nonadopted children (Miller et al., 2000). It is not surprising that there is no controlled evidence that attachment therapies are efficacious (Mercer, 2002).

Despite Candace Newmaker's and other cases and a virtually wholesale lack of scientific validation, attachment therapy appears to be increasingly accessible to practitioners and the public. More than fifty Web sites either offer or promote attachment therapy, and attachment therapy workshops have been approved for continuing education credits by the National Association of Social Workers and the APA.

Critical Incident Stress Debriefing Shortly after the September 11 terrorist attacks, approximately 9000 well-intentioned psychotherapists descended on Manhattan in an effort to forestall post-traumatic stress reactions among traumatized New Yorkers. A large proportion of these therapists administered critical incident stress debriefing (CISD)—also known as crisis debriefing—or its variants. CISD, which was developed to assist emergency responders (e.g., firemen) to cope with the immediate aftermath of trauma, has become immensely popular as a method of warding off posttraumatic stress symptoms among individuals exposed to trauma. This single-session procedure is typically conducted in groups (Mitchell, 1983). It proceeds according to a standardized set of steps—including strongly encouraging group members to discuss and "process" their negative emotions, delineating the posttraumatic symptoms that group members are likely to experience, and strongly discouraging group members from discontinuing participation once the session has begun. CISD is usually administered within twenty-four to seventy-two hours of the traumatic event (Gist & Lubin, 1999; Lohr, Hooke, Gist, & Tolin, 2003).

Controlled studies suggest that CISD is ineffective. Litz, Gray, Bryant, and Adler's (2002) meta-analysis of randomized controlled trials of CISD versus no treatment or alternative treatment control conditions yielded an overall effect size of $d = -.11$ for posttraumatic stress symptoms, suggesting either no effect or even a slight negative effect (although the confidence interval surrounding this effect size included zero).

Moreover, two controlled studies suggest that CISD has harmful long-term effects, perhaps by impeding natural recovery processes. Bisson, Jenkins, Alexander, and Bannister (1997) found that burn victims randomly assigned to CISD evidenced significantly higher posttraumatic stress disorder, general anxiety, and depression scores at a thirteen-month follow-up than did burn victims randomly assigned to an assessment-only control group. Mayou, Ehlers, and Hobbs (2000) performed a three-year follow-up from a randomized control group of motor vehicle accident victims. Individuals who received CISD exhibited significantly higher levels of global psychopathology and travel anxiety (but not posttraumatic stress symptoms per se) than did individuals in an assessment-only control group. Victims with high levels of intrusion and avoidance symptoms tended to recover on their own, whereas victims who received CISD tended to remain symptomatic.

Both studies suggest the possibility of an iatrogenic effect for CISD, although they require independent replication. We concur with the conclusions of the Cochrane review of studies on CISD: "There is no current evidence that psychological debriefing is a useful treatment of posttraumatic stress disorder after traumatic incidents. Compulsory debriefing of victims should cease" (Wessley, Rose, & Bisson, 2000, p. 1).

It is worth noting that studies of grief therapy for individuals who have lost loved ones similarly suggest the possibility of adverse effects, at least among individuals experiencing relatively normal bereavement reactions. Neimeyer (2000) reported the results of a meta-analysis of twenty-three controlled studies of grief therapy. He found a mean effect size of $d = .13$, which was significantly different from zero. This effect suggests that the effects of grief therapy, although positive, tend to be weak. Moreover, Neimeyer found that thirty-eight percent of clients who received grief therapy would actually have achieved superior end-state functioning had they been assigned to the no-treatment control condition, suggesting the distinct possibility of iatrogenic effects among a sizeable subset of individuals exposed to grief counseling. Given the prevalence of these negative effects, there is ample reason to question the wisdom of administering grief therapy, especially to individuals who are not severely depressed.

Peer Group Interventions for Conduct Problems Dishion, McCord, and Poulin (1999) reported that a disturbing twenty-nine percent of published intervention studies of adolescent problem behavior report negative effects. There is compelling evidence that at least some of these adverse effects are attributable to peer group interventions. The results of several quasi-experimental studies suggest that "deviancy training" (i.e., the reinforcement of antisocial behavior by peer discussions) is associated with significant increases in adolescent antisocial behavior (e.g., Dishion et al., 1997). Dishion and Andrews (1995) found that adolescents enrolled in peer groups—in contrast to those enrolled in parent-focused groups—exhibited increases in externalizing behaviors and tobacco use at one-year follow-up. A three-year follow-up revealed similar negative effects (Dishion et al., 1999).

Not all treatments for adolescent antisocial behavior produce negative effects. For example, group treatments for conduct problems have shown promising results when prosocial children are included in the group (Feldman, 1992). Nevertheless, the results of studies of peer group interventions point to a straightforward conclusion: it is generally best not to introduce conduct-disordered children to one another.

Scared Straight Programs for Conduct Problems Deterrence-oriented programs for delinquent youth have a long and checkered history. Although these programs originated within forensic rather than clinical psychology, they frequently target clients seen by clinical psychologists. "Scared Straight," perhaps the best known program, began in the 1970s with a group of New Jersey prisoners serving lifetime sentences. The prisoners attempted to discourage at-risk adolescents from a life of crime by exposing them to the harsh realities of prison life. A critically lauded and widely viewed television documentary on the program aired in 1979. According to Scared Straight, sixteen of seventeen youths enrolled in the program remained crime free in the ensuing three months (Petrosino & Turpin-Petrosino, 2000). Despite its almost exclusive reliance on informal testimonials derived from small samples, the program was adopted in numerous jurisdictions. They are popular for at least two reasons: they are inexpensive, and they are in accordance with the popular notion that getting tough on at-risk individuals is an effective approach to crime prevention.

In 1982, a randomized controlled trial examining the New Jersey program revealed a significant increase in arrests among those in the Scared Straight condition, compared with the no-treatment controls. Several reviewers reported similar results when evaluating comparable "kids-spend-the-day-in-prison" programs (e.g., Shermer, 1997). A more recent comprehensive meta-analytic review of Scared Straight programs by the Campbell Collaboration revealed negative findings in eight of nine quasi-experimental studies. The results further demonstrated that Scared Straight programs increased the odds of criminal behavior by a ratio of between 1.6 and 1.7 to 1 (Petrosino & Turpin-Petrosino, 2002).

It is disheartening that Scared Straight-type programs remain in use despite clear indications of potential negative effects. When the negative evaluation results from the California SQUIRES program (a program similar to Scared Straight) appeared, the response was to end the study rather than the program (Finckenauer et al., 1999).

Preliminary evaluations of related treatments for troubled youth, such as boot camps and wilderness therapies, have yielded equally dismal, if not more disturbing, results. Like Scared Straight, boot camps have been touted widely as a cost-effective get-tough approach to delinquent youth. However, data indicates that although boot camps are more costly than alternative treatments, they do not reduce recidivism. Moreover, in some studies they have been shown to increase it (Bottcher & Isorena, 1994; Peters, Thomas, & Zamberlan, 1997; Zhang, 1999; Parent, 2003).

Wilderness therapies, which have not received extensive research scrutiny, and boot camps often require intense physical exertion on the part of clients. Those in charge of these programs have occasionally abused this requirement, making demands on their charges that have led to the deaths of a number of healthy adolescents from heat exhaustion, blood clots, dehydration, suffocation, and drowning (*Salt Lake Tribune*, 2003).

Recovered Memory Interventions As noted earlier, surveys indicate that approximately one-fourth of American and Canadian therapists (e.g., Poole et al., 1995) regularly use suggestive techniques such as hypnosis, guided imagery, and dream interpretation to recover purported memories of child sexual abuse. Laboratory studies demonstrate that many of these techniques can implant false memories in some individuals, especially among those prone to fantasy and exaggeration (Lynn & Rhue, 1986).

For example, numerous laboratory studies have found hypnosis to increase the sheer volume of memory recall, both accurate and inaccurate. Hypnosis is also associated with an increased proportion of false memories, without an accompanying increase in the proportion of accurate memories, although it typically increases participants' confidence in their memories, even false ones (Lynn et al., 2003, Lynn, Lock, Myers, & Payne, 1997). Nor does hypnotic age regression accurately reinstate past memories (Nash, 1987).

Studies using the "imagination inflation" paradigm demonstrate that merely thinking about a previous (nonexistent) event increases the probability that this event will be reported as having occurred (e.g., Garry, Manning, Loftus, & Sherman, 1996). These investigations raise serious questions concerning the use of guided imagery, whereby therapists encourage clients to imagine various events that may or may not have occurred (e.g., child abuse). In addition, studies demonstrate that interpreting a dream as symbolic of a past experience (e.g., being lost in a public place in childhood) increases the likelihood that participants will report that experience as having occurred (Mazzoni, Loftus, Seitz, & Lynn, 1999). These study results raise the disquieting possibility that therapists who use suggestive techniques to recover traumatic memories are inadvertently creating, not discovering, these memories in their clients. Some may even be inducing variants or full-blown forms of posttraumatic stress disorder (Lilienfeld, 2002a).

Although critics (e.g., Brown, Scheflin, & Hammond, 1998) have questioned the relevance of laboratory studies of memory reconstruction to false memory creation in the real world, there is ample reason to believe that these studies markedly *underestimate* the likelihood of false memory implantation. Clinicians frequently prompt clients repeatedly for past memories, both within and across psychotherapy sessions. Moreover, the social pressures and demand characteristics of the modal therapy session are almost certainly higher than those of a one-shot laboratory study in which participants interact only briefly and superficially with an experimenter whom they have never met. Some critics (e.g., Olio, 1994) have further alleged that traumatic memories are extremely difficult or impossible to implant. However, researchers have found that suggestive memory procedures led approximately twenty to twenty-five percent of college participants to report having experienced a serious animal attack or a serious injury (Porter, Yuille, & Lehman, 1999). Cases in which clients report alien abductions following suggestive procedures (e.g., hypnosis) furnish a virtual proof for the assertion that such procedures can produce false memories in at least some clients.

The question of whether some recovered memories of trauma are genuine remains unresolved and should not be confused with the question of whether some of these memories are false. The answer to the latter question appears to be an unequivocal yes.

DID-Oriented Therapy Dissociative identity disorder (DID), formerly known as multiple personality disorder, is one of the most controversial conditions in psychopathology (Gleaves, 1996; Lilienfeld, Lynn, et al., 1999; Lilienfeld & Lynn, 2003; Spanos, 1994). Although there is little question that most individuals with DID genuinely suffer from symptoms of psychopathology, significant questions remain about the etiology of this condition. Proponents of the posttraumatic model of DID (e.g., Ross, 1997) maintain that DID is a consequence of childhood sexual abuse and other early trauma. Other proponents of this model (e.g., Gleaves, 1996) go further, arguing that DID is largely independent of sociocultural expectations and social psychological influences such as suggestive questioning by therapists.

In contrast, proponents of the sociocognitive model of DID (e.g., Lilienfeld, Lynn, et al., 1999; Lilienfeld & Lynn, 2003; McHugh, 1993; Spanos, 1994; Stafford & Lynn, 2002) contend that DID is largely a socially constructed condition resulting from iatrogenic influences—for example, inadvertent therapist prompting and cueing of purported "alters"—and sociocultural perceptions and expectations. This model does not exclude the possibility that early sexual abuse plays a causal role in certain cases of DID or deny that individuals with DID often enter psychotherapy with high levels of pre-existing psychopathology such as borderline personality disorder and bipolar disorder (Ganaway, 1995; Lilienfeld, Lynn, et al., 1999). Rather, the sociocognitive model posits that suggestive questioning on the part of therapists (e.g., "Is there another part of you to whom I have not spoken?") can inadvertently trigger the emergence of alters, especially among fantasy-prone individuals (see Lynn, Rhue, & Green, 1988, for a discussion of the relation between fantasy-proneness and alter formation) who are seeking an explanation for seemingly inexplicable psychological phenomena such as sudden mood changes and unstable relationships.

Numerous lines of converging quasi-experimental and epidemiological evidence strongly suggest that many or most cases of DID are partly iatrogenic in origin (see Lilienfeld, Lynn, et al., 1999; Lilienfeld & Lynn, 2003):

- The number of DID patients has increased dramatically over the past several decades, as have the number of alters among DID patients, although the number of alters at initial diagnosis has remained essentially constant. Both increases coincide with enhanced therapist awareness of DID and DID features.
- DID-oriented therapists reify and reinforce patients' displays of multiplicity by treating alters as discrete personalities and encouraging patients to call forth previously undiscovered alters. Many DID patients enter psychotherapy with no reported alters and begin to display alters only following DID-oriented psychotherapy.
- Therapists who use hypnosis to summon ostensibly undiscovered alters have more patients with DID in their caseloads than do other therapists.

- Most diagnoses of DID are made by a small number of therapists specializing in DID.
- Laboratory studies demonstrate that nonclinical individuals furnished with relevant cues and prompts (see Spanos, Weekes, & Bertrand, 1985) readily reproduce many of the typical signs and symptoms of DID.
- Diagnoses of DID were until recently limited largely to North America, where DID has received extensive media coverage in the past few decades, although such diagnoses have now begun to spread to countries (e.g., the Netherlands) in which DID has been more widely publicized.

Taken together, these lines of evidence provide a powerful circumstantial case for the iatrogenic origin of some cases of DID (cf., Brown, Frischholtz, & Scheflin, 1999). Indeed, even some influential proponents of the posttraumatic model of DID (e.g., Ross, 1997) acknowledge that DID can be largely iatrogenically produced by suggestive therapist procedures.

Facilitated Communication Facilitated communication is premised on the notion that communication defects of autistic children are attributable to motor rather than cognitive problems (Biklen, 1990). Hence, with the aid of a facilitator who guides the child's hands, autistic children (as well as children with similar developmental disabilities) purportedly can communicate by using a computer keyboard. However, there is compelling evidence from controlled studies that the "facilitated communications" ostensibly produced by autistic children are in fact unintentionally and unknowingly generated by the facilitators guiding the autistic children's hands. This remarkable phenomenon is known as the idiomatic effect (Wegner, 2002). As a consequence, there is no support for the claim that facilitated communication helps to elicit language among previously uncommunicative autistic children (see Herbert, Sharp, & Gandiano, 2002; Romanczyk, Arnstein, Soorya, & Gillis, 2003, for reviews).

Facilitated communication has been associated with numerous uncorroborated reports of child sexual abuse by the parents of autistic children. One widely publicized case involved Jenny Starch, a 14-year-old autistic girl who typed out approximately 200 allegations of vaginal and anal rapes against her father. Although these allegations were never corroborated, Jenny Starch was temporarily removed from her home (*Rocky Mountain Skeptic*, 1995).

CONSTRUCTIVE EFFORTS TO ADDRESS PSEUDO- AND UNSCIENTIFIC CLAIMS

Until recently, the field of clinical psychology has largely turned a blind eye to the threats posed by pseudoscientific and unscientific claims. As the late Paul Meehl (1993) observed,

> It is absurd, as well as arrogant, to pretend that acquiring a Ph.D. somehow immunizes me from the errors of sampling, perception, recording, retention, retrieval, and interference to which the human mind is subject. In earlier times, all introductory psychology courses devoted a lecture or two to the classic studies in the psychology of testimony, and one mark of a good psychologist was hard-nosed skepticism about folk beliefs. It seems that quite a few clinical psychologists never got exposed to this basic feature of critical thinking. My teachers at [the University of] Minnesota ... shared what Bertrand Russell called the dominant passion of the true scientist—the passion not to be fooled and not to fool anybody else ... all of them asked the two searching questions of positivism: "What do you mean?" "How do you know?" If we clinicians lose that passion and forget those questions, we are little more than be-doctored, well-paid soothsayers. I see disturbing signs that this is happening and I predict that, if we do not clean up our clinical act and provide our students with role models of scientific thinking, outsiders will do it for us (pp. 728–729).

Meehl's warnings, issued over a decade ago, are proving to be prescient. Increasing pressure to reform our practices has come not from inside the profession but from the outside in the form of lawsuits and the often draconian restrictions imposed by managed care companies. Nevertheless, the past decade has witnessed a number of constructive efforts within the profession to address the threats posed by unscientific methods. Two of these efforts have originated within the APA, an organization that has been frequently criticized for its complacency in the face of widespread pseudoscience (e.g., Dawes, 1994; Lilienfeld, 2002a).

Division 12 of the APA has advanced a set of criteria for empirically supported treatments (ESTs) for adult and childhood disorders, along with provisional lists of therapeutic techniques that satisfy these criteria (Chambless & Ollendick, 2001). Vigorous and healthy debate surrounds the criteria, as well as the EST list (Garske & Anderson, 2003;

Herbert, 2000;). Legitimate concerns have been raised that some practitioners and educators may adhere to the provisional EST list too rigidly, thereby prematurely reifying and deifying it (Westen, Morrison, & Thompson-Brenner, 2004). Despite this controversy, it is difficult to deny that the movement toward the specification of ESTs reflects a heightened emphasis on distinguishing interventions that have undergone scientific scrutiny from those that have not, clearly a positive development.

In addition, there is evidence suggesting that certain APA committees have begun to move in the direction of addressing threats posed by unsubstantiated psychotherapies. For example, several years ago the APA Continuing Education (CE) Committee denied support of workshops on Thought Field Therapy for CE credit on the grounds that the scientific evidence for this treatment was not sufficiently compelling to warrant its dissemination to practitioners (Lilienfeld & Lohr, 2000; Lohr et al., 2003; Singer & Nievod, 2003).

Furthermore, the Committee for the Scientific Investigation of Claims of the Paranormal (a group of scientists dedicated to the rigorous examination of untested and unorthodox claims) recently established a new subcommittee. The function of the Council for Scientific Medicine and Mental Health includes the evaluation of questionable or untested mental health claims. The establishment of this council coincided with the launching in 2002 of an interdisciplinary journal, *The Scientific Review of Mental Health Practice* (edited by the first author of this chapter), which is devoted to distinguishing scientifically supported from scientifically unsupported claims in clinical psychology, psychiatry, social work, and allied professions.

Prescriptive Remedies

The rampant promotion of scientifically questionable claims in clinical psychology poses a grave threat to both consumers of mental health services and the integrity of the profession (Lilienfeld & Lynn, 2003). We propose six straightforward remedies that should help bridge the scientist–practitioner gap (Tavris, 2003a,b) and combat the growing problems generated by the marketing and dissemination of pseudoscientific and nonscientific claims in clinical psychology.

1. The APA and other accrediting agencies must insist that clinical psychology training programs require formal training in critical thinking skills, particularly those needed to distinguish scientific from pseudoscientific methods of inquiry. Programs should

emphasize such issues as: (a) fundamentals in the philosophy of science, particularly the distinction between scientific and unscientific epistemologies (Lilienfeld, Lynn, & Lohr, 2003); (b) clinical judgment and prediction, and the processes (e.g., heuristics and biases) that can lead clinicians astray when evaluating assessment and therapy data (Garb, 1998; Garb & Boyle, 2003; Grove et al., 2000); (c) research methodologies required to evaluate the psychometric properties of assessment instruments (Hunsley, Lee, & Wood, 2003) and the efficacy and effectiveness of psychotherapies (Garske & Anderson, 2003); (d) issues in the psychology of human memory, particularly the reconstructive nature of memory and impact of suggestive therapeutic procedures on memory (Lynn et al., 2003; McNally, 2003); and (e) behavior–genetic methods necessary for disentangling genetic from environmental influences on individual differences. Moreover, the accreditation committee of the APA must be willing to withhold approval of doctoral programs that do not place substantial emphasis on these domains, which should be presumed in the education and training of all clinical psychologists.

In our view, the APA has inadvertently exacerbated the scientist–practitioner gap by encouraging clinical programs to adopt their own training models. According to the APA's new accreditation standards, clinical programs are evaluated by how well they adhere to their own training criteria, rather than by how well they satisfy a priori consensually adopted educational and training criteria (American Psychological Association, Committee on Accreditation, 2002).

Although we welcome creativity and innovation in how clinical psychology programs elect to meet fundamental educational goals, this does not mean that the nature of these goals should be left largely to programs themselves. We believe that psychology has advanced to the point where at least the rudiments of a core "critical thinking curriculum in clinical science" can be identified for all clinical programs. By permitting clinical programs to select their own training models and evaluating how well they hew to these models, accreditation bodies are abdicating their responsibility to ensure that future generations of clinical psychologists become thoughtful and informed consumers of the scientific literature.

We agree with O'Donohue (1989), who argued that the optimal model for clinical psychologists should not be the scientist–practitioner (i.e., the Boulder Model), but rather the "philosopher–scientist–practitioner," a model that O'Donohue playfully termed the "Even Bolder Model." As O'Donohue notes, clinical researchers and practitioners must be trained to evaluate evidence and to distinguish between more and less trustworthy knowledge claims. The "critical curriculum thinking in clinical science" we propose would be a helpful start in that direction.

Again, we turn to the history of medicine as an example. Prior to the early 1900s, medical education in the United States was in disarray. Many medical schools were of distressingly low quality and/or were proprietary institutions that emphasized financial profit more than rigorous medical training. This troubling situation was not rectified until 1910, when educational reformer Abraham Flexner issued his scathing indictment of the state of medical education. Flexner argued that medical schools must tighten their academic standards and that practitioners must be trained in university settings. Following the appearance of the Flexner Report, numerous substandard medical schools closed, and still others promptly ratcheted up their educational standards (see Bonner, 2002).

In our view, the field of clinical psychology is in dire need of its own Flexner Report. Accreditation bodies charged with the task of evaluating clinical psychology programs should insist that all students graduating from Ph.D. and Psy.D. programs be educated and scientifically discriminating consumers of the psychological research literature. The hundredth anniversary of the Flexner Report in 2010 would be a fitting date for a report that delineates a new set of rigorous educational and training criteria for clinical psychology programs.

2. In addition to developing criteria for and specification of empirically supported therapies, the field of clinical psychology must identify treatments that are patently devoid of empirical support or that have been found to be harmful either psychologically or physically. Developing a list of "Psychological Treatments to Avoid" is as important as developing a list of ESTs. Based largely on the evidence reviewed in this chapter, we propose a tentative list of potentially hazardous treatments (see Table 10.1), which like the list of ESTs, should be regarded as provisional and open to revision based on new evidence. Future research will almost surely lead to certain treatments being added to this list, and perhaps to others being removed. Nevertheless, practitioners should

TABLE 10.1 Psychological Treatments to Avoid

Intervention	Potential Harm
Attachment therapies (e.g., rebirthing)	Death and serious injury to children
Critical incident stress debriefing	Heightened risk for posttraumatic stress symptoms
Grief therapy for normal bereavement	Heightened risk for depressive symptoms
Suggestive techniques for memory recovery	Production of false memories of trauma; possible iatrogenic induction of posttraumatic stress disorder
DID-oriented therapy	Iatrogenic induction of "alters" (purported multiple personalities)
Peer group interventions for conduct problems	Exacerbation of conduct problems
Scared Straight and boot camp interventions for conduct problems	Exacerbation of conduct problems
Facilitated communication for infantile autism and developmental disabilities	False accusations of child abuse against family members

be exceedingly cautious about administering these treatments without compelling justification and ensure that their clients possess sufficient information for fully informed consent, including a discussion of the potential hazards of these treatments. For several of these treatments—particularly attachment therapies, critical incident stress debriefing, suggestive techniques for memory recovery, and facilitated communication for infantile autism—we would be hard-pressed to generate any compelling justification at the present time, given the unambiguous absence of scientific support and evidence of potential harm.

3. The APA and other psychological organizations must institute safeguards to require that the continuing education of practitioners be grounded in adequate scientific evidence. For example, the APA should terminate approval of CE workshops on techniques that are largely or entirely devoid of scientific support. These include Imago Relationship Therapy, calligraphy therapy, psychological theatre therapy, and Jungian sand play therapy (see Lilienfeld, 1998). Moreover, an APA-approved sponsor has recently offered CE credit for rebirthing (as noted earlier) and for CISD, two techniques that have been found to be potentially harmful. However, efforts by several clinical psychologists to work with APA to terminate CE approval for a CISD workshop proved unsuccessful.

By continuing to accept such practices, the APA is implicitly encouraging the use of techniques that are either ineffective or harmful. This concern is rendered all the more pressing when a major APA official responsible for the advancement of professional practice (and a former APA president!) opines in print that "Psychologists do not have to apologize for their treatments. Nor is there an actual need to prove their effectiveness" (Fox, 2000, pp. 1–2). We believe this attitude to be fundamentally destructive to the evidentiary bases of clinical psychology.

4. The APA and other professional psychological organizations must play a more active role in combating erroneous claims made in the popular press, radio, television, and the Internet regarding psychological services. Such claims are increasingly widespread. For example, in the absence of compelling evidence, ABC's *20/20* uncritically promoted EMDR for anxiety disorders (see Lilienfeld, 1996) and goggle therapy for clinical depression (see Lilienfeld, 1999) as breakthrough interventions. Psychological organizations have traditionally been reluctant to hold the media accountable for the popularization of unsubstantiated mental health methods. Given the influence of the media in shaping public perceptions of efficacious treatments, this reluctance must cease. We recommend that the APA, the American Psychological Society, and other psychological organizations develop coordinated networks of experts who can address media claims regarding questionable or unsubstantiated mental health services.

   Moreover, we recommend that these organizations institute formal programs of public relations training for officials who interact regularly with the news media. The APA has occasionally failed to communicate effectively with the news media in response to scientific controversies involving psychological issues (see Lilienfeld, 2002b, for an example of the APA's inadequate response to a controversial meta-analysis concerning the relation between child sexual abuse and adult psychopathology). By preparing officials to deal with such controversies pre-emptively, the APA and other psychological organizations should be in a far better position to head off likely misinterpretations of psychological findings.

5. The APA and other professional organizations (e.g., state and provincial licensing boards) must be willing to impose meaningful sanctions on practitioners who provide clinical services that are patently devoid of scientific support or that have been shown to be potentially harmful. We are well aware of the formidable

pragmatic obstacles involved in such an endeavor. Moreover, we are sensitive to the possibility that overzealous licensing boards could sanction practitioners for administering empirically promising, although still scientifically preliminary, interventions. Nevertheless, we believe that an initial focus on the most egregious offenses by clinicians would represent a crucial step toward safeguarding the public against pseudoscientific and unscientific practices.

The APA Ethics Code offers some guidance in this regard. It makes clear in several places (e.g., Rule 1.06) that psychologists must rely on the best available scientific knowledge when making professional judgments. We should note, however, that there is substantial ambiguity in the Code (Rule 1.14) regarding harm incurred to the public: "Psychologists take reasonable steps to avoid harming their patients or clients, research participants, students, and others with whom they work, and to minimize harm where it is foreseeable and unavoidable." We believe that the code should be revised to make more explicit the responsibilities of mental health professionals to be familiar with the scientific evidence regarding the costs and potential dangers of their services. At a minimum, service providers must be willing to assume responsibility for actions that result from ignorance of the scientific evidence or acceptance of pseudoscientific and unscientific claims.

6. The APA must make the combating of ineffective and harmful practices its number one priority. In recent years, the APA, especially its Practice Directorate, has expended considerable time, money, and energy in the effort to extend clinical psychologists' practice into a new domain, namely, psychopharmacology. Although there are reasonable arguments both for and against psychologist prescriptive authority (see Hayes & Heiby, 1998, for a discussion), we respectfully suggest that the APA should first ensure that the overwhelming majority of clinical psychologists are delivering scientifically informed interventions in the domains in which they are currently practicing.

First things should come first. The debate over psychologist prescription privileges should come later. Our first priority is to reestablish clinical psychology as a scientifically sound discipline.

REFERENCES

American Psychological Association (2002). *Report of the Committee on Accreditation.* Washington, DC: Author.

Austin, J. (2000). *Multisite Evaluation of Bootcamp Programs: Final Report.* Washington, DC: George Washington University, Institute on Crime, Justice, and Corrections.

Azrin, N.H. & Foxx, R.M. (1974). *Toilet Training in Less Than One Day.* New York: Simon & Schuster.

Bass, E. & Davis, L. (1988). *The Courage to Heal.* New York: Harper & Row.

Beutler, L.E. & Harwood, T.M. (2001). Antiscientific attitudes: What happens when scientists are unscientific? *Journal of Clinical Psychology, 57,* 43–51.

Beyerstein, B.L. (2001). Fringe psychotherapies: The public at risk. *The Scientific Review of Alternative Medicine, 5,* 70–79.

Biklen, D. (1990). Communication unbound: Autism and praxis. *Harvard Educational Review, 60,* 291–314.

Bisson, J.L., Jenkins, P.L., Alexander, J., & Bannister, C. (1997). A randomized controlled trial of psychological debriefing for victims of acute harm. *British Journal of Psychiatry, 171,* 78–81.

Bonner, A. (2002). *Iconoclast: Abraham Flexner and a Life in Learning.* Baltimore; MD: Johns Hopkins University Press.

Bottcher, J. & Isorena, T. (1994). *LEAD: A Boot Camp and Intensive Parole Program: An Implementation and Process Evaluation of the First Year.* Washington, DC: *NCJ 150513.* California Youth Authority and U.S. Department of Justice, National Institute of Justice.

Brown, D., Frischholtz, E.J., & Scheflin, A.W. (1999). Iatrogenic dissociative identity disorder: An evaluation of the scientific evidence. *Journal of Psychiatry and the Law, 27,* 549–637.

Brown, D., Scheflin, A.W., & Hammond, D.C. (1998). *Memory, Trauma Treatment, and the Law.* New York: Norton.

Bunge, M. (1984). What is pseudoscience? *Skeptical Inquirer, 9,* 36–46.

Callahan, R.J. (1995, August). A Thought Field Therapy (TFT) algorithm for trauma. Paper presented at the *105th Annual Convention of the American Psychological Association,* San Francisco.

Callahan, R.J. (2001). Thought Field Therapy: Response to our critics and a scrutiny of some old ideas of science. *Journal of Clinical Psychology, 57,* 1154–1170.

Chambless, D.L. & Ollendick, T.H. (2001). Empirically supported psychological interventions: Controversies and evidence. *Annual Review of Psychology, 52,* 685–716.

Chapman, L.J. & Chapman, J.P. (1967). Genesis of popular but erroneous psychodiagnostic observations. *Journal of Abnormal Psychology, 72,* 193–204.

Cook, T.D. & Campbell, D.T. (1979). *Quasi-Experimentation: Design and Analysis Issues for Field Settings.* Boston: Houghton Mifflin.

Corsini, R.J. (2001). *Handbook of Innovative Therapy* (2d ed.). New York: Wiley.

Davey, R.I. & Hill, J. (1999). The variability of practice in interviews used by professionals to investigate child sexual abuse. *Child Abuse and Neglect, 23,* 571–578.

Davidson, P.R. & Parker, K.C.H. (2001). Eye movement desensitization and reprocessing: A meta-analysis. *Journal of Consulting and Clinical Psychology, 69,* 305–316.

Dawes, R.M. (1994). *House of Cards: Psychology and Psychotherapy Built on Myth.* New York: Free Press.

Dawes, R.M., Faust, D., & Meehl, P.E. (1989). Clinical versus actuarial judgment. *Science, 243,* 1668–1674.

Dishion, T.J. & Andrews, D.W. (1995). Preventing escalation in problem behaviors with high-risk young adolescents: Immediate and 1-year outcomes. *Journal of Consulting and Clinical Psychology, 63,* 538–548.

Dishion, T.J., Eddy, J.M., Haas, E., Li, F., & Spracklen, K. (1997). Friendships and violent behavior during adolescence. *Social Development, 6,* 207–223.

Dishion, T., McCord, J., & Poulin, F. (1999). When interventions harm: Peer groups and problem behavior. *American Psychologist, 54,* 755–754.

Dolnick, E. (1998). *Madness on the Couch: Blaming the Victim in the Heyday of Psychoanalysis.* New York: Simon & Schuster.

Drabick, D.A. & Goldfried, M.R. (2000). Training the scientist-practitioner for the 21st century: Putting the bloom back on the rose. *Journal of Clinical Psychology, 56,* 327–340.

Eisner, D.A. (2000). *The Death of Psychotherapy: From Freud to Alien Abductions.* Westport, CT: Praeger.

Feldman, R.A. (1992). The St. Louis Experiment: Effective treatment of antisocial youths in prosocial peer groups. In J. McCord & R.E. Tremblay (Eds.), *Preventing Antisocial Behavior: Interventions from Birth through Adolescence* (pp. 233–252). New York: Guilford.

Finckenauer, J.O., Gavin, P.W., Hovland, A., & Storvoll, E. (1999). *Scared Straight: The Panacea Phenomenon Revisited.* Prospect Heights, IL: Waveland.

Fox, R.E. (1996). Charlatanism, scientism, and psychology's social contract. *American Psychologist, 51,* 777–784.

Fox, R.E. (2000, Winter). The dark side of evidence-based treatment. *Practitioner Focus.* Available online at: http/www.apa.org/practice/pf/jan00/cappchair.html.

Ganaway, G.K. (1995). Hypnosis, childhood trauma, and dissociative identity disorder: Toward an integrative theory. *International Journal of Clinical and Experimental Hypnosis, 43,* 127–144.

Garb, H.N. (1998). *Studying the Clinician: Judgment Research and Psychological Assessment.* Washington, DC: American Psychological Association.

Garb, H.N. & Boyle, P.A. (2003). Understanding why some clinicians use pseudoscientific methods: Findings from research on clinical judgment. In S.O. Lilienfeld, S.J. Lynn, & J.M. Lohr (Eds.), *Science and Pseudoscience in Clinical Psychology* (pp. 17–38). New York: Guilford.

Garry, M., Manning, C., Loftus, E.F., & Sherman, S.J. (1996). Imagination inflation: Imagining a childhood event inflates confidence that it occurred. *Psychonomic Bulletin and Review, 3,* 208–214.

Garske, J.P. & Anderson, T. (2003). Toward a science of psychotherapy research: Present status and evaluation. In S.O. Lilienfeld, S.J. Lynn, & J.M. Lohr (Eds.), *Science and Pseudoscience in Clinical Psychology* (pp. 145–175). New York: Guilford.

Gist, R. & Lubin, B. (Eds.). (1999). *Response to Disaster: Psychosocial, Community, and Ecological Approaches.* Philadelphia: Brunner/Mazel.

Gleaves, D.H. (1996). The sociocognitive model of dissociative identity disorder: A reexamination of the evidence. *Psychological Bulletin, 120,* 42–59.

Goisman, R.M., Warshaw, M.G., & Keller, M.B. (1999). Psychosocial treatment prescriptions for generalized anxiety disorder, social phobia, and panic disorder, 1991–1996. *American Journal of Psychiatry, 156,* 1819–1821.

Gould, R.A. & Clum, G.A. (1993). A meta-analysis of self-help treatment approaches. *Clinical Psychology Review, 13,* 169–186.

Griffin, N. & Goldsmith, L. (1985, March). The charismatic kid: Tony Robbins, 25, gets rich peddling a hot self-help program. *Life, 8,* 41–46.

Gross, P.R. & Levitt, N. (1994). *Higher Superstition: The Academic Left and Its Quarrels with Science.* Baltimore: Johns Hopkins University Press.

Grove, W.M. (Chair). (2000). *APA Division 12 (Clinical) Presidential Task Force "Assessment for the year 2000": Report of the Task Force.* Washington, DC: American Psychological Association, Division 12.

Grove, W.M. & Lloyd. M. (in preparation). *Survey on the Use of Mechanical Prediction Methods in Clinical Psychology.*

Grove, W.M. & Meehl, P.E. (1996). Comparative efficiency of informal (subjective, impressionistic) and formal (mechanical, algorithmic) prediction procedures: The clinical-statistical controversy. *Psychology, Public Policy, and Law, 2*, 293–323.

Grove, W.M., Zald, D.H., Lebow, B.S., Snitz, B.E., & Nelson, C. (2000). Clinical versus mechanical prediction: A meta-analysis. *Psychological Assessment, 12*, 19–30.

Hayes, S. & Heiby, E. (1998). *Prescription Privileges for Psychologists: A Critical Reappraisal*. Reno, NV: Context.

Heaton, J. & Wilson, N. (1995). *Tuning in Trouble: Talk TV's Destructive Impact on Mental Health*. San Francisco: Jossey-Bass.

Herbert, J.D. (2000). Defining empirically supported treatments: Pitfalls and possible solutions. *The Behavior Therapist, 23*, 13–122, 134.

Herbert, J.D., Lilienfeld, S.O., Lohr, J.M., Montgomery, R.W., O'Donohue, W.T., Rosen, G.M., & Tolin, D.F. (2000). Science and pseudoscience in the development of eye movement desensitization and reprocessing. *Clinical Psychology Review, 20*, 945–971.

Herbert, J.D., Sharp, I.R., & Gaudiano, B.A. (2002). Separating fact from fiction in the etiology and treatment of autism: A scientific review of the evidence. *Scientific Review of Mental Health Practice, 1*, 23–43.

Hibbard, S. (2003). A critique of Lilienfeld et al.'s "The scientific status of projective techniques." *Journal of Personality Assessment, 80*, 260–271.

Hunsley, J., Lee, C.M., & Wood, J.M. (2003). Controversial and questionable assessment techniques. In S.O. Lilienfeld, S.J. Lynn, & J.M. Lohr (Eds.), *Science and Pseudoscience in Clinical Psychology* (pp. 39–76). New York: Guilford.

Kalal, D.M. (1999). Critical thinking in clinical practice: Pseudoscience, fad psychology, and the behavior therapist. *The Behavior Therapist, 22*, 81–84.

Koocher, G.P., Goodman, G.S., White, C.S., Friedrich, W.N., Sivan, A.B., & Reynolds, C.R. (1995). Psychological science and the use of anatomically detailed dolls in child sexual abuse assessments. *Psychological Bulletin, 118*, 199–222.

Kvale, S. (1992). Postmodern psychology: A contradiction in terms? In S. Kvale (Ed.), *Psychology and Postmodernism* (pp. 31–57). London: Sage.

Lilienfeld, S.O. (1996). EMDR treatment: Less than meets the eye? *Skeptical Inquirer, 20*, 25–31.

Lilienfeld, S.O. (1998). Pseudoscience in contemporary clinical psychology: What it is and what we can do about it. *The Clinical Psychologist, 51*, 3–9.

Lilienfeld, S.O. (1999). ABC's 20/20 features segment on "goggle therapy" for depression and anxiety. *Skeptical Inquirer, 23*, 8–9.

Lilienfeld, S.O. (2001, August 25). Fringe psychotherapies: Scientific and ethical implications for clinical psychology. In S.O. Lilienfeld (Chair), Fringe psychotherapies: What lessons can we learn? Presentation at invited symposium, *Annual Convention of the American Psychological Association*, San Francisco.

Lilienfeld, S.O. (2002a). The scientific review of mental health practice: Our *raison d'etre*. *Scientific Review of Mental Health Practice, 1*, 5–10.

Lilienfeld, S.O. (2002b). When worlds collide: Social science, politics, and the Rind et al. child sexual abuse meta-analysis. *American Psychologist, 57*, 176–188.

Lilienfeld, S.O. & Lohr, J.M. (2000). Thought field therapy practitioners and educators sanctioned. *Skeptical Inquirer, 24*, 5.

Lilienfeld, S.O. & Lynn, S.J. (2003). Dissociative identity disorder: Multiple personalities, multiple controversies. In S.O. Lilienfeld, S.J. Lynn, & J.M. Lohr (Eds.), *Science and Pseudoscience in Clinical Psychology* (pp. 109–142). New York: Guilford.

Lilienfeld, S.O., Lynn, S.J., Kirsch, I., Chaves, J.F., Sarbin, T.R., Ganaway, G.K., & Powell, R.A. (1999). Dissociative identity disorder and the sociocognitive model: Recalling the lessons of the past. *Psychological Bulletin, 125*, 507–523.

Lilienfeld, S.O., Lynn, S.J., & Lohr, J.M. (Eds.). (2003). *Science and Pseudoscience in Clinical Psychology*. New York: Guilford.

Lilienfeld, S.O., Wood, J.M., & Garb, H.N. (2000). The scientific status of projective techniques. *Psychological Science in the Public Interest, 1*, 27–66.

Litz, B.T., Gray, M.J., Bryant, R.A., & Adler, A.B. (2002). Early intervention for trauma: Current status and future directions. *Clinical Psychology: Science and Practice, 9*, 112–134.

Lohr, J.M., Fowler, K.A., & Lilienfeld, S.O. (2002). The dissemination and promotion of pseudoscience in clinical psychology: The challenge to legitimate clinical science. *The Clinical Psychologist, 55*(3), 4–9.

Lohr, J.M., Hooke, W., Gist, R., & Tolin, D.F. (2003). Novel and controversial treatments for trauma-related stress disorders. In S.O. Lilienfeld, S.J. Lynn, & J.M. Lohr (Eds.), *Science and Pseudoscience in Clinical Psychology* (pp. 243–272). New York: Guilford.

Lohr, J.M., Tolin, D.F., & Lilienfeld, S.O. (1998). Efficacy of eye movement desensitization and reprocessing: Implications for behavior therapy. *Behavior Therapy, 26*, 123–156.

Lynn, S.J., Lock, T.G., Loftus, E.F., Krackow, E., & Lilienfeld, S.O. (2003). The remembrance of things past: Problematic memory recovery techniques in psychotherapy. In S.O. Lilienfeld, S.J. Lynn, & J.M. Lohr (Eds.), *Science and Pseudoscience in Clinical Psychology* (pp. 205–239). New York: Guilford.

Lynn, S.J., Lock, T.G., Meyers, B., & Payne, D.G. (1997). Recalling the unrecallable: Should hypnosis be used to recover memories in psychotherapy? *Current Directions in Psychological Science, 6*, 79–83.

Lynn, S.J. & Rhue, J.W. (1986). The fantasy-prone person: Hypnosis, imagination, and creativity. *Journal of Personality and Social Psychology, 51*, 404–408.

Lynn, S.J., Rhue, J.W., & Green, J.P. (1988). Multiple personality disorder and fantasy proneness: Is there an association or dissociation? *British Journal of Experimental and Clinical Hypnosis, 5*, 138–142.

Marano, H.E. (1997, May–June). When planets collide. *Psychology Today, 30* (3), 28–33.

Matson, J.L. & Ollendick, T.H. (1977). Issues in toilet training normal children. *Behavior Therapy, 8*, 549–553.

Mayou, R.A., Ehlers, A., & Hobbs, M. (2000). Psychological debriefing for road and traffic accident victims. *British Journal of Psychiatry, 176*, 589–593.

Mazzoni, G.A., Loftus, E.F., Seitz, A., & Lynn, S.J. (1999). Creating a new childhood: Changing beliefs and memories through dream interpretation. *Applied Cognitive Psychology, 13*, 125–144.

McFall, R.M. (1991). Manifesto for a science of clinical psychology. *The Clinical Psychologist, 44*, 75–88.

McHugh, P.R. (1993). Multiple personality disorder. *Harvard Mental Health Newsletter, 10*, 4–6.

McNally, R.J. (2003). *Remembering Trauma*. Cambridge, MA: Belknap/Harvard University Press.

Meehl, P.E. (1954). *Clinical versus Statistical Prediction*. Northvale, NJ: Jason Aronson.

Meehl, P.E. (1993). Philosophy of science: Help or hindrance? *Psychological Reports, 72*, 707–733.

Mercer, J. (2002). Attachment therapy: A treatment without empirical support. *Scientific Review of Mental Health Practice, 1*, 105–112.

Mercer, J., Sarner, L., & Rosa, L. (2003). *Attachment Therapy on Trial*. Westport, CT: Praeger.

Miller, R., Fan, X., Christensen, M., Grotevant, H., & van Dulmen, M. (2000). Comparisons of adopted and non-adopted adolescents in a large, nationally represented sample. *Child Development, 71*, 1458–1473.

Mitchell, J.T. (1983). When disaster strikes…the critical incident stress debriefing process. *Journal of Emergency Medical Services, 8*, 36–39.

Myers, D.G. (2002). *Intuition: Its Powers and Perils*. New Haven, CT: Yale University Press.

Nash, M.R. (1987). What, if anything, is regressed about hypnotic age regression? A review of the empirical literature. *Psychological Bulletin, 102,* 42–52.

Neimeyer, R. (2000). Searching for the meaning of meaning: Grief therapy and the process of reconstruction. *Death Studies, 24,* 541–558.

Norcross, J.D., Sanrock, J.W., Campbell, L.F., Smith, T.P., Sommer, R., & Zuckerman, E.L. (2000). *Authoritative Guide to Self-Help Resources in Mental Health.* New York: Guilford.

O'Donohue, W. (1989). The (even) bolder model: The clinical psychologist as metaphysician–scientist–practitioner. *American Psychologist, 44,* 1460–1468.

Olio, K.A. (1994). Truth in memory. *American Psychologist, 49,* 442–443.

Parent, D. (2003). Correctional boot camps: Lessons from a decade of research. *National Institute of Justice Journal.*

Peters, M., Thomas, D., & Zamberlan, C. (1997). *Boot Camps for Juvenile Offenders.* Program Summary, NCJ 164258. Washington, DC: U.S. Department of Justice, Office of Juvenile Justice and Delinquency Prevention.

Petrosino, A. & Turpin-Petrosino, C. (2000). "Scared Straight" and other prison tour programs for preventing juvenile delinquency. *The Cochrane Library,* Issue 4.

Piper, A. (1993). "Truth serum" and "recovered memories" of sexual abuse: A review of the evidence. *The Journal of Psychiatry and Law, 21,* 447–471.

Polkinghorne, D.E., (1992). Postmodern epistemology of practice. In S. Kvale (Ed.), *Psychology and Postmodernism* (pp. 146–165). London: Sage.

Polusny, M.A. & Folette, V.M. (1996). Remembering childhood sexual abuse: A national survey of psychologists' clinical practices, beliefs, and personal experiences. *Professional Psychology: Research and Practice, 27,* 41–52.

Poole, D.A., Lindsay, D.S., Memon, A., & Bull, R. (1995). Psychotherapists' opinions, practices, and experiences with memories of incestuous abuse. *Journal of Consulting and Clinical Psychology, 68,* 426–437.

Porter, S., Yuille, J.C., & Lehman, D.R. (1999). The nature of real, implanted, and fabricated childhood emotional events: Implications for the recovered memory debate. *Law and Human Behavior, 23,* 517–537.

Reichenbach, H. (1938). *Experience and Prediction.* Chicago: University of Illinois Press.

Rocky Mountain Skeptic (1995, September). *Exploring facilitated communication* [online at http://bcn.boulder.co.us/community/rms/rms-fc1.html].

Romanczyk, R.G., Arnstein, L., Soorya, L.V., & Gillis, J. (2003).The myriad of controversial treatments for autism: A critical evaluation of efficacy. In S.O. Lilienfeld, S.J. Lynn, & J.M. Lohr (Eds.), *Science and Pseudoscience in Clinical Psychology* (pp. 363–398). New York: Guilford.

Rosen, G.M. (1987). Self-help treatment books and the commercialization of psychotherapy. *American Psychologist, 42,* 46–51.

Rosen, G.M., Glasgow, R.E., & Moore, T.E. (2003). Self-help therapy: The science and business of giving psychology away. In S.O. Lilienfeld, S.J. Lynn, & J.M. Lohr (Eds.), *Science and Pseudoscience in Clinical Psychology* (pp. 399–424.). New York: Guilford.

Ross, C.A. (1997). *Dissociative Identity Disorder: Diagnosis, Clinical Features, and Treatment of Multiple Personality.* New York: Wiley.

Ruscio, J. (2001). *Clear Thinking with Psychology: Separating Sense from Nonsense.* Pacific Grove, CA: Wadsworth.

Sagan, C. (1995, January/February). Wonder and skepticism. *Skeptical Inquirer, 19,* 24–30.

Salt Lake Tribune (2003, July 13). Utah wilderness therapy deaths. Available at http://www.sltrib.com/2003/jul/07132003/utah/75064.asp.

Schon, D. (1983). *The Reflexive Practitioner: How Professionals Think in Action.* New York: Basic.

Shannon, S. (Ed.) (2002). *Handbook of Complementary and Alternative Therapies in Mental Health*. San Diego, CA: Academic.

Shapiro, F. (1995). *Eye Movement Desensitization and Reprocessing: Basic Protocols, Principles, and Procedures*. New York: Guilford.

Shapiro, F. & Forrest, M.S. (1997). *EMDR: The Breakthrough Therapy for Overcoming Anxiety, Stress, and Trauma*. New York: Basic.

Shermer, M. (1997). *Why People Believe Weird Things: Pseudoscience Superstition and Other Confusions of our Time*. New York: Freeman.

Shermer, M. (2001). *The Borderlands of Science: Where Sense Meets Nonsense*. New York: Oxford University Press.

Singer, M. & Lalich, J. (1996). *Crazy Therapies: What Are They? How Do They Work?* San Francisco: Jossey-Bass.

Singer, M. & Nievod, A. (2003). New age therapies. In S.O. Lilienfeld, S.J. Lynn, & J.M. Lohr (Eds.). *Science and Pseudoscience in Clinical Psychology* (pp.176–204). New York: Guilford.

Smith, M.L., Glass, G.V., & Miller, T.I. (1980). *The Benefits of Psychotherapy*. Baltimore: Johns Hopkins University Press.

Spanos, N.P. (1994). Multiple identity enactments and multiple personality disorder: A sociocognitive perspective. *Psychological Bulletin, 116*, 143–165.

Spanos, N.P., Weekes, J.R., & Bertrand, L.D. (1985). Multiple personality: A social psychological perspective. *Journal of Abnormal Psychology, 94*, 362–376.

Stafford, J. & Lynn, S.J. (2002). Cultural scripts, memories of childhood abuse, and multiple identities: A study of role-played enactments. *International Journal of Clinical and Experimental Hypnosis, 50*, 67–85.

Stanovich, K. (2001). *How to Think Straight about Psychology* (6th ed.). New York: HarperCollins.

Sternberg, R.J. (2003). Analyzing the relationship between therapists and research psychologists. *The Chronicle Review*, 17–25 April 4th.

Strupp, H.H., Hadley, S.W., & Gomez-Schwartz, B. (1978). *Psychotherapy for Better or Worse: The Problem of Negative Effects*. New York: Wiley.

Tavris, C. (2003a). Mind games: Psychological warfare between therapists and scientists. *The Chronicle Review*, February 28, B7–B9.

Tavris, C. (2003b). The widening scientist-practitioner gap. In S.O. Lilienfeld, S.J. Lynn, & J.M. Lohr (Eds.), *Science and Pseudoscience in Clinical Psychology* (pp. ix–xvii). New York: Guilford.

Tsoi-Hoshmand, L.T. & Polkinghorne, D.E. (1992). Redefining the science–practice relationship and professional training. *American Psychologist, 47*, 55–66.

Wampold, B.E., Mondin, G.W., Moody, M., Stich, F., Benson, K., & Ahn, H. (1997). A meta-analysis of outcome studies comparing bona fide psychotherapies: Empirically, "All have won and all must have prizes." *Psychological Bulletin, 122*, 203–215.

Watkins, C.E., Campbell, V.L., Nieberding, R., & Hallmark, R. (1995). Contemporary practice of psychological assessment by clinical psychologists. *Professional Psychology: Research and Practice, 26*, 54–60.

Wegner, D.M. (2002). *The Illusion of Conscious Will*. Cambridge, MA: MIT Press.

Wessley, S., Rose, S., & Bisson, J. (2000). Brief psychological interventions ("debriefing") for trauma-related symptoms and the prevention of posttraumatic stress disorder (Cochrane Review). *The Cochrane Library, 4* [on-line].

Westen, D., Morrison, C., & Thompson-Brenner, H. (2004). The empirical status of empirically supported therapies: Assumptions, methods, and findings. *Psychological Bulletin, 126*, 133–151.

Wilson, N. (2003). Commercializing mental health issues: Entertainment, advertising, and psychological advice. In S.O. Lilienfeld, S.J. Lynn, & J.M. Lohr (Eds.). *Science and Pseudoscience in Clinical Psychology* (pp. 425–460). New York: Guilford.

Wolfner, G., Faust, D., & Dawes, R.M. (1993). The use of anatomically detailed dolls in sexual abuse evaluations: The state of the science. *Applied and Preventive Psychology, 2,* 1–11.

Wood, J.M., Nezworski, M.T., Lilienfeld, S.O., & Garb, H.N. (2003). *What's Wrong with the Rorschach? Science Confronts the Controversial Inkblot Test.* San Francisco: Jossey-Bass.

Wright, R., & Cummings, N. (2000). *The Practice of Psychology: The Battle for Professionalism.* Phoenix, AZ: Zeig, Tucker, and Theisen.

Zeiss, R.A. (1978). Self-directed treatment for premature ejaculation. *Journal of Consulting and Clinical Psychology, 46,* 1234–1241.

Zhang, S.C. (1999). *An Evaluation of the Los Angeles Country Drug Treatment Boot Camp.* Final Report, NCJ 189787. San Marco, CA: California State University and the U.S. Department of Justice, National Institute of Justice.

11

THE DISEASING OF AMERICA'S CHILDREN: THE POLITICS OF DIAGNOSIS

John K. Rosemond

I have been conducting an informal poll for the past five years. When a parent tells me that her child has been diagnosed as "having" attention deficit (hyperactivity) disorder, oppositional defiant disorder, and/or childhood-onset bipolar disorder (ADD, ODD, COBD), I ask, "And what did the diagnosing therapist tell you caused your child's problems?" The words vary, but the answer does not: genes.

- "He told me my child was born with a biochemical imbalance. He determined that that sort of thing runs in my family."
- "She said my child's brain is wired differently from most kids' brains, and that he probably inherited this from his father."
- "We were told that his problems were genetic."

This contention—that dysfunctional behavior is inherited—is unproven. Worse, no good scientific evidence supports it. Although some researchers are convinced that a biological smoking gun will eventually be found, the fact remains that one has not been found. Pediatrician and author William Carey (2002; Carey & Jablow, 1999) says, "The assumption that ADHD symptoms arise from cerebral malfunction has not been supported even after extensive investigations," and "No consistent structural, functional, or chemical neurological marker is found in children with the ADHD diagnosis as currently formulated." Carey is but one of many investigators who have arrived at this conclusion.

Although therapists continue to make claims about the genetic component of ADHD as if they are established and incontrovertible, they are nothing more than speculation. Furthermore, they are speculation that flies in the face of established fact, not to mention plain old common sense.

It is a fact that from generation to generation, genes work in a reliably predictable fashion. In popular parlance, they are "passed on," such that within any population group a trait that is characteristic of one generation inevitably shows up in the next, and to approximately the same extent. For example, if it could be determined that twenty-five percent of American children born in 2003 to American-born parents who were born to American-born parents (we've gone back two generations now) came to us with brown eyes, then we absolutely know that if we examine all American birth records from 1945 to 1955, we will find that very close to twenty-five percent of children born during that ten-year period sported brown eyes. New genes that suddenly emerge in a population group are called "mutations," and even assuming that a mutation is favored, it takes a long, long time for any mutation to become significantly widespread.

The question now becomes: if genes cause ADD, ODD, and COBD where is the evidence that significant numbers of American children born from 1945 to 1955 exhibited the symptoms associated with these supposed "disorders?" After all, no informed person would deny that these diagnoses are significantly widespread among American children.

There is no such evidence. Indeed, there is a wealth of evidence to the contrary. During the peak years of the baby boom, America suffered a teacher and classroom shortage that resulted in an embarrassment of what today would be considered horribly overcrowded classrooms. An elementary school classroom of forty to fifty students taught by one teacher was not at all unusual. My first-grade classroom at a Catholic school in Charleston, SC, in the early 1950s held fifty students. Sister Mary was the sole adult in the room. My second-grade classroom in the suburbs of Chicago consisted of thirty-seven children, again taught by one teacher. My third-grade class picture shows forty-two children, and three are listed as absent. Again, we're talking about one teacher, no aide.

Although first and second grades are a bit fuzzy, I remember third grade fairly well. Mrs. Hoy did not have to deal with many discipline problems. She occasionally sent a child outside to sit in the hall, but occasionally is the operative word. (I remember sitting in academic purgatory once or twice myself.) She undoubtedly reprimanded a child or two on any given day. But I most clearly remember an orderly yet exciting learning environment. When Mrs. Hoy taught, we listened. When she gave an instruction, we followed it. I would certainly remember if four or five children (approximately ten percent, the proportion of today's school-age children who supposedly have ADD, ODD, and/or COBD) presented major behavior problems.

To check out the unthinkable possibility that my experience might be unique and my memory failing me, I have asked others of my generation who attest to having attended overcrowded (by today's standards) classrooms if they recall teachers spending significant amounts of time on disciplinary matters. No, they answer. We fifty-something boomers all remember the occasional child whose desk abutted the teacher's, the occasional child who got into more than his (it was always a boy) fair share of trouble. But no peer among the hundred or more to whom I've spoken remembers children who were hopelessly incorrigible, much less out of control. No one remembers a child who openly defied adult authority. No one remembers a child who threw classroom tantrums. No one remembers a child who talked back insultingly to a teacher, much less reared back to hit her when she upset him. Are all of our memories failing equally rapidly?

I doubt it. A good number of the women who taught in America's schools during that time are still with us. In my capacity as a public speaker on "parenting" issues, I give two hundred-plus presentations yearly across the United States, and occasionally abroad. In the course of my travels, I frequently encounter these women (and the occasional male), now well into their retirement. I have met:

- A woman in Miami who taught seventy first-graders by herself in 1950, her third year teaching, who told me, "They were going to eventually split them between me and another teacher, but when they realized I was having no problems at all, they decided to save money and left me with them all year long. And I really had no problems. Oh, you know, the occasional outburst of mischief, but no outstanding difficulties with any one child." And these were children, mind you, who came from all walks of life.
- A Hartford, CT, woman who in 1956, her first year teaching, presided over a class of sixty first-graders. She said, "They came;

they sat; they paid attention; they did what I told them to do. I disciplined hardly at all." These children, too, came from all walks of life.

- An Atlanta woman who, by herself, taught a second-grade class of sixty-five children in 1955. Her teaching day began at 8:15 A.M. and ended at 3:15 P.M. Her testimony: "I didn't have to discipline much at all. They came to me already disciplined. Praise God, because I had not been trained to discipline. I'd been trained to teach, and that's what I was able to do."

- A man who in 1962 taught sixty sixth-graders in a self-contained class. He reported to me that not one of these sixty children presented any significant problem. Discipline was a nonissue in his class, he said.

Over the years, I have collected numerous testimonies from long-retired veterans of the teaching profession. The not-so-remarkable thing—to a person my age, that is, who was taught by these people—is that these testimonies are virtually interchangeable. In one voice, they attest to calm orderly classrooms. Not classrooms that were problem free, but "overcrowded" classrooms that were orderly and in which discipline was a relatively easy matter.

The statistics not only bear this out, but belie the idea that children learn better in smaller classes. Historical data is clear on this: effective learning is not a matter of small class size, but of good behavior. In the early 1950s, when the average elementary classroom in America held thirty-five children and one teacher, achievement at every grade level was considerably higher than is the case today (National Center for Education Statistics, 2000; Gatto, 2000), when the average adult/child ratio in a public elementary school is one to twelve. I'm sure the National Education Association does not want the American public to know that.

A mental health professional once told me that the reason retired teachers don't remember kids who, by today's standards, were ADD/ADHD, ODD, and/or COBD is "they weren't in school because the schools could not accommodate them." Where were they? He said that parents kept them at home. Really? If any child in the neighborhoods I grew up in were being kept at home during the day, I would have known about it. You couldn't keep that sort of thing a secret. Let me assure you, there were no such children. I've asked numerous people my age if they knew of such homebound kids. No one remembers any, save the occasional child who was severely handicapped, which is not the case with behavior disorders.

These disorders are supposed to be caused by genes, remember? That would predict that one in ten school-age children in the 1950s was not in school. For those of you who weren't there, this was a time when every school system employed at least one truant officer. If you were absent from school for more than a day, these very scary people were likely to pay a visit to your house just to make sure you were genuinely sick. They patrolled shopping centers and other known gathering places, nabbing kids who were playing hooky.

Concerning the preposterous idea that "these kids" weren't in school in the '50s, I'm reminded of a child who tells a lie, then has to tell another to cover the first, then has to tell another to cover the first two, and so on. These people, professionals in name only, have lied to the American public about the genes thing. Now they have no choice but to either admit the lie or invent even more lies.

The perpetuators of the disease model of behavior disorders engage in disingenuous misleading arguments. They must, because the position they have staked out cannot be supported with fact. A psychologist and a psychiatrist recently debated this issue in a professionals-only Web chat room. The exchange was telling. The psychiatrist compared "mental illness" (a broad category that includes, in the thinking of people who employ such terminology, childhood behavior disorders) to Alzheimer's disease. The psychologist astutely pointed out that the problem with this argument is that although it has been established beyond doubt that Alzheimer's has a biological basis, this is not the case for *any* psychiatric disorder listed in the DSM-IV. Telling us about the biological basis of Alzheimer's, therefore, tells us nothing about the supposed biological basis of, say, attention deficit disorder. The psychiatrist then said that the psychologist was "ignoring conclusive findings about brain structure and related cognitive and behavioral problems," but cleverly omitted any citations of such "conclusive" research.

This reminded me of the manner in which a former president of Children and Adults with Attention Deficit Disorder (CHAADD) responded to my claim in my syndicated newspaper column that at age ten my son, Eric (now thirty-five), had been completely cured, in less than three months, of what today would be diagnosed as a serious case of ADD/ADHD. The cure consisted of discipline of the old-fashioned sort (i.e., psychologically incorrect, yet a discipline that did not involve spankings). In a letter to me, the CHAADD president asserted that ADD/ADHD is a biological disorder that requires medical treatments. If Eric was relieved of symptoms without drugs, she said, then he did not have ADD/ADHD. Inasmuch as Eric exhibited all the defining symptoms, her assertion does nothing but call into question the value of the DSM-IV criteria. Without meaning to do so, she admitted that the criteria define nothing whatsoever; they merely constitute a list of problem behaviors.

In 1979, my wife and I reverted in our parenting practices. We decided to begin raising our kids the way our parents had raised us. We began disciplining in compelling ways (e.g., we stopped using time-outs), we assigned the children to significant household responsibilities, and we removed television and video games from their lives. The effect, especially on Eric, was remarkable. In January of 1979, his third-grade teacher had told us that he would not be able to go to the fourth grade. In April, she told us she had seen a minor miracle. "Whatever you are doing, Mr. and Mrs. Rosemond," she said, "keep on doing it."

Eric was promoted to the fourth grade and had no significant problems from that point on. I began to realize that in child-rearing matters, my profession was not the solution; it was the problem. This caused me not only to revise my thinking about children but to revise my professional practice. Since then, I have been witness to the testimonies of hundreds of parents who, by employing simple, old-fashioned child-rearing methods, have likewise "cured" their children of severe cases of what professionals have called ADD/ODD/COBD. I once pointed this out to a nationally known expert in ADD/ADHD. He told me that some children had "real" ADD and some children had behavior problems that mimicked ADD. I asked him how he could determine the difference. He told me that the real-ADD kids responded to Ritalin. This from a man who portrays himself as a scientist.

Disease model advocates make several outrageous claims about central nervous system (CNS) stimulants such as Ritalin, one such claim/canard being that these drugs will "slow down" a person with ADD/ADHD but will "speed up" a person who is ADD-free. As anyone familiar with the pharmacology of drugs such as Ritalin knows, therapeutic levels of these drugs do not cause users to run around like Keystone Kops. Nor do they cause a reduction in activity level. Indeed, children who take these drugs are able to sit in one place for longer periods of time because the drugs increase attention span. Quite simply, the more focused you are, the less active you are. But the "Ritalin slows down ADD kids/speeds up non-ADD kids" myth supports the equally fictitious notion that ADD/ADHD kids are physiologically different in significant ways from non-ADD/ADHD kids. Like I said, one lie leads inevitably to another, then another, and then another.

Furthermore, as anyone with pharmacological knowledge knows, one hundred people given a therapeutic dose of Ritalin will respond in pretty much the same way (excepting the occasional pronounced side effect). Nonetheless, we are to believe that when a child whose behavior fits the description for one of these disorders as presented in the DSM is subsequently cured by nonmedical means, that child did not really have a disorder. In other words, the fact that the child's behavior improves when he or she is administered a CNS stimulant (a virtual given) is proof the child has a disease. Methinks this is a prime example of fuzzy logic and circular reasoning, which characterize the thinking of the self-deluded people in question.

No, this ADD/ODD/COBD business is not a matter of genes. The issue of genes becomes moot when the behaviors in question can be controlled by proper (i.e., old-fashioned) discipline. What, then, is the explanation for the rash of children who earn these diagnoses?

Before I answer that question, let me answer another: do I believe that ADD, ODD, and COBD are over-diagnosed? No, I do not. I maintain that if, through some Orwellian Act of Congress, a research team were able to assess every school-age child in America and adhered strictly to the definitions provided in the DSM-IV, they would find that more than half of all children in America merit one or more of these diagnoses. Furthermore, I believe that the percentage is inching up with every passing year. That the DSM criteria—objectively and dispassionately applied—capture so many of today's kids is chilling to anyone familiar with Aldous Huxley's *Brave New World*. The way things are shaping up, the not-so-distant prospect of most of America's children on one drug or another—administered for the supposedly altruistic purpose of helping them "function" more effectively—is hardly preposterous.

So, having addressed the over-diagnosis issue, what is the explanation for the rash of children who exhibit the glaring deficiencies in self-control described in the DSM-IV? If not genes, biochemical imbalances, or faulty "wiring," then what explains the obvious fact that a disproportionate number of today's kids do indeed display the diagnostic criteria? The answer can be easily found in the criteria themselves, a summary of which follows:

- Short attention span
- Impulsive
- Unfocused, fails to finish tasks
- Has difficulty waiting his or her turn

- Easily distracted
- Intrusive
- Belligerently defiant
- Easily frustrated
- Loses temper easily
- Denies responsibility for wrongdoing
- Oppositional
- Aggressive reactions to frustration
- Attention-seeking
- Rages and explosive tantrums

The above list describes a pathological antisocial condition traditionally known as "the terrible twos." In fact, nearly every child ever born has and does exhibit many, if not most, of those "symptoms" during his or her toddlerhood. Quite obviously, the above list does not describe a biological condition; rather, it describes a developmental condition, one that is ubiquitous. Furthermore, this developmental condition existed in 1950, just as it existed in 50 B.C. and will typify toddlers one thousand years from now (assuming we don't find a way to annihilate ourselves before then).

Now we're getting somewhere! The very simple notion that ADD, ODD, and COBD are developmental phenomena explains the ease with which teachers taught grossly overcrowded classrooms during the peak years of the baby boom. To wit: in the 1960s, a culturewide paradigm shift occurred. America entered this decade a culture informed by tradition and respectful of traditional authority. America exited the '60s a culture informed by the new electronic media, disdainful of tradition, and cynical and rejecting of traditional authority, including parental authority. During that tumultuous decade, we became a fully postmodern society.

The rise of clinical psychology coincided with this paradigm shift, and psychologists (and other mental health professionals) did more than any other professional group to demonize the traditional marriage (supposedly bad for women), the traditional family (supposedly inherently pathological), and traditional child rearing (supposedly bad for children). As a consequence of this disingenuous, cut-from-whole-cloth propaganda, America embraced a nouveau "parenting" ethic that bore absolutely no resemblance to the one that had preceded it.

Until this happened, it was axiomatic that parents reared their children much the same way they themselves had been reared. My generation—the baby boomers—put an end to that. I am a member of the last generation of American children to be raised the "old" way, and a member of the first generation of American parents to raise their children the new way. The traditional paradigm emphasized character development, with the goal of good citizenship. The new paradigm (I call it postmodern psychological parenting) emphasizes supposedly healthy psychological development, with the goal of instilling high self-esteem, which recent research by Professor Roy Baumeister (Baumeister, Smart, & Boden, 1996) has confirmed is associated with self-centered, impulsive, antisocial behavior, that is, extended toddlerhood. The traditional paradigm emphasized the discipline of the child's behavior, with the goal of teaching self-control. The postmodern paradigm emphasizes the need to understand and communicate with the child about his or her feeling state, with the goal of helping the child "get in touch with his feelings."

Within the context of the traditional premodern paradigm, when a child misbehaved, he was punished. The new paradigm prescribes that adults talk to the misbehaving child (I call this "yada-yada discipline"), to explain why he should not have done what he did and what he should do next time a similar situation arises. It cannot be emphasized strongly enough that these are two entirely different points of view concerning the child. One presumes that the child is inherently disposed to misbehave (a Biblical view, therefore, antithetical to postmodernity); the other assumes that the child is inherently disposed to be good. One presumes that the child can be turned from his original nature only through a combination of powerful love and equally powerful discipline (not physical, necessarily, but compelling nonetheless); the other presumes that the child can be talked, distracted, and gently prodded into behaving properly.

The premodern point of view is realistic, the postmodern idealistic. Symptomatic of the postmodern paradigm are ineffectual discipline practices, the most glaring example being time-outs, the most ineffectual discipline method ever devised. From the premodern point of view, there is nothing as tragically absurd as a mom making a seven-year-old who has just hit her in a fit of pique, sit in a chair for five minutes and "think about it." The premodern knows that under the circumstances, the child will almost certainly hit his mother again. And he does. (The child is later discovered to have childhood-onset bipolar disorder, of course.)

The premodern parent understood, intuitively, that the most advantageous time to deal with bad behavior—tantrums, belligerent defiance, disrespect, destructiveness—was when it first began to emerge during toddlerhood. This early intervention was called "nipping it in the bud." Between the premodern child's second and third birthdays, he or she was disciplined in a powerful resolute fashion. In so doing, the parents led the child out of toddlerhood into creative childhood.

In the process, the child's mother redefined herself to the child. By age two, he had every reason to believe his mother was his personal servant for life, there to do his bidding and cater to his every whim. By age three he saw her as a commanding, formidable (yet loving and approachable, take it from one who was there) authority figure, a person with whom he felt completely secure but whom he also knew was not to be trifled with. Simultaneously, the parents made it clear to the child that their relationship with one another, as opposed to their individual relationships with him, was paramount in the family. Everything changed during that critical transitional period, and toddlerhood was cured.

Postmodern psychological parenting does not and cannot cure toddlerhood. Compelling cultural and peer pressures encourage today's mother to perform as a servant to her child for the whole of his or her tenure at home (which begins to explain, in part, why the average age of emancipation in America has been inching ever upward since the early 1970s). In fact, servant in perpetuity is the new ideal in American motherhood. The message on today's "mother bar" reads thusly: The Mother Who Serves Her Child in the Busiest and Greatest Variety of Ways is the Best Mother. Today, the marriage is secondary to the mother–child relationship, and the perpetual toddler rules the home.

Whereas fifty years ago, it was "unheard of" (the words of many who were raising children at the time) for a child who had reached his or her third birthday to still be throwing tantrums, openly defying parental authority, and hitting parents in rages (all typical toddler behaviors), it is not at all unusual today to see school-age children exhibiting such behaviors when their parents displease them. These same children are likely to have problems paying attention in school, organizing schoolwork, staying on task, remembering things, and so on. This is not ADD, ODD, or COBD, and this sure as shootin' isn't about genes. This is toddlerhood in perpetuity, or TIP, the predictable result of parents—mothers mostly, although the "new" dad, in an effort to be his kids' best buddy, is close to catching up—lying in their children's beds, fighting their children's battles, paddling their children's canoes, and stewing in their children's juices.

Quite simply, you cannot raise children in two entirely different ways and expect to arrive at the same outcome. Premodern, traditional child rearing cured toddlerhood by age three. Postmodern psychological "parenting" perpetuates toddlerhood indefinitely. There is no mystery here, and there is no place in this equation for drugs. But I run ahead of myself.

A prime example of the toll postmodern psychological parenting has taken on both parenthood and childhood is the difference in average age of toilet training from 1958 to 2003. In the former year, a team of researchers from Harvard University (1958) determined that ninety-plus percent of children were toilet trained and virtually accident-free at twenty-four months. How does that possibly square with the contention of pediatrician/author T. Berry Brazelton (Brazelton & Sparrow, 2004) and others that it is difficult, at best, to toilet train a child below age two? Brazelton contends that trying to train a pre-two is possible but will likely result in the development of "toileting issues," which presumably last a lifetime. This is hogwash, psychobabble. Brazelton's propaganda, which serves no good except to increase the value of disposable diaper company stock, has the sole effect of extending toddlerhood, and often disastrously so. In addition to three-year-olds in diapers, other symptoms of extended toddlerhood in postmodern America include the preponderance of:

- Children older than thirty-six months being rolled through public places in portable thrones, otherwise known as strollers
- Children older than twenty-four months with pacifiers protruding prominently from the lower middle of their faces
- Children older than eighteen months drinking from "sippee cups" or, worse yet, bottles
- Elementary-age children who are still hitting their parents (their moms, mostly) when they become upset
- Children older than thirty-six months who are still biting other children

What purpose is served when mental health professionals manufacture and disseminate the lies in question? The answer has to do with the character of postmodernism, one feature of which is pragmatism. The nature of pragmatism was eloquently stated by popular psychologist Dr. Phil, who was recently quoted on Oprah Winfrey's Web site as saying that "It's not a matter of right or wrong; it's a matter of what works." (In contrast, the premodernist, of which I am one, would say, "It's not a matter of what works; it's a matter of what's right versus what's wrong.")

In the case of ADD, AHDH, and COBD, it matters not that the biogenetic hypothesis is unproven, unsupported by good science, and just downright illogical; it is functional. It serves a purpose; several in fact, all of which accrue, in the final analysis, to the benefit of the treating professional.

1. The child's parents, more specifically, the child's mother, is absolved of all responsibility for the problem. The postmodern mother—because her thinking about her child and childrearing is contaminated by a confusion of behavioral, Freudian, and humanistic ideas (i.e., psychobabble)—tends to believe that she is the cause and her child is the effect, that everything her child does or fails to do is the consequence of something she has done or failed to do in his life. His acceptance into the gifted and talented program is a testament to her dedication (she played Mozart to him when he was in her womb) and the sacrifices she has made for his intellectual betterment. The flip side of this, of course, is the fear that any problem her child develops is a result of some egregious mistake or failing on her part. So, the mother of a child whose behavior earns a ten on the vexing scale fears, more than anything, that *she* is the real culprit. If she had only let him sleep with her/not let him sleep with her, toilet trained him earlier/later, held him out of kindergarten for a year/not held him out of kindergarten, and so on, and so on, and so on, he would not have the problems in question.

2. The therapist, having magically lifted the parents'/mother's guilt, becomes, in their/her eyes, a "savior." This ensures that the parents will accept the therapist's recommendations, virtually without question.

3. Having nullified the possibility that the parents might bring some skepticism to the analysis/recommendations, the therapist is able to mystify the child's problems, a process that began with the unethical claim that tests were needed to confirm a diagnosis of ADD/ODD/COBD (need I remind that the DSM lists no test-based criteria for any of the foregoing?). This sells the parents on the spurious notion that the child's problems are the consequence of an inherited disease process or state that cannot be cured; rather, it can only be treated. The child's problems, from the parents' point of view, become unfathomable.

4. It follows that the therapist is able to "capture" the child and his parents as long-term clients and sell the parents on the notion that expensive medical therapies, that is, drugs, are necessary.

5. This leaves the therapist free to conduct time- and cost-inefficient individual therapy sessions with the child, wasting the parents' time and money.

6. The child, about whom the parents once said "drives us crazy," is redefined as a victim, now deserving special consideration, most especially from his teachers.
7. The child's parents have a "cause" they can champion, thus further mitigating the guilt they feel at having misunderstood, and therefore mishandled, their child.
8. The child is further insulated from responsibility for his behavior once he is placed on a "treatment program" involving drugs. Any subsequent upswing in bad behavior will simply be attributed to the need for an "adjustment" in his medication. Needless to say, this also serves to maintain the family's expensive relationship with the child's therapist.

A soap opera is born, with a cast of characters that features a gene (from the father, no doubt) as villain, mother and child as victims/sympathetic characters, the school as unsympathetic and insensitive (i.e., the child's teachers didn't recognize his "special needs" and therefore punished him when he did bad things), and the therapist as savior, redeemer, knight in shining armor. In short, the biogenetic hypothesis serves the interests of the mother, the therapist, the prescribing physician, and the manufacturer(s) of the drug(s) prescribed. The only person the biogenetic hypothesis does not benefit is the child.

One of the more stupid things professionals who specialize in the diagnosis and "treatment" of ADD, AHDH, and COBC tell me is that I am "blaming parents." In fact, the only blame I am assigning is to a mental health community that, with the help of a most cooperative media, sold postmodern psychological childrearing to American parents. Just as a culture can embrace a dysfunctional political philosophy (e.g., Germany, 1932), a culture can embrace a dysfunctional parenting philosophy, and America did exactly that in the 1960s and 1970s. Under the circumstances, today's parents cannot be "blamed" for thinking that the manner in which ninety-eight percent of their friends and neighbors are raising their kids is The One True and Right Way.

The charge that I am "blaming parents" is a clever means of reminding the mothers of the children in question that the disease model relieved them of their worst fear. Do they really want to listen to the likes of me? The problem, as the mental health community well knows by now, is that many of America's parents do take me seriously when I tell them that they should not trust the very profession that created the problem and that profits from the problem to solve the problem. The real issue is not that I am a threat to parents. The real issue is that I am a threat to a professional community that is out of control.

CODA

A friend of mine participates in a national network of pediatricians who share information and advice with one another through the Web. Certain of the exchanges leave him amused whereas others provoke his outrage. In the latter category was the recent response of a "highly thought of developmental/behavioral pediatrician" to another physician who asked about a twenty-six-month-old youngster who was keeping his parents up much of the night, most every night. In addition, the child was "very active" and prone to tantrums during the day.

The pediatrician in question responded to the effect that a diagnosis of ADHD might be appropriate, as lots of kids who are so diagnosed during their school years have similar histories. Excuse me? In the first place, it is equally true that a good number of kids who do just fine in school have similar histories. In addition, as I've pointed out, nearly every two-year-old exhibits the symptoms associated with and necessary to a diagnosis of attention deficit disorder. With few exceptions, two-year-olds are active and prone to fits when they don't get their way. The fits in question may even be wildly destructive. They are impulsive, often defiant, and "bounce" from one thing to another like pinballs. Problems with sleeping through the night are also common at this age. A two-year-old who may have slept through the night since the age of three months may suddenly begin waking up several times a night, creating a major disturbance each time.

None of these behaviors indicates that anything is "wrong." The daytime behaviors at issue result from a combination of the developmental state of the brain at this age and narcissism (some prefer "egocentricity"). The immature brain cannot focus on any one thing for any length of time and lacks the capacity to think "ahead," and the narcissist that emerges from behind the mask of infancy at around eighteen months of age cannot tolerate anyone getting in her way or denying her what she thinks is her due.

It is disturbing, to say the least, that a highly respected pediatrician—one who calls himself a developmental/behavioral pediatrician, no less!—would suggest that behaviors which are by no means abnormal at this age, behaviors which simply signal a need for powerful disciplinary measures grounded in an abundance of love, are cause for a diagnosis of any sort, much less ADHD. This implies that the child is a possible candidate for medication. As my friend pointed out, should the child wind up on the receiving end of one of the drugs used to "treat" ADHD, the child's parents will undoubtedly report fewer daytime discipline problems, including tantrums. That leaves the sleeping problems, for which the child's pediatrician might prescribe a second medication to which the child might well respond "positively." And in no time at all, we have yet another set of parents who are on their way to becoming addicted to giving their child drugs whenever a behavior problem rears its ugly little head.

This speaks to a dangerous drift in modern pediatrics: the tendency to isolate a child's behavior from its context and judge the behavior, rather than the parents' management of it, as the problem. If this drift continues we face a future where not only relatively few parents practice old-fashioned (i.e., effective) discipline, but one in which discipline itself has become old fashioned.

REFERENCES

Baumeister, R.F., Smart, L., & Boden, J.M. (1996). Relation of threatened egotism to violence and aggression. *Psychological Review, 103*, 5–33.

Brazelton, T. & Sparrow, J. (2004). *Toilet Training: The Brazelton Way.* New York: De Capo.

Carey, W. (2002). Patterns of childrearing. In R. Jensen & D. Cooper (Eds.) *Attention Deficit Disorder—State of the Science.* Kensington, NY: Civic Research Institute.

Carey, W. & Jablow, M.M. (1999). *Understanding Your Child's Temperament.* Philadelphia: Hungry Minds.

Gatto, J.T. (2000). *The Underground History of American Education.* New York: Oxford Village.

National Center for Education Statistics (2000, August). *Results Over Time: NAEP 1999 Long-Term Trend Summary Data Tables.* http://nces.ed.gov/nationalreportcard/tables/Ltt1999/(accessed July 6, 2003).

12

ABORTION, BOXING, AND ZIONISM: POLITICS AND THE APA

William T. O'Donohue and Christopher Dyslin

This chapter examines a number of resolutions issued by the American Psychological Association (APA), often through its Public Interest Directorate, that define the organization's stance on a wide range of political issues. A sampling of these resolutions appears throughout the text. The APA resolutions reflect positions on topics such as limiting access to abortions, AIDS education, the legality of boxing, corporal punishment, prevention of motor vehicle trauma, television violence and children, academic freedom, the Vietnam War, apartheid, condemning dissenters to mental hospitals, nuclear freeze, a federally funded peace academy, actions of UNESCO against the state of Israel, handgun control, usage of "Dr.," the Equal Rights Amendment, and a resolution expressing the APA's (1988, p. 43) "relief at the release of the American hostages from Iran."

PROPER CONDITIONS FOR APA-ISSUED POLITICAL RESOLUTIONS

The first question this chapter addresses is: to what extent is it proper and reasonable for the APA to articulate a position on these issues?

Politics has a direct impact on the ability of psychologists to do research and practice. For example, politics plays a major role in determining how much and what research is funded. Moreover, the government's recent involvement in healthcare reform involves the question of the reimbursibility of psychologists. Thus, although it would be imprudent for the APA to be entirely apolitical, the APA itself recognizes that an organization may be "politic[ized] and diver[ted] from its original principles and purposes" (1988, p. 48). This raises another aspect of the question: by taking these positions has the APA become politicized and diverted from its legitimate principles and purposes?

The APA sees itself as broadly committed to enhancing human welfare (e.g., APA, 1992), and this may be part of the rationale to become involved in these issues, which obviously can have a strong impact on human well-being. Raymond Fowler, in his capacity as the chief executive officer of the APA, has stated:

> Few would deny that in keeping with our mission of promoting human welfare, APA has a responsibility to share the literature of psychology. However, the membership has long debated whether our responsibility extends to taking a more active stance, passing resolutions and advocating for our positions. Over the years, interpretations of our mission have been debated, broadened and narrowed several times. (1993, p.2)

Psychological Issues in the Abortion Debate

Whereas, in 1969, the APA identified freedom of reproductive choice as a mental health and child welfare issue; whereas, the APA Council of Representatives decries the uninformed movement in many state legislatures to recriminalize abortion or limit access to the full range of reproductive options, especially to poor women who use publicly funded health services; whereas, erroneous assertions about widespread severe negative psychological effects of abortion are being used to argue for laws that restrict reproductive freedom; whereas, a review of the best scientific evidence by an APA panel of experts finds these assertions to be without basis in fact; whereas, uninformed public statements and a lack of understanding about psychological responses after unwanted pregnancy and abortion can themselves create emotional distress; whereas, "the weight of the evidence is that legal abortion as a resolution to an unwanted pregnancy, particularly in the first trimester, does not create psychological hazards for most women undergoing the procedure"; and, whereas, the preponderance of scientific data supports the conclusion that freedom of choice and a woman's control over her critical life decisions promote psychological health; therefore, be it moved that the Council of Representatives of the APA directs the Executive Vice President and Chief Executive Officer to undertake an immediate initiative to disseminate scientific information on reproductive freedom to policy-makers, to the public, and to state psychological associations and APA divisions. This initiative will have top priority and will include suggestions for action to be presented to state associations and divisions. In order to implement this resolution, the Council directs the development of a staff working group, including representatives of each Directorate and the Media Relations office, to gather the scientific data and disseminate it to the public and to the state associations and divisions.

Adler (1989)

The standards for promoting human welfare are so broad that they lack any real substance. Would any organization commit itself to indifference or resistance to the promotion of human welfare? Moreover, enhancing human welfare would appear to require the APA to do more than simply take a position on a political question. Two other conditions also need to be met: (1) The position taken by the APA needs to be the correct position, because incorrect positions could negatively affect human welfare, and (2) the negative collateral effects (e.g., alienating dissenters) of the APA's position need to be less than the advantages.

What is the evidence that the APA has actually taken the correct position on political issues? Unfortunately, there is little. This is not to say that the APA has taken the incorrect position, but rather that in many cases the evidence is such that informed and reasonable people can formulate diverse positions on the issue. Abortion is a case in point. The APA has taken a strong stance in supporting the "reproductive rights" of women and calling efforts in state legislatures to restrict abortions "uninformed" (APA Council of Representatives, 1989, p. 1). However, the APA does not cite any—yet alone compelling—evidence that suggests its position on this divisive issue is the obviously "informed" and correct one.

Stances Need Strong Research Backup

Our point is not that the APA has taken the wrong position on issues, but that it is incumbent upon the association to offer strong evidence for asserting its position (particularly before pejorative attributions are published about opposing positions. Unfortunately, the APA usually offers no supporting evidence, which leads to a number of negative consequences: the possibility of error and attendant harm; the impression of an epistemological irrationalism or dogmatism by failing to cite or search for evidence that bears on the question; and the failure to educate.

At this juncture it is important to raise another question: why has the APA made resolutions on these particular issues? The association has been conspicuously silent on other issues that affect human welfare such as the environment, education reform, capital punishment, and international monetary policy. We suggest that an excellent reason for choosing particular issues to address would be that psychologists have expertise relevant to the controversy. This is consistent with the Tyler (1969) report, which suggests that the APA confine its political activities to positions where there is "solid supporting research data" (Fowler, 1993, p. 2).

Boxing

In 1985, the Council adopted the following resolution:

WHEREAS, recent studies show that existing medical controls and safety measures have not prevented chronic brain damage in boxers who have fought in recent years (after 1960), and WHEREAS, neuropsychological testing is a highly sensitive and accurate means of detecting brain damage in fighters and others with head injuries, and WHEREAS, many psychologists educate the public and especially young people through courses and textbooks, and WHEREAS, resolutions calling for the elimination of both amateur and professional boxing have been passed recently by the American Medical Association and the British Medical Association, BE IT RESOLVED that the American Psychological Association: encourage the elimination of both amateur and professional boxing, a sport in which the objective is to inflict injury; communicate its opposition to boxing to appropriate regulating bodies; assist state psychological societies to work with their state legislatures to enact laws to eliminate boxing in their jurisdictions; educate the American public, especially children and young adults, about the dangerous effects of boxing on the health of participants; specifically, psychologists who give courses and who write textbooks that take up relations between behavior and the nervous system are asked to consider including material on boxing and brain damage in their courses and textbooks; encourage neuropsychological evaluations of boxers be given on a periodic (one to two year) basis; and encourage ring-side evaluations during bouts be done by individuals who are trained to perform neurocognitive investigations of acute mental status change.

However, as the examples sprinkled throughout this chapter show, the APA's resolutions egregiously omit any direct citation of the literature with one noteworthy exception, that of the insanity defense. Rather, the resolutions tend to offer very sweeping and vague summaries: for example, "Whereas, unfortunately *unsubstantiated psychological theories and research* have, nevertheless, been misused to justify discrimination against women and to oppose the Equal Rights Amendment" (APA, 1988, p. 59, italics added); and "Whereas, erroneous assertions about widespread severe negative psychological effects of abortion are being used to argue for laws that restrict reproductive freedom" (APA Council of Representatives, 1989, p. 1).

This is obscurantist. What exactly is this "unsubstantiated research?" And, for that matter, what exactly is unsubstantiated research? For its resolutions to be anything more than pejorative rhetoric, the APA needs to document the research to which these vague claims actually refer. If this research is published, are we to assume that the peer review process failed in that it is actually without any merit? The APA should be consistent with its stated policy and explicitly substantiate its claims by reviewing relevant psychological research. This would have all the advantages that typically accrue to a well-documented and well-argued case, including enabling others to learn their own errors and exposing the APA's evidence to the light of criticism so that improvements can be made. If psychologists fail to do this, how are they acting consistently as scientists and scholars?

The most cynical reason that can be given for the general absence of cited research is that there is simply no relevant research that can be brought to bear on the question. For example, in its resolution equating Zionism with racism, the APA states that the United Nation's General Assembly resolution is a "political distortion of the meaning of racism" (APA, 1988, p. 49). How are psychologists experts on the meaning of racism? What data bear on this? Moreover, this resolution goes on to state:

> Wishing to continue its support of the principles on which the United Nations was founded, and concerned about the divisive effects of the process of politicalization, the American Psychological Association joins with other professional, scholarly,

and scientific bodies calling on the United Nations to *reassert its ideals, return to its original goals, and halt the destructive politicalization of its specialized agencies.*

APA (1988, p. 49, emphasis added)

How are we as psychologists experts on the ideals and original goals of the United Nations?

Children

Corporal punishment

In 1974, the Council adopted the following resolution on corporal punishment:

WHEREAS: The resort to *corporal* punishment tends to reduce the likelihood of employing more effective, humane, and creative ways of interacting with children; WHEREAS: It is evident that socially acceptable goals of education, training, and socialization can be achieved without the use of physical violence against children, and that children so raised, grow to moral and competent adulthood; WHEREAS: *Corporal* punishment intended to influence "undesirable responses" may create in the child the impression that he or she is an "undesirable person"; and an impression that lowers self-esteem and may have chronic consequences; WHEREAS: Research has shown that to a considerable extent children learn by imitating the behavior of adults, especially those they are dependent upon; and the use of *corporal* punishment by adults having authority over children is likely to train children to use physical violence to control behavior rather than rational persuasion, education, and intelligent forms of both positive and negative reinforcement; WHEREAS: Research has shown that the effective use of punishment in eliminating undesirable behavior requires precision in timing, duration, intensity, and specificity, as well a considerable sophistication in controlling a variety of relevant environmental and cognitive factors, such that punishment administered in institutional settings, without attention to all these factors, is likely to instill hostility, rage, and a sense of powerlessness without reducing the undesirable behavior; THEREFORE BE IT RESOLVED that the American Psychological Association opposes the use of *corporal* punishment in schools, juvenile facilities, child care nurseries and all other institutions, public or private, where children are cared for or educated.

In other cases, the APA has taken positions not only on desirable political ends but also on the means by which these ends should be pursued. For example, "….the American Psychological Association deplore and reject the apartheid system; *support efforts of institutions to divest themselves of holdings in companies which do business in South Africa….*" (APA, 1988, p. 39, italics added). In this case the APA conflates the ends of eliminating apartheid with the much more controversial methods of economic sanctions. Again, what data or expertise do psychologists have that bears on the merits of economic divestment as the best means by which to end apartheid?

In fact, in the most egregious example, the APA states a position while simultaneously asserting the irrelevancy of psychological theories and research: "Whereas, *psychological theories and research* should have no bearing upon the desirability of the Equal Rights Amendment, which is a matter of human rights rather than of scientific fact; … " but then "resolves to support the passage of the Equal Rights Amendment" (APA, 1988, p. 59). The question then becomes: on what grounds does the APA offer its support?

It appears that the APA has not decided to confine its political commitments to issues upon which psychologists have some legitimate expertise. Rather, the association has given itself great latitude in weighing in on a number of issues on which it has no legitimate expertise. One possible unwanted outcome of this political promiscuity is that when psychologists take a stand on issues about which they actually do have legitimate expertise, the impact or perception of this position might be negatively affected. A further problem is that when its resolutions are tenuously or not at all based on data, errors are more likely. The APA has to countenance the possibility that these resolutions are wrong, and that in being wrong harm can be done. Thus, it becomes vital for the APA to minimize error by explicitly considering data and argument when making its resolutions.

Television Violence and Children

In 1984, the Council adopted the following resolution on television violence and children:

WHEREAS, the great majority of research studies have found a relationship between televised violence and behaving aggressively, and WHEREAS, the conclusion drawn on the basis of 25 years of research and a sizable number of experimental and field investigations is that viewing televised violence may lead to increases in aggressive attitudes, values, and behavior, particularly in children, and WHEREAS, many children's programs contain some form of violence, BE IT RESOLVED that the American Psychological Association (1) encourages parents to monitor and to control television viewing by children (2) requests industry representatives to take a responsible attitude in reducing direct imitatable violence on "real-life" fictional children's programming or violent incidents on cartoons, and in providing more programming for children designed to mitigate possible effects of television violence, consistent with the guarantees of the First Amendment; and (3) urge industry, government, and private foundations to support relevant research activities aimed at the amelioration of the effects of high levels of televised violence on children's attitudes and behaviors.

The Truth about Consequences

We also suggest that another criterion needs to be met in order for the APA to make a resolution on a political issue: that is, the collateral effects of the position taken need to be outweighed by the advantages of taking the position. By collateral effects we mean the consequences for dissenting psychologists when their professional organization takes a political stance that they do not agree with, the effects on the public's perceptions of the organization, and the effects on the political issue.

Political commitments by a professional organization have consequences for professionals who participate in the organization. Psychologists may have an interest in becoming APA members for the professional benefits that are gained by this association, for example, access to information, professional insurance, and the like. However, the APA's political positions can result in alienating or placing dissenting psychologists in a difficult bind. The APA's position on what it biasedly and tendentiously calls "reproductive choice" is a case in point. The association states that it has "identified freedom of reproductive choice as a mental health and child welfare issue" and resolves that the "termination of pregnancy be considered a civil right of the pregnant woman" (APA Council of Representatives, 1989, p. 1).

Abortion is a divisive and controversial issue. The APA's resolution obviously places those who hold a dissenting view (including but not limited to practicing Roman Catholics) in a difficult position. Do they want to belong to an organization that advocates a position that they consider immoral? Or, as they might phrase it, should they be a member of an organization that condones the "killing of babies?" Unless the APA has extremely compelling data to show the utter illegitimacy of the anti-abortion stance, it might be prudent not to take a position on this divisive issue, both out of respect for the diversity of opinion surrounding this issue and to avoid placing member-psychologists in an unnecessarily difficult situation.

In addition, by taking these positions, the APA might be undercutting its credibility. Failure to insist upon compelling evidence before taking political positions may give the APA the appearance of a quasipolitical organization rather than a scientific and professional organization. It should be noted that psychologists *qua* concerned citizens can express their political views through genuinely political organizations or can form separate political organizations that deal with political issues in the mode of Physicians for Social Responsibility.

International

Apartheid

In 1986, the Council adopted the following resolution:

WHEREAS, the government of South Africa has persistently denied basic human rights to Black South Africans, and, in fact, has encouraged arbitrary arrests, brutal beatings, and the detention of Blacks for purposes of political repression; and WHEREAS, the government of South Africa has intentionally disrupted Black family life through the practice of forceable relocation and separation; and WHEREAS, the government of South Africa has legislated censorship and repression of national and international communications; and WHEREAS, the government of South Africa has through its police incursions on college campuses revoked the academic freedom which is essential to university life; BE IT RESOLVED that the American Psychological Association deplores and rejects the apartheid system; supports efforts of institutions to divest themselves of holdings in companies which do business in South Africa; encourages the United States government to develop meaningful sanctions against the White minority government in South Africa with the intention of motivating political and social reforms; and urges American psychologists to refuse to collaborate in projects sponsored by the South African government until human rights reforms are instituted.

In various places the APA Ethical Code (APA, 1992) makes reference to limiting the psychologists' behavior to the boundaries of their competence. For example, Principle F states that "psychologists try to avoid misuse of their work" (p. 1600). Standard 1.06 states that "psychologists rely on scientifically and professionally derived knowledge when making scientific or professional judgments or when engaging in scholarly or professional endeavors" (p. 1600). Principle 3.03 states that "psychologists do not make public statements that are false, deceptive, misleading, or fraudulent, either because of what they state, convey, or suggest or because of what they omit concerning their research, practice, or other work activities or those of person or organization with which they are affiliated" (p. 1604). This raises the question of whether the APA's resolutions rely on scientific and professional knowledge, misuse the research of psychologists, or are false and misleading because of what they state or omit.

A case in point is the resolution on psychological issues in the abortion debate: "The APA Council of Representatives decries the *uninformed movement* in many state legislatures to recriminalize abortion or limit access to the full range of reproductive options ..." (APA Council of Representatives, 1989, p. 1). On what scientific basis does the APA indicate that certain movements by democratically elected officials are *uninformed?* Does this go beyond the scientific data?

It also is noteworthy that the resolutions of the APA tend to represent only a select portion of the political spectrum. This was recognized by Fox (1993), who indicated that the APA tends to advocate liberal/leftist positions and suggested that the APA move toward a more radical leftist position. This raises the possibility that the APA has become illegitimately politicized by those who have a certain agenda. There are better avenues of expressing this viewpoint other than a professional scientific organization that should be open to individuals of all political persuasions.

This raises the third issue: the relationship between the APA's resolutions and the democratic procedures that comprise the American constitutional political process. For example, if individuals in certain states have elected individuals based partly on their promises to enact certain legislation regarding abortion, what basis does the APA have for calling this "uninformed?" This may simply be the democratic process at work: the will of the people being expressed. Psychologists are not a representative sample of Americans and, therefore, may have political interests and biases different from those expressed through democratically determined processes. If the APA truly regards this as uninformed, then perhaps it needs to explicate the information that it feels is missing. Its role is more properly one of teaching (where knowledge exists) rather than pejorative name calling. One also might wonder whether an authoritarian, antidemocratic element drives the APA's actions when it directly opposes and in some cases attempts to sanction (e.g., not holding its meetings in states whose democratically elected representatives did not pass the Equal Rights Amendment) the resolutions of democratic processes.

Moreover, the possibility exists that the APA's resolutions might have some influence on the political process. How does the nonpsychologist react when he or she hears that the APA has taken these stands? It is reasonable to hypothesize that at least a certain subset of individuals may interpret the resolutions as indicating that there is compelling psychological evidence behind these positions. For example, a nonpsychologist might interpret the resolution concerning reproductive rights as a psychological fact that efforts at legislating restrictions are uninformed. Lacking such evidence, these resolutions then distort the political process by creating misinformation. These issues are important and should be considered clearly and accurately. Thus, although the APA takes issue with "political interference" in awarding research funds, (APA Council of Representatives, 1989, p. 1), it does not seem to view its own behavior as "interference" in the political process.

Nuclear Freeze

In 1982, the Council adopted the following statement:

The American Psychological Association (1) calls upon the President of the United States to propose to the U.S.S.R. that together both countries negotiate an immediate halt to the nuclear arms race. Specifically, we call upon each country to adopt an immediate mutual freeze on all further testing, production, and deployment of all nuclear warheads, missiles, and delivery systems; and (2) calls upon the Administration and the Congress to transfer the funds saved to civilian use. Concurrently, they should work jointly with labor, management, and local communities to develop plans to convert the nuclear arms industry to civilian production, thus protecting jobs and strengthening our national economy. We hereby call upon elected officials at local, state, and federal levels publicly to endorse this resolution.

SCRUTINIZING THE APA'S OWN POLITICAL PROCESS

Before examining how just and reasonable APA's resolution process is, it is necessary to examine the stated purpose of the APA, the organization's structure, how its elected officers represent the membership, and the process by which the organization develops, approves, and publishes its resolutions.

The Purpose of the APA

The purpose of the organization is stated as Article One of the APA's *Bylaws:*

> The objects of the American Psychological Association shall be to advance psychology as a science and profession and as a means of promoting human welfare by the encouragement of psychology in all its branches in the broadest and most liberal manner; by the promotion of research in psychology and the improvement of research methods and conditions; by the improvement of the qualifications and usefulness of psychologists through high standards of ethics, conduct, education, and achievement; by the establishment and maintenance of the highest standards of professional ethics and conduct of the members of the Association; by the increase and diffusion of psychological knowledge through meetings, professional contacts, reports, papers, discussions, and publications; thereby to advance scientific interests and inquiry, and the application of research findings to the promotion of the public welfare.

> *APA, Council of Representatives (1989, p. 1)*

U.N. General Assembly Resolution Equating Zionism with Racism

In 1977, the Council adopted the following statement:

The Council of Representatives of the American Psychological Association shares the widely expressed distress with the United Nations General Assembly Resolution which holds that Zionism is a form of racism and racial discrimination. This political distortion of the meaning of racism is unacceptable to scientific researchers and professional practitioners in psychology. Wishing to continue its support of the principles on which the United Nations was founded, and concerned about the divisive effects of the process of politicization, the American Psychological Association joins with other professional, scholarly, and scientific bodies calling on the United Nations to reassess its ideals, return to its original goals, and halt the destructive politicization of its specialized agencies. In addition, as an indication of its vigilance and concern, the Council urges the Board of Directors through its Committee on International Relations in Psychology to continue monitoring the evolving United Nations scene and to present periodically to the Council a status report with recommendations as appropriate.

The Organization's Structure

The structure of the APA, as articulated in its bylaws (APA Council of Representatives, 1989), consists of its membership, several elected officers (past president, president, president-elect, recording secretary, treasurer, and chief-staff officer), a board of directors (comprising the aforementioned elected officers and six other members elected by and from the previous Council of Representatives), and the Council of Representatives. The elected Council of Representatives is the legislative body with "full power and authority over the affairs and funds of the Association ... including the power to review upon its own initiative the actions of any board, committee, Division, or affiliated organization" (p. 7).

The Representation of Members

Members of the APA are allowed input in the decision-making process of the organization. Any member can petition one percent of the voting membership to request that the Council of Representatives generate a mail vote on any issue that does not contradict the APA bylaws (APA Council of Representatives, 1989). The petition process is the only avenue available to APA members who are not also members of a state psychological association or division of the APA but wish to be involved in the organization's decision-making and legislation. Because members of the Council of Representatives, which creates all APA resolutions, are elected by state and division votes, the many psychologists who are members only of the national organization have no representation when it comes to policy-making other than the APA president, who is elected by the voting membership of the national organization.

Women

Equal Rights Amendment

In 1975, the Council adopted the following resolution statement on the ERA:

WHEREAS, psychological theories and research should have no bearing upon the desirability of the Equal Rights Amendment, which is a matter of human rights rather than of scientific fact; WHEREAS, unfortunately, unsubstantiated psychological theories and research have, nevertheless, been misused to justify discrimination against women and to oppose the Equal Rights Amendment; BE IT RESOLVED that the American Psychological Association (a) asserts that arguments linking sex differences and their origins to the desirability of the Equal Rights Amendment are specious and without foundation; (b) deplores these misuses of psychological theories; (c) supports the passage of the Equal Rights Amendment.

The Policy-Making Process

An APA resolution developed by the Council of Representatives or by a board or committee of the governance structure must be approved by the Board of Directors before going to the Council for the final vote. The Council meets at the annual convention and or at special meetings arranged in advance by a majority vote. Resolutions are passed by a majority vote of the Council, and proceedings of the Council's meetings are published in the APA Council policy reference book as well as in press releases. The APA bylaws point out that "meetings of Council except those specifically designated as executive sessions, shall be open to members of the Association, but they may not speak or otherwise participate in the meeting unless specifically invited to do so by the President" (APA Council of Representatives, 1989, p. 8).

Is the Process Just?

When one considers a just process for legislation, the U.S. political system can arguably be used as a paradigmatic example. Some of the things that make the U.S. government's legislative system just are: a system of checks and balances (e.g., the countervailing powers of the three branches of government); the use of debate and hearings on legislative issues that are open to the public; a process that is open to expert testimony (e.g., *amicus* briefs); and the individual accountability derived from making voting records of the elected legislators available to the public.

An examination of the APA's process for developing resolutions indicates a discrepancy between the existing process and what most would consider a just and reasonable process. There are a number of areas where the organization falters. APA members who do not belong to an APA division or a state psychological association are not equally represented on the Council of Representatives, which formulates and votes on resolutions. The presidents of the APA, who do sit on the Council of Representatives and are elected by the general membership, have not publicly presented their ideas in official statements released during the elections on the political issues that are voted on by the Council.

A perusal of the pre-election statements in the May 1993 issue of the *APA Monitor on Psychology* (American Psychological Association, 1993) shows that only one of the five candidates made specific reference to their positions on any political issue and that election guidelines require candidates to confine their statements to psychological issues. A look at every subsequent election issue of the APA *Monitor* reveals that in most years not one of the five candidates addressed any political issue other than that of defeating managed care—which is more of a practice issue than a political one.

Although some Council meetings are open to the general membership, the membership does not have the right to participate. Because the voting records of Council members are not published and distributed to members, and because the APA's resolutions are not published or distributed to prospective members, it is difficult for members and potential members to access the actual proceedings of previous Council meetings and the APA resolutions approved. Thus, new members may be unaware of the political positions of the organization they are joining.

In 1977, the Council Adopted the Following Resolution

The Council reaffirms its action of January 1977 declaring that the APA shall not hold its convention in states that have not ratified the equal rights amendment (ERA). In view of ambiguities concerning the contractual status of agreements with Atlanta, New Orleans, and Las Vegas at the time of that vote, the Council now declares that the policy applies regardless of understandings of commitments undertaken prior to the establishment of this policy. The Board of Directors, with the advice of the Board of Convention Affairs, is instructed to implement this policy with practical regard for the necessary timing of commitments to alternate sites. Further, Council directs the Board of Directors to terminate existing letters of agreement with the cities of Atlanta, New Orleans, and Las Vegas following the close of the next scheduled session of the Georgia legislature and the winter 1978 and 1979 sessions of the Louisiana and Nevada legislatures, should any or all of those state legislatures fail to reverse their previous votes on the equal rights amendment.

PROPOSALS

First, we recommend that the APA constrain its political activity to issues in which psychologists have legitimate expertise. Defining "legitimate expertise" can be partly accomplished by following a second recommendation: that in taking a political position the APA adhere to its own ethical stipulations regarding public statements and the description of research findings. The evidence available on the issue should be honestly and fairly presented, including its weaknesses and alternative interpretations. This would prevent the APA from taking a partisan position and ensure that resolutions are committed to the search for an accurate understanding of the phenomenon in question. Documents supporting the resolutions might take the form of critical literature reviews. This approach would allow the APA to offer evidence for its position and offer an opportunity for others to respond substantively to the data and arguments.

This approach would be more consistent with an educative, rather than a politically partisan, role. Moreover, it might serve as an impetus for psychologists to conduct research and seek relevant information, therefore adding knowledge rather than more opinion to the political process. For example, we could argue that it is good to take a position opposing apartheid; however, if an APA resolution opposing apartheid is not based on research evidence, it has no value other than political opinion. As psychologists we should be taking a scientific approach and issuing data-based resolutions that would provide added value to the public.

The following motion, said to have been adopted by unanimous consent at the August 1977 Council meeting, was noted

Assuming passage by a state of the ERA, and given that the APA is a national association, it is moved that the annual convention of the Association may be held in any state of the Union that has passed the ERA or, on occasion, in view of the substantial relationship with Canada (Article XII, Section I of the APA Bylaws states that "the provinces of Canada are to be regarded as the equivalent of states"), in any major metropolitan area of Canada.

Implementation of our proposed solution may have the "unwanted" consequence of constraining the range of political issues on which the APA takes positions. However, psychologists must be reminded that there are other political organizations in which they can participate, and there is always the possibility of forming a separate politically oriented organization for psychologists.

In order to respect diversity of opinion, it is recommended that the APA encourage the expression of minority and dissenting opinions. These opinions should be given similar opportunities to be expressed and published.

Finally, the constraints proposed in the Tyler (1969, p. 1) report still seem appropriate, although not practiced:

> In considering which particular action to take among those within the permissible range, the decision makers would use criteria that constitute additional constraints: 1. The importance of the problem area (primarily to psychologists, but also to society as a whole). 2. The amount of research-based information available. 3. The extent of value agreement on the issue among APA members. 4. The probability that the action will be effective.

It seems that only the first criterion affects current practice inasmuch as we have previously documented the disjunction of resolutions and research data. Moreover, plebiscites of APA members have not been taken regarding these issues so the degree of value consensus is unknown, and there is no outcome data on the impact and/or effectiveness of these resolutions. Thus, it appears that the APA utilizes these sound constraint criteria for rhetorical value and not for guiding its political involvement. The APA would better serve its members and the public if it brought its actions in line with these constraints and proposals.

REFERENCES

Adler, N.E. (1989) The medical and psychological impact of abortion on women. Testimony on behalf of the American Psychological Association before the U.S. House of Representatives, Committee on Government Operations, Subcommittee on Human Resources and Intergovernmental Relations, 16 March, 1989. Washington, DC: APA Council of Representatives.

American Psychological Association. (1988). *APA Council Policy: Reference Book*. Washington, DC: Author.

American Psychological Association. (1989). *Bylaws*. Washington, DC: Author.

American Psychological Association. (1992). Ethical principles of psychologists and code of conduct (revised). *American Psychologist, 47*, 1597–1611.

American Psychological Association (1993). In APA annual election, five go the distance. *APA Monitor*, May, p. 4.

American Psychological Association Council of Representatives (1989). Psychological issues in the abortion debate. Unpublished manuscript.

Carter, L.F. (1956). Proceedings of the sixty-fourth annual business meeting of the American Psychological Association, Chicago, IL. *American Psychologist, 11*, 595–603.

Fowler, R.D. (1993). Social issues stances: Why APA takes them. *APA Monitor,* April, p. 2.

Fox, D.R. (1993): Psychological jurisprudence and radical social change. *American Psychologist, 48,* 234–241.

Miller, G.A. (1969). Psychology as a means of promoting human welfare. *American Psychologist, 24,* 1063–1075.

Tyler, L. (1969). An approach to public affairs: Report of the Ad Hoc Committee on Public Affairs. *American Psychologist, 24,* 1–4.

13

THE DUMBING DOWN OF PSYCHOLOGY: FAULTY BELIEFS ABOUT BOUNDARY CROSSINGS AND DUAL RELATIONSHIPS

Ofer Zur

This chapter investigates the nature of commonly held and misguided beliefs regarding the "evils" of boundary crossings and dual relationships in psychotherapy: that they are essentially unethical, illegal, harmful, and likely to lead to exploitation of clients (Bersoff, 1999; Koocher & Keith-Spiegel, 1998; Pope & Vasquez, 1998). Boundary issues and dual relationships in psychotherapy have been highly controversial subjects among psychotherapists for a long time. Ethics and law courses and risk management seminars have warned about the quicksand of dual relationships and instructed therapists to avoid them like the plague (Lazarus & Zur, 2002). Despite there being no credible evidence to support the belief in the depravity of boundary crossings and dual relationships, these terms have been used synonymously with harm and exploitation and have been baselessly linked to sex.

Nonsexual relationships in psychotherapy, our focus here, include situations where multiple roles exist between a therapist and a client. Such relationships are normal, healthy, and unavoidable elements of country and small town living and reflect the natural intimacy of many other societal groups with a shared culture, including the disabled, gays, and closed minority groups (e.g., American Indians). Other dual relationships occur when the psychotherapy client and the therapist are fellow students or members of the same church, synagogue, AA fellowship, or political party action group. They can be academic or professional colleagues, friends, parents of children who attend the same school, or fellow players in a local recreational league.

Boundary crossings in psychotherapy encompass any deviation from traditional, rigid, strict, "only in the office," antiquated, emotionally distant forms of therapy that were established by classic psychoanalysis almost a century ago. They refer to issues of self-disclosure, length, and place of sessions, physical touch, activities outside the office, gift exchange, social, and other forms of dual relationships. Boundary crossings are often part of well-formulated treatment plans or evidence (research)-based treatments (EBT). Examples include flying in an airplane with a patient who suffers from a fear of flying, having lunch with an anorexic patient, making a home visit to a bedridden patient, going for a vigorous walk with a depressed patient, or accompanying a patient to a dreaded but medically essential doctor's appointment to which he or she would not go alone. Robin Williams, playing the counselor in the movie *Good Will Hunting*, uses boundary crossing when he decides to break the ice by taking the highly resistant and distrustful young client, played by Matt Damon, to the riverbank for a walk. Other potentially helpful boundary crossings include giving a nonsexual hug, sending cards, exchanging appropriate gifts, lending a book, attending a wedding, confirmation, Bar Mitzvah, or funeral, or going to see a client-actor perform in a show.

Boundary violations, unlike boundary crossings, refer to situations where therapists violate clients' boundaries by physically, financially, or sexually exploiting them. Accepting a large sum of money as a gift or having sexual relations with a current client are clearly boundary violations, however, it is very tricky to define most other boundary violations because the harm or violation is frequently in the eye of the beholder, especially in a culture like ours that seems to encourage and support those who perceive themselves as victims.

Although the common advice from most ethicists, supervisors, risk management instructors, and attorneys is to avoid all boundary crossings and dual relationships, the reality is that in many situations it is neither advisable nor possible to do so. Often such boundary crossings as hugging a grieving mother or going to an open space with an agoraphobic patient constitute the most helpful, effective, and reasonable interventions. In many settings such as rural areas, military bases, and religious communities, dual relationships are impossible to avoid; in fact, it would be unwise to do so (Lazarus & Zur, 2002). Nevertheless, many psychotherapists hold the persistent, unrealistic, and irrational belief that boundary crossings and dual relationships are inherently harmful and exploitative, and should, therefore, be scrupulously avoided.

The boundary-crossing dogma and the dual relationships prohibition are examples of how self-serving dogmas are justified, rationalized, popularized, perpetuated, and enforced in the field of psychology and counseling. Our goal is to shed light on how and why the dogma concerning the depravity of boundary crossings and dual relationships has taken hold of the entire profession and why the rigid, analytic-risk-management approach to therapy and ethics has come to dominate. It is fascinating to observe that a profession composed mostly of nonpsychoanalytic practitioners has come to abide by strict or even cartoon-like versions of psychoanalytic theory. Of even greater concern is that educated and intelligent professionals have been transformed into frightened clinicians who too often unprofessionally, unethically, and even immorally place their own fears ahead of the care of clients.

Nonanalytic, intrinsically communal, and relationally oriented professionals have come to endorse separation, segregation, and isolation as the basis for their practices. It is also noteworthy that psychology, which has a widely advertised and highly visible commitment to cultural diversity, actually mandates rigid adherence to mainstream Western culture's emphasis on separation, individualism, and independence over connection, mutuality, and interdependency. Another interesting peculiarity is that therapists, who are often hired to challenge their clients' flawed cognitions and help them think critically, have developed an uncritical and self-serving tunnel vision when it comes to boundary crossings and dual relationships.

This chapter does not intend to give a blanket endorsement to dismantling therapeutic boundaries or promote the indiscriminant employment of dual relationships in therapy. Its intention is to emphasize that the goal of the therapist should be the client's care, healing, dignity, and well-being rather than the avoidance of risk or blind adherence to a certain treatment dogma. Like any clinical intervention, dual relationships and boundary crossings should be intentionally employed only when they are likely to increase therapeutic effectiveness, and as an integral part of a well-articulated, flexible treatment plan based on each client's specific problem, situation, and needs.

ETHICS CODES FOR DUAL RELATIONSHIPS

The ethics codes of most professional psychotherapist organizations frown on dual relationships. Although they do not declare dual relationships unethical, they are bluntly biased against them (Zur, 2002). The American Psychological Association (2002), and all other major professional psychotherapy associations—including the American Association for Marriage and Family Therapists (2001), American Counseling Association (1996), and the National Association of Social Workers (1999)—have very slowly and grudgingly changed their ethical guidelines in the last two decades to reflect the reality that dual relationships are inevitable in many settings. Still, all these codes are very wary about dual relationships, and several mandate the avoidance of dual relationships when possible (Lazarus & Zur, 2002). The codes encourage cultural diversity and sensitivity, but on the other hand, they indirectly view cultures that uphold values such as mutuality, interdependence, and familiarity between caretakers and clients as inferior.

Part of the dumbing down of psychology is that we enshrine ethics codes as sacred documents rather than examine them critically. "I say read the code weekly, but if not weekly, at least monthly," states Ed Nottingham, an associate member of APA's Ethics Committee, who was lauded by the *APA Monitor* (Smith, 2003, p.61). Canter and her coauthors, Bennet, Jones, and Nagy (1996), like most experts on ethics, list knowledge of the Ethics Code as a starting point for ethical decision making. Knowing the Code is important, however, the priorities should be to train ourselves in critical thinking and calibrate our moral compasses. We must explore the relevant cultural issues involved and identify our biases and self-serving beliefs. The Code of Ethics should be treated as a professional and political work in progress, not as a sacred document.

In fact, we have allowed the trivialization of the codes of ethics by including a special section that cautions therapists about dual relationships. This is utterly unnecessary because the codes already lay out the mandate to avoid exploitation and do no harm. It is demeaning and patronizing to presume that therapists are incapable of making clinical or treatment decisions on their own, that they cannot apply the "no harm" mandate to dual relationships without committing some egregious sin.

THE MISGUIDED REJECTION OF DUAL RELATIONSHIPS

A stubborn and irrational perception regarding the so-called evils of boundary crossings and dual relationships persists throughout the profession. Dual relationships, in particular, have been considered illegal (California Board of Psychology, 2001; Evans, 1997; Strasburger, Jorgenson, & Sutherland, 1992), unethical (Austin, 1998; Bennett, Bricklin, & VandeCreek, 1994; Bersoff, 1999; Claiborn, Berberoglu, Nerison, & Somberg, 1994; Epstein, Simon, & Kay, 1992; Gutheil & Gabbard, 1993; Pope, 1988), harmful (Brown, 1994; Epstein & Simon, 1990; Doverspike (1999); Kitchener, 1988; Koocher & Keith-Spiegel, 1998), and exploitative (Austin, 1998; Craig, 1991; Keith-Spiegel & Koocher, 1985; Lakin, 1991; Simon, 1989; St. Germaine, 1996).

These same widespread beliefs aver that dual relationships also interfere with clinical work (Bersoff, 1996; Borys, 1994; Faulkner & Faulkner, 1997; Gottlieb, 1993; Langs, 1974; Pepper, 1991) and violate professional boundaries (Borys & Pope, 1989; Kagle & Geibelhausen, 1994; Kitchener, 1988; Nagy, 2000; Simon, 1995; Sonne, 1994). Furthermore, dual relationships have been cited as proof of therapists' pathology, such as lack of integrity (Kitchener, 1996; Pope, 1991), propensity to rationalization (Borys, 1992; Pope & Vasquez, 1998), tendencies toward narcissism and self-aggrandizement (Pepper, 1991), and opening the way to sexual intimacy (Doverspike, 1999; Epstein et al., 1992; Gabbard, 1994; Pope, 1990).

Chomsky's Model and Psychology's "Core Group"

Noam Chomsky's (1988) widely used model of manufactured consent offers help in the exploration of how nonsensical, unrealistic, and self-serving beliefs have come to dominate the field of psychotherapy, especially around the issues of boundary crossings and dual relationships. Manufactured consent has been described as the process whereby relatively few people have overwhelmingly influenced public opinion and decision making, as well as the worldview and functions of a culture or organization. The inflated power of these individuals, who represent and embody certain interests and beliefs, is derived from their control over the dissemination of information and is often fueled by self-interest and dogmatism.

Applying this understanding to the field of psychotherapy and dual relationships makes it clear that a handful of people in key professional positions have held sway over the profession and have controlled and manipulated the dissemination, flow, and types of information available to other professionals. As with manufactured consent in political arenas, the driving force in the field of psychotherapy derives from people who are not necessarily conscious of or deliberately conspiratorial in their manipulations. They are mostly committed professionals who seek power and control, and hold strong and rigid beliefs in the righteousness of their ideas and combine this with a great determination to convince, frighten, intimidate, or coerce others to do the "right thing."

People in this "core group" hold influential gatekeeping positions in the field of psychotherapy as book and journal editors; members of ethics committees, boards, and task forces; attorneys for professional organizations; forensic consultants; and expert witnesses for boards and courts. The top tier of this core group is composed of Koocher (Koocher & Keith-Spiegel, 1998), Pope (1986, 1988, 1989, 1990, 1991), Bersoff (1999), Epstein (Epstein & Simon, 1990), Langs (1974), and Simon (1991, 1992, 1995). Historically, two women, Bouhoutsos (Pope & Bouhoutsos, 1988) and Keith-Spiegel (Keith-Spiegel & Koocher, 1985; Koocher & Keith-Spiegel, 1998; Pope, Tabachnick, & Keith-Spiegel, 1987) have played an important role in cementing the rigid dogma professing the depravity of dual relationships.

The second tier within this group is composed of Borys (Borys & Pope, 1989), Brown (1991), Gabbard (Gabbard & Nadelson, 1995), Gutheil (Gutheil & Gabbard, 1993), Kitchener (1988), Sonne (1994), Younggren (Younggren & Skorka, 1992), and Woody (1998). In the third tier are Doverspike (1999), Faulkner and Faulkner (1997), Gottlieb (1993), Lakin (1991), Nagy (2000), Pepper (1991), Vasquez (Pope & Vasquez, 1998), and Strasburger and Jorgenson (Strasburger, Jorgenson, & Sutherland, 1992). A more recent addition to the group is Mary Beth Kenkel, editor of the journal *Professional Psychology: Research and Practice*.

The power of three highly influential members of the core group seems to be particularly far-reaching. Gerald Koocher, coauthor of the widely used text *Ethics in Psychology* (Koocher & Keith-Spiegel, 1998), is highly critical of dual relationships. Koocher has held numerous positions with the APA, the most recent being a two-term stint as treasurer. He has also been the editor of the influential journal *Ethics and Behavior*. Like Koocher, Donald Bersoff has held several APA positions, including APA attorney and member of the Council of Representatives. Although, to my knowledge, he has never practiced psychotherapy, experienced dual relationships as a therapist, or struggled with conflict with his own patients, he nevertheless wrote a widely used text—*Ethical Conflicts in Psychology* (1999)—that is heavily biased against dual relationships. Bersoff's numerous powerful positions within the APA and the fact that the APA published his book constitute an intriguing multiple relationship in itself. Kenneth Pope, the third example, is the most prolific writer and quoted author on the topic of dual relationships, and probably the most powerful and feared champion of the conservative view of dual relationships. Among many other influential positions, he has served as the chair of the APA Ethics Committee and coauthored a popular text on ethics (Pope & Vasquez, 1998), also published by the APA. Vasquez also has held several prominent positions within the APA.

In a fascinating and profoundly ironic twist of multiple relationships, several members of the core group not only serve on ethics committees and are involved in writing and revising ethics codes but also simultaneously serve as highly paid expert witnesses against therapists who, in their opinion, have violated the codes, laws, or beliefs that they themselves manufactured and put in place. If it were not for the numerous therapists who have lost their licenses, livelihoods, reputations, and dignity, this huge irony would be great material for a third-rate comedy.

Forces Fueling the Aversion to Boundary Crossings and Dual Relationships

A number of forces have fueled the faulty beliefs surrounding the issue of boundary crossings and dual relationships. Psychoanalytic theory emphasizes the importance of the analyst establishing neutrality and clear and rigid boundaries with the client to effectively manage transference, the hallmark of analytic work. Simon, a top member of the core group, epitomizes the analytic case against boundary crossings and dual relationships when he prescribes these supposedly universal rules for therapy: "Maintain therapist neutrality. Foster psychological separateness of the patient … Interact only verbally with clients. Ensure no previous, current, or future personal relationships with patients. Minimize physical contact. Preserve relative anonymity of the therapist." (Simon, 1995, p. 514). Langs (1974), a prominent psychoanalyst and equally prominent member of the core group, like most traditional analysts who ignore other therapeutic approaches, views all boundary crossings and dual relationships as having a significant negative impact on the therapeutic process.

Blinded by worship of their analytic dogma, these writers seem to make universal therapeutic proclamations that, although often being out of touch with reality, nevertheless have been adopted by many ethicists and courts. The original intent of consumer protection agencies and professional organizations to protect the welfare of clients by issuing a straightforward ban on sexual relationships between therapists and clients has mushroomed into a massively broad prohibition of boundary crossings and dual relationships in an attempt to ward off any and all possible harm to patients involved in therapeutic treatment.

Risk management is viewed as sufficient reason for professionals to avoid boundary crossings, dual relationships, and other often positive interventions, despite their therapeutic benefits. Therapists refrain from engaging in certain behaviors and interventions not because they are clinically ill-advised, harmful, or wrong but because they may *appear* wrong in court (Williams, 1997, 2000). Boundary crossings and dual relationships are considered high risk; therefore, most attorneys and risk management experts advise therapists to avoid them. Gutheil & Gabbard (1993) clarified the situation accurately with this chilling statement: "From the viewpoint of current risk management principles, a handshake is about the limit of social physical contact at this time" (p. 195).

Risk management may sound like pragmatic advice, but in fact it is a misnomer for a practice in which fear of licensing boards and attorneys, rather than clinical and client considerations, determine the course of therapy. A big part of the dumbing down in our field can be traced to the fear imposed by those who frighten us into disregarding science and decency for the sake of protecting ourselves. Unethically and callously, most risk management presentations warn against providing care to the homebound sick, disabled, or elderly and warn us against self-disclosure and other humanistic, cognitive, family, behavioral, or group therapy-based interventions. Therapists are supposedly trained, hired, and paid to provide the best care possible for clients. This includes the employment of dual relationship interventions when appropriate. Therapists are not paid to act defensively. Lazarus (1994) pronounces that "one of the worst professional or ethical violations is that of permitting current risk management principles to take precedence over humane interventions" (p. 261).

Feminist therapists seem split on the issue of dual relationships. The more vocal politically and professionally active faction focuses on issues of power, male dominance, sexuality, and patriarchal values. Predictably, they take a strong stance against boundary crossings and dual relationships and fight for the protection of what they see as vulnerable female clients sexually exploited by powerful male therapists. Borys, Bouhoutsos, Keith-Spiegel, Jorgenson, Kitchener, Sonne, and Vasquez are members of the core group representing this ideology. Their influence seems to penetrate important ethics committees, boards, and the legislative arena.

The much less vocal feminist faction centers on essential issues of inclusion, connection, mutuality, self-disclosure, and equality. Predictably, the focus of these writers, as manifested in the important work of Greenspan (1995) and the Feminist Therapy Institute (1987), is how healing often entails tearing down rigid, arbitrary, professional boundaries rather than erecting them. The prolific writer Laura Brown (1989, 1990, 1991, 1994) seems to play both sides of the net as she focuses obsessively on male power and power issues in general, intermittently condemning boundary crossings and dual relationships and at other times acknowledging the importance of feminist principles such as mutuality, self-disclosure, flexible boundaries, and familiarity as aids to healing.

Manufacturing Consent on the Depravity of Dual Relationships

There are numerous ways in which consent on the immorality of dual relationships has been contrived and manipulated.

Repetitive Misinformation That Dual Relationships Are Unethical and Harmful Frequent, repetitive, and persistent dissemination of the flawed idea that dual relationships are inherently unethical and harmful has been one of the most powerful tools for manufacturing consent on this issue (Zur, 2002). The often-quoted ethicist Kitchener (1988) erroneously claims, "all dual relationships can be ethically problematic and have the potential for harm" (p.217). Pope (1990) made a frightening and nonsensical declaration that has become a kind of standard for many professionals: "…. non-sexual dual relationships, while not unethical and harmful per se, foster sexual dual relationships" (p. 688). These incessant ubiquitous messages by the core group demonstrate an effective, proven propaganda technique widely used by politicians, the military, and cults (Keen, 1986), aimed at convincing the message recipients that even baseless and irrational assertions are true.

Exclusive Reliance on the Writings of the Core Group: Creating the Illusion of Unanimity Core group writers tend to quote each other relentlessly and almost exclusively. This is exemplified in Borys (1994) and Gutheil (1994), in which the core group writers composed eighty-three percent and seventy-five percent of the citations, respectively. In Bersoff's (1996) widely used ethics textbook, all nine entries on dual relationships in therapy were by members of the core group, and four were authored or co-authored by Pope. Such repetitive and at times exclusive circulation of a set of references promotes a sense that this is the only valid position available in professional literature. This cultivates an illusion that dissent does not exist and that condemnation of dual relationships is universal.

Exclusion and Suppression of Opposing Viewpoints: The Power of Disinformation Very few propaganda techniques are more effective to persuade, manipulate, and distort a situation as disinformation, the suppression of relevant information. This exclusionary form of "spin" is notoriously successful at creating uninformed consent. Dual relationships have systematically and consistently been suppressed, excluded, and censored. Articles that represent a more positive attitude towards nonsexual dual relationships—for example, Barnett (1992), Barnett and Yutrzenka (1994), Hedges (1993), Jennings 1992), Lazarus, (1994), Sears (1990), Smith (1990), Stockman (1990), and Tomm (1993)—have largely been ignored and excluded by most books and articles, even though they appear to offer a balanced discussion of dual relationships. Conspicuously, Bersoff (1996), Gabbard and Nadelson (1995), Kitchener (1996), Nagy (2000), Simon (1995), Sonne (1994), and St. Germaine (1996) failed to mention any of the above referenced articles of which, as knowledgeable scholars, they must have been fully aware.

Perhaps the most outstanding example lies in the extensively cited ethics text by Pope and Vasquez (1998), which includes forty-eight citations of Pope's own work but none of the above references. A more recent example surfaced in an *APA Monitor* article (Smith, 2003) on dual relationships. The article adheres to the "anti-dual relationships" APA party line and quotes an old 1993 article; however, it conspicuously fails to mention a whole body of published articles, especially a book by Lazarus and this author (Lazarus & Zur, 2002), that takes a more balanced view of dual relationships. When a protesting Letter to the Editor regarding this omission was finally published, the name of the book was edited out. Our letter to APA included this statement:

> …In our view, your reports on multiple relationships do not concur with APA's own Ethical Principles and its overall Code of Ethics. These principles and codes emphasize integrity, responsibility, and the commitment to present unbiased, complete, and updated information. You boldly elect to neglect the most comprehensive and most updated texts and articles on the topic of multiple or dual relationships… [and] fail to mention that

there is a growing body of knowledge that asserts that multiple relationships can increase therapeutic effectiveness....

Zur and Lazarus (2003, p. 5)

Another example of blunt exclusion is an article by Campbell and Gordon (2003) describing the inevitability of dual relationships in rural areas and concluding that "Although the best practice is to abstain from multiple roles and boundary compromises.... " This article clearly suppresses an entire body of knowledge not in support of its conclusion.

Disinformation also takes the form of excluding references to orientations and practices that support boundary crossings and dual relationships. The core group and their followers systematically ignore behavioral, cognitive-behavioral, humanistic, group, family, feminist, and existential orientations, which currently are the most practiced orientations and tend to regularly employ clinically beneficial boundary crossings such as self-disclosure and "out-of office" exposure therapies for anxiety and phobias (Lazarus, 1994, 1998; Williams, 1997; Zur, 2001). Unaccountably, these research-supported interventions are considered violations by many ethicists, psychoanalysts, and risk management advocates and are glaringly absent from papers written by authors who oppose dual relationships. Humanistic orientations and a segment of feminist orientations tend to look favorably on deliberate and strategic implementation of helpful dual relationships (Greenspan, 1995; Williams, 1997) and predictably are almost entirely absent from core group publications.

This systematic suppression extends to the censorship of case studies or clinical examples of beneficial dual relationships. A classic example is the chapter in Koocher and Keith-Spiegel's (1998) textbook that includes fifty-one vignettes of dual relationships, not one of which has a positive outcome. Nagy's (2000) extensive case study list has the same perfect rate of exclusion. Almost all writing by the core group fails to present cases of clinically beneficial dual relationships, although they abound.

In addition, opposing viewpoints are suppressed through denial of the inevitable, normal, and healthy aspects of dual relationships in rural and other communities. More than eighty percent of the U.S. land area is rural, and twenty percent (55 million) of the U.S. population lives, works, or serves in rural areas (Stamm, 2003), a fact that has been conspicuously ignored by most writers from the core group. The majority of literature on the topic is silent on the inevitable, normal, and healthy aspects of dual relationships in small, tightly knit, interconnected groups of people, such as those in rural areas (Barnett, 1996; Barnett & Yutrzenka, 1994; Hargrove, 1986; Jennings, 1992; Schank, 1998; Schank & Skovholt, 1997).

It is important to emphasize that "small communities" also exist within metropolitan areas, including church communities (Geyer, 1994; Llewellyn, 2002; Montgomery & DeBell, 1997), lesbian communities (Brown, 1989; Sears, 1990; Smith, 1990), deaf communities (Guthmann & Sandberg, 2002), and feminist and other communities (Brown, 1991; Harris, 2002; Lerman & Porter, 1990). Military communities are another rarely mentioned example of an environment in which dual relationships are not only normal but, in fact, even mandated by military law (Staal & King, 2000; Zur & Gonzalez, 2002).

Although mentioning the inevitability of dual relationships, the APA-published book *Rural Behavioral Health Care* (Stamm, 2003) also largely and conspicuously ignores the richness of interwoven lives of caregivers and patients in rural areas. Nagy (2000), a prominent member of many APA and CPA ethics committees, seems to deny the reality of millions of Americans living in rural areas when he ludicrously claims that "There are usually plenty of other therapists you can refer them to …" (p. 99). The oddest aspect is that such bizarre, out-of-touch, and unrealistic advice goes largely unchallenged or, even worse, is embraced and adopted by journal and book editors, ethicists, boards, courts, and, most disturbing, by therapists themselves.

Disinformation is also fostered by denial of non-Western traditional cultural values of interdependence, mutuality, and dual relationships. Conflicting traditions govern how our society deals with the morass surrounding boundary crossings and dual relationships. The traditional ethnocentric Western view has been one of the most dominant contributors to the condemnation of both boundary crossings and dual relationships. Therapies practiced by non-Western cultures and ethnic groups that do not subscribe to the rigid isolation and segregation forms of therapy are seen as substandard, unethical, and even illegal.

Psychotherapists and counselors pride themselves on being culturally sensitive but, as the imbroglio of dual relationships clearly reveals, the ethnocentric view prevails. Idealizing traditional western values of independence, privacy, and isolation over traditional non-Western values of interconnectedness, mutuality, and interdependence is a key facet of this propaganda campaign (Lazarus & Zur, 2002; Lerman

& Porter, 1990). In a McDonald's-like phenomenon, it seems that the toxicity of individualization, separation, and segregation is being exported all over the world, even in much more communally oriented cultures (Slack & Wassenaar, 1999).

Most ethics codes advocate strongly for rigid boundaries and give mere lip service to cultural diversity. Greenspan's (1995) penetrating analysis on values and therapy—which found Grunebaum's (1986) findings that distant, rigid, and uninvolved therapists have been reported by patients themselves to be actually detrimental—has effectively been ignored by almost all of those opposing the value of dual relationships. Also systematically disregarded have been Sears' (1990) article on dual relationships in the Native American community, Kertesz's (2002) work on dual relationships in Latin America, Lerman and Porter's (1990) emphasis on cultural sensitivity, and Thomas (2002) on bartering.

Extensive Reliance on Psychoanalytic Theory Precluding a Balanced View of the Issue The endlessly cited works of the analytically oriented members of the core group—Epstein (Epstein & Simon, 1990), Langs (1974), Lakin (1991), and Simon (1991, 1995)—dominate the articles that demonize dual relationships. According to these authors, any deviation from the psychoanalytic blank-screen isolation stance that they so strictly endorse is likely to result in the absolute nullification of therapeutic effectiveness and even cause harm. The rigid analytic orientation of these authors blinds them and their adherents to the fact that most practitioners do not adhere to, believe in, or practice psychoanalysis. To add insult to injury, the works of these writers have been used to justify the imposition of strict rules on the entire field, and administrative and civil penalties on many nonanalytic practitioners (Lazarus, 1994; Williams, 1997, 2000).

Tilting the Playing Field: Conjuring the Illusion of Balanced Perspectives In the few instances where the opposing view is given a voice, authors who promote the extinction of dual relationships compromise the opposition's validity by giving it minimal space and no serious consideration. In 1994, Koocher, as editor of *Ethics & Behavior,* published an invited article by Arnold Lazarus entitled "How Certain Boundaries and Ethics Diminish Therapeutic Effectiveness." In a perfectly executed spin, the editor then invited six high-profile discussants to respond to the single article. Predictably, none of the respondents was supportive of Lazarus' approach, nor did any come from cognitive-behavioral or humanistic approaches that are likely to endorse boundary crossings and embrace appropriate dual relationships. Six experts used thirty-three pages to denounce what one expressed in seven pages. By inviting Lazarus, Koocher created the illusion of open-mindedness. In reality, he orchestrated an uneven playing field in which Lazarus' approach ended up being slammed by six highly regarded professionals. The illusion of balanced representation was achieved, and the dogma was preserved and even fortified.

Portrayal of Dual Relationships as Synonymous with Harm, Exploitation, and Sex Many writers not only view dual relationships as leading to harm and exploitation but, most disturbing, use the term interchangeably with harm, exploitation, and even sex. In Austin's (1998) book, the dual relationships chapter opens with: "Any relationships with a client other than the therapeutic relationships constitute a dual relationship. A client has the right to be treated by a therapist who will not exploit their trust" (p. 450). Kitchener (1996) links dual relationships with lack of integrity, betrayal, and untrustworthiness. Grosso (1997) includes socializing with clients among his examples of harmful dual relationships. Sonne (1994), rather strangely, cites a resemblance of dual relationships to drunk driving. Doverspike (1999) associates dual relationships with sleeping at the wheel, and Koocher and Keith-Spiegel (1998), like Pope and so many other writers, baselessly associate dual relationships with inherent harm and conflict of interest.

Viewing Dual Relationships as a Prime Risk Management Concern
For professionals, risk management seems to constitute a valid reason to avoid dual relationships. Boundary crossings and dual relationships are considered high risk and, therefore, not advisable according to attorneys and risk management experts. This dogma was installed by the core group and others who often also serve and are paid as risk management and forensic experts in litigation. This same group has instigated a fear of lawsuits and of hypervigilant regulatory and consumer protection agencies. This has created an atmosphere of anxiety for therapists, particularly around the issues of boundary crossings and dual relationships. This fear has altered the way many therapists conduct therapy and steered them away from utilizing proven effective treatments that may include boundary crossings or helpful, healthy dual relationships.

Cognitive Dissonance as a Contributing Dynamic to Belief in the Evils of Dual Relationships Therapists are continuously exposed to warnings about the dangers of dual relationships. These warnings come from many sources: risk management workshops, analytic sources, graduate classes, supervision, ethics and law seminars, attorneys' advice columns, newsletters, and so on. The fear of licensing boards, attorneys, and litigation has led most therapists to avoid not only dual relationships but also any behavior that resembles boundary crossing (e.g., home visits). As the cognitive dissonance theory (Festinger, 1957) predicts, such fear-based avoidance behaviors also alter clinicians' attitudes toward dual relationships, even among those who do not believe that dual relationships are inherently wrong. Consent in this case, has been manufactured by instilling fear; this results in alteration of behavior and the subsequent change of attitudes to justify the behavior.

The Fallacy of the "Slippery Slope" Myth Surrounding Dual Relationships One of the main arguments against dual relationships is the snowball effect described by Gabbard (1994): "....the crossing of one boundary without obvious catastrophic results (making) it easier to cross the next boundary" (p. 284). In a classic example, Sonne (1994) details how a therapist and client who play tennis together can easily begin to carpool or drink together. But it is Pope (1990) who has been a one-man juggernaut in the popularization of the slippery slope idea, transmogrifying it into something like a professional ethical standard. Clearly, scholars from the core group sexualize any deviation from strict analytic practices and make a direct causal link not only between dual relationships and harm but also between nonsexual and sexual dual relationships.

Although the slippery slope claim is clearly illogical, fear-based, and syllogistic, it is nevertheless referred to extensively and presented as if it were evidence-based and factual. Almost all core group members have found support for their dogmatic stance in the fact that a boundary crossing always precedes sexual exploitation of clients. Confusing such sequential relationships with causal ones is like saying that doctors' visits cause death because most people see a doctor before they die. To assert that hugging a child or mourning mother or a visit to a elderly client are likely to lead to harm, exploitation, or sex is illogical and paranoid (Lazarus & Zur, 2002).

It is insulting for educated psychotherapists to be repeatedly lectured on the paranoid notion of the slippery slope. It is intellectually demeaning to claim that a handshake between a therapist and client is likely to lead to sex, or a gift to exploitative business relationships. Nevertheless, if repeated often enough by enough experts, ethicists, and attorneys, it becomes the dumbed-down professional standard.

Burning the Heretics: Depiction of the Opposition as Unethical and Pathological Therapists involved in dual relationships are generally accused of lacking integrity and of being unethical and immoral by many members of the core group and their followers. The work of Pope (1988) especially denigrates therapists' arguments for the curative power of dual relationships as self-deceiving and self-serving rationalizations. Therapists who believe that dual relationships can be beneficial to clients are said to employ defense mechanisms such as rationalization and exploit clients for their own needs and gratification. Members of the core group describe the narcissistic, self-deceptive, egocentric, self-aggrandizing, delusional, and pathological characteristics of therapists who violate the supposedly universal, rigid analytic boundaries. Craig (1991) makes a frightening inference worthy of a witch hunt: "Ethical counselors cultivate unambiguous relationships. ... Unethical counselors cultivate dual relationships" (p. 49). Attributing such ugly character flaws to therapists who disagree with mainstream traditions is one of the most dangerous abuses of psychology, similar to that used in totalitarian regimes such as the USSR.

A debate on the merits of dual relationships during the APA's annual convention in Chicago in 2002 revealed yet a new tactic in the fight to protect the dogma. What was meant to be a scholarly debate between invited top experts on the subject of dual relationships was moderated by a former APA president in front of hundreds of psychologists, including members of the APA Ethics Committee, the APA's attorney, and the director of the APA's Insurance Trust, the director of the APA Office of Ethics, and many other prominent APA members. Without intervention from the moderator or protest from the audience, one panelist launched a vicious personal attack on two of the participants, Dr. Lazarus and this author, questioning our credentials and integrity and criticizing our professionalism and judgment, among other things. The attack astounded many of the attendees, at least one of whom—Cyril Franks, Distinguished Professor Emeritus of Psychology, Rutgers University—wrote to the APA to complain about this unprecedented behavior of bypassing "all the significant issues that had been raised" and instead impugning the integrity of other panelists. Franks was also very disturbed at the unprofessional behavior of the monitor in refusing to stop "this unseemly development" (Franks, 2002).

Of course, this letter never saw the light of day. Censorship is a relentless and consistent force in these circles. Refusing to condemn this outrageous conduct was tantamount to approval by the APA Ethics Committee and many other APA officials who were present at the debate. This, combined with the *APA Monitor's* refusal to publish Franks' letter, indirectly encourages such vicious personal attacks on those who will not toe the party line.

Publication of Flawed and Biased Research Research on dual relationships inspires methodological concerns stemming primarily from the ideological biases of researchers (Williams, 1992). For example, a number of surveys conducted on dual relationships in therapy have had significantly low return rates that put the validity of the findings into question. The miserably low return rates reported by Epstein, Simon, and Kay (1992), Ramsdell and Ramsdell (1993), and Sharkin and Birky (1992) were twenty-one, twenty-six, and thirty-two percent, respectively. This kind of invalid meaningless research should have never been published.

Given the witchhunt-like atmosphere surrounding the issues of boundaries and dual relationships, most therapists who believe that crossing traditional boundaries can be curative are, in spite of promises of anonymity, highly unlikely respond to such surveys. This creates a heavily biased sample that in turn nullifies the validity of the research. Biased survey instruments developed by Pope et al. (1987) have been repeatedly cited and used by many researchers despite questions about the validity and reliability of the questionnaire. For example, a question like, "Your therapist hugs you in the session" gets perilously close to, "When did you stop beating your wife?" and could have been presented as, "Your therapist holds you at a time of deep distress and grief."

Similarly, the assessment of harm to clients and its alleged causal link to boundary crossings and dual relationships has also been criticized for methodological reasons (Williams, 1995). The admitted biases of researchers, combined with the dread of persecution, has in essence nullified the possibility that any significant and valid data might be collected about the effect or value of nonsexual dual relationships. In his novel *Lying on the Couch*, the renowned group therapist, existentialist, and psychiatrist Irvin Yalom (1997) makes clear that those who have benefited from dual relationships are not likely to appear in research statistics. Yalom argues that those who have profited from dual relationships may be doing so well that they no longer seek counseling and are consequently unavailable to researchers.

Another possibility is that although the dual relationship experience was positive, the client is likely aware that the relationship was also regarded by some as illicit, and might, therefore, try to protect the therapist with silence. "The truth is, we just don't have the data," Yalom claims through one of his characters. "We know about the casualties only. In other words, we just know the numerator, but not the denominator" (p. 220). In an attempt to present a unified consent about the evils of dual relationships, researchers continue to present flawed, biased, and, above all, misleading "scientific" conclusions.

The core group and their supporters have used their influence and gatekeeping positions in the field of psychotherapy and counseling to manipulate, influence, and ultimately manufacture consent about the depravity of boundary crossings and dual relationships. They have employed misinformation, disinformation, and distortion of facts to reach their goal. They have excluded those who differ with them from voicing their opinions while forming their own consensual choir by quoting one another incessantly and at times exclusively. They have silenced the opposition by introducing fear (preaching "risk management"), intimidation (pathologizing those who do not share their views), and coercion (serving on punitive ethics committees and boards). They have profited from the rules they themselves created by serving as expert witnesses and helping indict those who did not follow their rules.

Worst of all, members of the core group have succeeded in demonizing and sexualizing what has always been normal and human behavior, such as laughter and sharing. The therapeutic aspects of touch in therapy (Smith, Clance, & Ames, 1998) have been demonized and sexualized in similar fashion. They have been able to pathologize what is healthy and what we have considered essential to human survival throughout most of human history: a sense of mutuality, familiarity, communion, interdependence, and connectedness.

Self-Serving Motives behind the Condemnation of Boundary Crossings and Dual Relationships

The obvious question that follows the discussion of how consent has been manufactured is why such nonsensical concepts have been so readily accepted. The common reason given for the ban on boundary crossings and dual relationships is that it protects clients from exploitative therapists. However, this "for-your-own-good" argument is not as simple as it sounds. The passive acceptance of boundary crossings and dual relationships as bad by almost all psychotherapists and counselors, regardless of their venue or treatment orientations, cannot be fully explained by the manipulations of the core group. For such an irrational myth to exist and find professional acceptance despite its unrealistic demands to rigidly isolate and fanatically segregate, it must serve the therapists themselves in some professional, emotional, or financial way.

Promotion of an Isolated Therapeutic Environment Increases Therapists' Influential Power The private nature of psychotherapy has been known to enhance clients' self-disclosure, reduce feelings of shame, and increase their sense of trust and safety. However, these same attributes may also exponentially increase the power of therapists over their patients. In the isolation of the office, clients are left to rely on their imaginations and, as a result, many tend to unrealistically idealize their therapists and attribute great power, wisdom, and beauty to them. Such idealization or projection without any real-life corroborative support is likely to gratify many therapists and give them power over their unrealistically adoring clients.

Psychoanalysis, in particular, has emphasized the importance of therapy in isolation and anonymity of the therapists for transferencial/clinical reasons. This may apply to psychoanalytic techniques, however, there is no therapeutic reason to make the "blank-screen" approach an industrywide standard. It is unpleasant to acknowledge but military basic training and cults are examples of institutions that, like psychotherapy, use isolation to increase influential power and conduct brainwashing. Although there are several compelling reasons for therapy to be conducted in a private and confidential environment, the obsession with privacy and the resultant rigidly imposed isolation may ultimately be more damaging than enhancing to the welfare of clients. This self-serving obsession with isolation unfortunately has been translated into laws, ethics codes, and guidelines that imbue therapists with undue power. This power can be used positively, but it may also increase the risk of exploitation and harm to clients.

Promoting the Illusion of Therapists' Omnipotence and Clients' Helplessness The inflated notion that therapists have extraordinary and unrealistic power to manipulate, control, exploit, and irreversibly harm consenting clients by a slight deviation from standard procedures is one of the most ludicrous, unfounded, and prevalent assumptions underlying the belief in the depravity of boundary crossings and dual relationships. Therapists' insidious belief in their own omnipotence has been a concern since the early days of therapy when Jones (1951) labeled it the "God Syndrome." Much has been written about the mental health of therapists and the often not-so-healthy reasons they turn to the psychotherapy or counseling professions.

There are some arrogant therapy teachers who even make their students sign a contract that the student will not divulge their methods to those who are not specially trained in them. The reason given is that these supposedly superpowerful techniques can severely harm clients treated by anyone who is not approved and trained by the master. That the master and his acolytes are handsomely paid for this "special" treatment may have something to do with it. In reality, the motivation is economic and self-aggrandizing.

The argument against dual relationships portrays patients as malleable, weak, and defenseless in the hands of their powerful and dominant therapists. Doverspike (1999), like most of his fellow members of the core group, lauds the concept of "once a client, always a client." The State of Florida Psychology Practices Code, chapter 21U, section 15.004, shockingly states: " For purpose of determining the existence of sexual misconduct as defined herein, the psychologist–client relationship is deemed to continue in perpetuity." The argument is that if a male therapist, for example, saw a woman in brief therapy discussing her concerns about her young child, twenty years later he would still have infinite power over this supposedly helpless and vulnerable female. According to this feminist-inspired, power-based, political ideology, because of the professional power discrepancy between a male therapist and a female client, consensual intimate relationships between therapist and clients can never take place.

This uncritical view of the disparity in power, besides being unrealistic, is highly demeaning to our clients in general, and insulting to women clients in particular. The myth presents a stereotypic view of women clients as hysterically amenable, emotionally helpless, and utterly vulnerable to their therapists' influence. In reality, many therapists work with some women clients who are much more powerful than they are—influential executives, powerhouse attorneys, inspired authors, and creative entrepreneurs. Many therapists with low self-esteem work hard at cultivating an aura of power to appear and feel credible. Healthier therapists focus on healing relationships and breaking down rigid boundaries rather than on the power relationships and inflexible boundaries in therapy. The rigid imposition of isolation and the myth of the depravity of boundary crossings and dual relationships purport to protect clients from exploitative therapists but, in fact, offer a way for therapists to promote a self-aggrandizing, unrealistic, anarchistic sense of power.

Protecting Therapists from Shame and Exposure The lives of many therapists are actually far from what clients imagine them to be or what the therapists pretend they are. Therapists who are poor, lonely, or depressed understandably attempt to disguise this situation. The ban on boundary crossings and dual relationships and the dogma of isolation allow therapists to rationalize and legitimize their concealment of distressing and shameful aspects of their lives. The question must always be, "Is the motivation selfish or benevolent?" Boundaries, confidentiality, and privacy can be appropriate but are not always clinically advised. Many clients respond better to flexibility, self-disclosure, familiarity, or dual relationships with the therapist (Greenspan, 1995; Lerman & Porter, 1990). Erecting a rigid, ideologically based fence around therapy and an artificial wall between therapists and clients—which might interfere with therapy—is a perfect way for therapists to legitimize their defenses and deal with any sense of shame and need to hide.

Allowing Incompetent Therapists to Stay in Business: The Resistance Excuse There are several less high-minded reasons for the pretense that rigid therapeutic boundaries must be maintained for clients' protection and privacy. These have to do with the professional, emotional, and financial benefits that therapists reap from the implementation of these beliefs. In the isolated setting, therapists can bask in their clients' idealization, experience the attendant increase in power and influence, and enjoy the therapeutic mystique that thrives in this environment. In rigidly segregated consulting rooms, therapists can also blame the client for lack of progress and use terms such as "resistance" to justify the continuation of charging clients, at times for many years, even though nothing is being accomplished. Such insulation allows therapists to stay in business regardless of their clinical effectiveness.

SUMMING IT UP

Like most professions, the mental health profession is deeply vested in protecting its turf (e.g., lobbying for parity law), enhancing its status (e.g., pushing for higher reimbursement rates), and increasing economic power (e.g., petitioning for prescription privileges). Imposing rigid isolation on psychotherapy is an additional aspect of efforts to enhance therapists' influence and power, even at the expense of client care. The processes that are fueled by the need for professional survival often fly in the face of reason, self-examination, and critical thinking.

The assault on boundary crossings and dual relationships provides us with a good case study of the dumbing down of psychology. The dogma persists even though many theoretical orientations support boundary crossings as being clinically helpful and at times the best intervention for the situation. The dogma persists even though trust and familiarity are fostered by dual relationships and less isolated environments are likely to reduce the possibility of exploitation rather than increase it.

The dumbing down of psychotherapy naturally starts in graduate schools where techniques, orientations, research methods, statistics, and risk management are the focus of learning without a balancing emphasis on anthropology, philosophy, comparative religions, critical thinking, or compassion, empathy, and intimacy. Although technical and scientific knowledge are an essential part of psychotherapy, we also know that techniques by themselves count for only a minimal variant in therapy (Lambert, 1992; Bergin & Garfield, 1994). Even though the literature has repeatedly concluded that the therapeutic relationship is the best predictor of clinical effectiveness (Frank, 1970; Norcross & Goldfried, 1992), courses that concentrate exclusively on the intimate relationships between therapist and client beyond concerns with transference and countertransference are rare.

Graduate school professors endlessly quibble about which orientation is superior rather than teach students to intervene according to the client's condition, situation, personality, and culture. As a result, instead of thoughtful, knowledgeable, and sensitive therapists who are able to think critically, form intimate connections with their clients, and effectively employ proven clinical interventions, graduate schools mostly spit out highly technical, ethically and morally insensate, frightened, and theoretically rigid therapists. In a similar manner, licensing focuses on abstract knowledge of research methodologies, techniques, and ethics and law rather than going through the much more difficult process of also evaluating therapists for the capacity for empathy, self-awareness, emotional health, and critical thinking. Given our graduate education and licensing methods, the dumbing down of our profession is virtually assured.

Although privacy, confidentiality, and appropriate boundaries are key elements in effective therapy and should be implemented appropriately and flexibly, we must refuse to suppress diverse opinions on any topic, including that of dual relationships and boundaries. That is a guaranteed way of dumbing down any field of knowledge. Psychologists have long studied the phenomenon of groupthink, obedience to authority, and authoritarianism; however, they fall into the same trap for which they criticize others. Our graduate schools and the entire profession should be celebrating a diversity of opinions; instead we see widespread suppression of any view that is not mainline, self-serving, or politically correct.

Burning the heretics, pathologizing and marginalizing those who disagree, and extirpating the dissenting view are only some of the techniques used to silence opposition. Hansen and Goldberg (1999) reflect on the presentation of boundary crossings and dual relationships as harmful and exploitative: "… when a psychologist sees professional behavior contrary to his or her personal values, the observer may well cry 'unethical,' when a more apt response might be 'I disagree'" (p. 499). The lack of differentiation between disagreement and what is unethical has led to uncritical acceptance of the party-line dogma and, hence, the dumbing down of our field.

The belief in the depravity of boundary crossings and dual relationships in psychotherapy is primarily based on the urban analytic risk-management model of psychotherapy. It baselessly claims that boundary crossings and dual relationships are essentially unethical, harmful, and lead to exploitation of and sex with clients. Even though most therapists are not psychodynamically oriented, boundary crossings are often part of evidence-based therapies, and dual relationships are a healthy and normal part of communal life and can enhance therapeutic effectiveness. Still, the irrational and unrealistic belief in the evils of boundary crossings and dual relationships prevails.

This essentially paranoid myth has primarily been disseminated by a core group of influential professionals who hold key gatekeeping positions in the field. They have manufactured consent through classic propaganda techniques such as incessant repetitions of the message, misinformation, disinformation, publication of biased research findings, concealment of information, and pathologizing and marginalizing the opposition. These techniques have proved very effective when employed for larger issues of war, economy, or social policy and have brought about the methodical demonization of boundary crossings and dual relationships in psychotherapy. Regardless of how unrealistic, illogical, or paranoid the dogma is, therapists seem to swallow it hook, line, and sinker.

But more than good propaganda techniques are at the root of such acceptance; there is a subtler, more insidious reason than a misguided belief in the immorality of boundary crossings and dual relationships. A deeper motive is that the ensuing mandated segregation of therapy and the avoidance of boundary crossings and dual relationships actually benefit therapists. Although the ban is claimed to be for the clients' "own good," in fact, the absence of all boundary crossings and dual relationships and the resulting isolation increase therapists' personal, professional, and economic power. In an ironic twist, the ban, which was supposed to protect clients from exploitative therapists, increases isolation of the clients, thereby increasing not only the therapists' influential power but the likelihood of exploitation. The most "beneficial" aspect of the imposed isolation is the therapists' ability to blame clients for lack of progress because of their "resistance" while continuing to charge for ineffective therapy.

Spreading the irrational, unrealistic, and paranoid message that boundary crossings and dual relationships are immoral is an affront to our professional judgment. Putting risk management and fear of speaking up for what we believe ahead of clinical considerations and care for our clients erodes our original commitment to healing. Rigidly employing "only in the office" emotional distance therapy impugns our professional integrity. Focusing on the codes of ethics as our exclusive guiding text to the exclusion of philosophical, cultural, and spiritual considerations dumbs down our moral and ethical judgment.

Although most of the professional literature on the topic of boundary crossings and dual relationships is dominated by the core group and their faction, a few professional journals have encouraged critical thinking about the complexities of boundary crossings and nonsexual dual relationships. They include: *Professional Psychology: Research and Practice*; *Psychotherapy: Theory, Research, Practice, and Training; The Independent Practitioner;* and *Voices.* There are also a limited number of books that support critical thinking and a balanced view of boundaries and dual relationships. These include Herlihy and Corey (1992), Heyward (1993), Howard (1986), Lazarus and Zur (2002), and Lerman and Porter (1990).

When is it appropriate to intentionally employ boundary crossings? The shortest, most comprehensive, and intelligent answer is provided by Lazarus (1994) when he says, "It depends." It depends on the client's situation, culture, socioeconomic class, presenting problem, personality, diagnosis, and background. It is essential to the welfare of clients that clinical decisions are based on these kind of considerations, instead of on ignorance, fear, dogma, or self-serving beliefs. Clinical interventions stemming from the rigid standpoint that dual relationships are inherently detrimental do not do justice to clients or the profession. Rather than avoiding boundary crossings and dual relationships on general principle, therapists can accept and welcome them as an effective therapeutic tool to be employed when clinically appropriate.

If the misinformation currently being disseminated succeeds in continuing to stop therapists from placing the best interests of clients first, then we all fall victim to blind compliance and fear-based avoidance behaviors. Ignorance of a truly broad and balanced array of perspectives or, even worse, the illusion that one possesses that knowledge, considerably compromises the potential for clinical effectiveness. To discard the option of healthy, helpful, nonsexual boundary crossings and dual relationships in psychotherapy is not only unjust to clients, but an insult to the profession.

It is our responsibility as therapists to maintain our personal and professional integrity by being truly informed, thinking critically, and being aware of our own biases, fears, self-serving attitudes, self-aggrandizing beliefs, and convenient behaviors. Ultimately, we alone can make the decision to eschew fear, self-interest, and dogma in order to put our clients' care above all else. It is at that moment that we truly act with integrity and become moral, ethical, and effective human beings and therapists.

REFERENCES

American Association for Marriage and Family Therapists (AAMFT). (2001). *AAMFT Code of Ethics.* Washington, DC: Author. Retrieved July 8, 2001, from: http://www.aamft.org/about/revisedcodeethics.htm.

American Counseling Association (ACA). (1996). *Code of Ethics and Standards of Practice.* Alexandria, VA: Author. Retrieved July 8, 2001, from: http://www.cacd.org/codeofethics.html.

American Psychological Association (APA). (1992). Ethical principles of psychologists and code of conduct. *American Psychologist, 47,* 1597–1611.

American Psychological Association (APA). (2002). Ethical Principles of Psychologists and Code of Conduct. Retrieved May 3, 2003, from: http://www.apa.org/ethics/code2002.pdf

Austin, K.M. (1998). *Dangers for Therapists.* Redlands: California Selected Books.

Barnett, J.E. (1992). Dual relationships and the federal trade commission. *The Maryland Psychologist, 3,* 12–14.

Barnett, J.E. (1996). Boundary issues and dual relationships: Where to draw the line? *The Independent Practitioner, 16* (3), 138–140.

Barnett, J.E. & Yutrzenka, B.A. (1994). Non-sexual dual relationships in professional practice, with special applications to rural and military community. *The Independent Practitioner, 14* (5), 243–248.

Bennett, B.E., Bricklin, P.M., & VandeCreek, L. (1994). Response to Lazarus's "How certain boundaries and ethics diminish therapeutic effectiveness." *Ethics & Behavior, 4* (3), 263–266.

Bergin, A.E. & Garfield, S.L. (Eds.). (1994). *Handbook of Psychotherapy and Behavior Change* (4th ed.). New York: Wiley.

Bersoff, D.N. (Ed.) (1996). *Ethical Conflicts in Psychology.* Washington, DC: American Psychological Association.

Bersoff, D.N. (Ed.) (1999). *Ethical Conflicts in Psychology.* Washington, DC: American Psychological Association.

Borys, D.S. (1992). Nonsexual dual relationships. In L. Vandecreek, S. Knapp, & T.L. Jackson (Eds.), *Innovations in Clinical Practice: A Source Book, Vol. 11.* (pp. 443–454). Sarasota, FL: Professional Resource Exchange.

Borys, D.S. (1994). Maintaining therapeutic boundaries: The motive is therapeutic effectiveness, not defensive practice. *Ethics and Behavior, 4* (3), 267–273.

Borys, D.S. & Pope, K.S. (1989). Dual relationships between therapist and client: A national study of psychologists, psychiatrists, and social workers. *Professional Psychology: Research and Practice, 20,* 283–293.

Brown, L.S. (1989). Beyond thou shalt not: Thinking about ethics in the lesbian therapy community. *Women and Therapy, 8,* 13–25.

Brown L.S. (1990). Ethical issues and the business of therapy. In H. Lerman & N. Porter (Eds.), *Feminist Ethics in Psychotherapy* (pp. 60–69). New York: Springer.

Brown, L.S. (1991). Ethical issues in feminist therapy. *Psychology of Women, 15,* 323–336.

Brown, L.S. (1994). Boundaries in feminist therapy: A conceptual formulation. *Women and Therapy, 15,* 29–38.

California Board of Psychology. (2001). *A Consumer Guide to Psychological Services.* Sacramento, CA: Author.

Campbell, C.D. & Gordon, M.C. (2003). Acknowledge the inevitable: Understating multiple relationships in rural practice. *Professional Psychology: Research and Practice, 34* (4), 430–434.

Canter, M.B., Bennett, B.E., Jones, S.E., & Nagy, T.F. (1996). *Ethics for Psychologists: A Commentary of the APA Ethics Code.* Washington, DC: American Psychological Association.

Chomsky, N. (1988). *Manufacturing Consent.* New York: Pantheon.

Claiborn, C.D., Berberoglu, L.S., Nerison, R.M., & Somberg, D.R. (1994). The client's perspective: Ethical judgments and perceptions of therapist practices. *Professional Psychology, Research and Practice, 25* (3), 268–274.

Craig, J.D. (1991). Preventing dual relationships in pastoral counseling. *Counseling and Values, 36,* 49–55.

Doverspike, W.F. (1999). *Ethical Risk Management: Guideline for Practice.* Sarasota: Professional Resource.

Epstein, R.S. & Simon, R.I. (1990). The exploitation index: An early warning indicator of boundary violations in psychotherapy. *Bulletin of the Menninger Clinic, 54,* 450–465.

Epstein, R.S., Simon, R.I., & Kay. G.G. (1992). Assessing boundary violations in psychotherapy: Survey results with the Exploitation Index. *Bulletin of the Menninger Clinic, 56,* 150–166.

Erickson, M. & Rossi, E. (1979). *Hypnotherapy: An Exploratory Casebook.* New York: Irvington.

Evans, D.R. (1997). *The Law, Standards of Practice, and Ethics in the Practice of Psychology.* Toronto: Mond Montgomery.

Faulkner, K.K. & Faulkner, T.A. (1997). Managing multiple relationships in rural communities: Neutrality and boundary violations. *Clinical Psychology: Science and Practice, 4* (3), 225–234.

Feminist Therapy Institute (1987), Feminist therapy code of ethics. Denver: Author.

Festinger, L. (1957). *A Theory of Cognitive Dissonance.* Evanston, IL: Row, Peterson.

Frank, J.D. (1970). *Persuasion and Healing.* New York: Schocken.

Gabbard, G.O. (1994). Teetering on the precipice: A commentary on Lazarus's "How certain boundaries and ethics diminish therapeutic effectiveness." *Ethics and Behavior, 4* (3), 283–286.

Gabbard, G.O. & Nadelson, C. (1995). Professional boundaries in the physician-patient relationship. *Journal of the American Medical Association, 273* (18), 1445–1449.

Geyer, M.C. (1994). Dual role relationships and Christian counseling. *Journal of Psychology and Theology, 22* (3), 187–195.

Gottlieb, M.C. (1993). Avoiding exploitative dual relationships: A decision-making model. *Psychotherapy, 30,* 41–48.

Greenspan, M. (1995). Out of bounds. *Common Boundary Magazine, July/August,* 51–58.

Grosso, F.C. (1997). *Ethics for Marriage, Family, and Child Counselors.* Santa Barbara, CA: Author.

Grunebaum, H. (1986). Harmful psychotherapy experience. *American Journal of Psychotherapy, 40,* 166–176.

Gutheil, T. & Gabbard, G.O. (1993). The concept of boundaries in clinical practice: Theoretical and risk management dimensions. *American Journal of Psychiatry, 150,* 188–196.

Gutheil, T.G. (1994). Discussion of Lazarus's "How certain boundaries and ethics diminish therapeutic effectiveness." *Ethics and Behavior, 4* (3), 295–298.

Guthmann, D. & Sandberg, A.K. (2002). Dual relationships in the deaf community: When dual relationships are unavoidable and essential. In A.A. Lazarus & O. Zur (Eds.) *Dual Relationships and Psychotherapy,* New York: Springer, pp. 298–297.

Hansen, N.D. & Goldberg, S.G. (1999). Navigating the nuances: A matrix of considerations for ethical–legal dilemmas. *Professional Psychology: Research and Practice, 30* (5), 495–503.

Hargrove, D.S. (1986). Ethical issues in rural mental health practice. *Professional Psychology: Research and Practice, 17,* 20–23.

Harris, R.S. (2002) Dual relationships and university counseling center environments. In A.A. Lazarus & O. Zur (Eds.) *Dual Relationships and Psychotherapy,* New York: Springer, pp. 337–347.

Hedges, L.E. (1993). In praise of the dual relationship. *The California Therapist, May/June,* 46–50.

Herlihy, B. & Corey, G. (1992). *Dual Relationships in Counseling.* Alexandria, VA: American Association for Counseling and Development.

Heyward, C. (1993). *When Boundaries Betray Us: Beyond What Is Ethical in Therapy and Life.* New York: HarperCollins.

Howard, D. (1986), *The Dynamics of Feminist Therapy.* New York: Haworth.

Jennings, F.L. (1992). Ethics of rural practice. *Psychotherapy in Private Practice (Special Issue: Psychological Practice in Small Towns and Rural Areas), 10* (3), 85–104.

Jones, E. (1951). The God Complex. In idem, *Essays in Applied Psychoanalysis,* 2, pp. 244–265. London: Hogarth.

Kagle, J.D. & Geilbelhausen, P.N. (1994). Dual relationships and professional boundaries. *Social Work, 39* (2), 213–220.

Keen S. (1986). *Faces of the Enemy: Reflections of the Hostile Imagination.* San Francisco: Harper & Row.

Keith-Spiegel, P. & Koocher, G.P. (1985). *Ethics in Psychology: Professional Standards and Cases.* New York: Random House.

Kertesz, R. (2002). Dual relationships in therapy in Latin America. In A.A. Lazarus & O. Zur (Eds.) *Dual Relationships and Psychotherapy,* New York: Springer, pp. 329–334.

Kitchener, K.S. (1988). Dual role relationships: What makes them so problematic? *Journal of Counseling and Development, 67,* 217–221.

Kitchener, K.S. (1996) Professional codes of ethics and ongoing moral problems in psychology. In W. O'Donohue & R.F. Kitchener (Eds.), *The Philosophy of Psychology* (pp. 361–370). London: Sage.

Koocher, G.P. & Keith-Spiegel, P. (1998). *Ethics in Psychology: Professional Standards and Cases.* New York: Oxford University Press.

Lakin, M. (1991). *Coping with Ethical Dilemmas in Psychotherapy.* New York: Pergamon.

Lambert, M.J. (1992). Psychotherapy outcome research: Implications for integrative and eclectic therapists. In J.C. Norcross & M.R. Goldfried (Eds.), *Handbook of Psychotherapy Integration* (pp. 94–129). New York: Basic.

Langs, R.J. (1974). The therapeutic relationship and deviations in technique. In R.J. Langs (Ed.), *International Journal of Psychoanalytic Psychotherapy: Vol. 4* (pp. 106–141). New York: Jason Aronson.

Lazarus, A.A. (1994). How certain boundaries and ethics diminish therapeutic effectiveness. *Ethics and Behavior, 4,* 255–261.

Lazarus, A.A. (1998). How do you like these boundaries? *The Clinical Psychologist, 51,* 22–25.

Lazarus, A.A. & Zur, O. (Eds.) (2002). *Dual Relationships and Psychotherapy.* New York: Springer,

Lerman, H., & Porter, N. (Eds.) (1990). *Feminist Ethics in Psychotherapy.* New York: Springer.

Llewellyn, R. (2002). Sanity and sanctity: The counselor and multiple relationships in the church. In A.A. Lazarus & O. Zur (Eds.) *Dual Relationships and Psychotherapy,* New York: Springer, pp. 298–314.

Montgomery, M.J. & DeBell, C. (1997). Dual relationships and pastoral counseling asset or liability? *Counseling and Values, 42* (1), 30–41.

Nagy, T.F. (2000). *Ethics in Plain English: An Illustrative Casebook for Psychologists.* Washington, DC: American Psychological Association.

National Association of Social Workers (NASW). (1999). *Code of Ethics.* Retrieved July 27, 2001, from http://www.naswdc.org/Code/ethics.htm.

Nietzsche, F. (1977) (Trans) *Portable Nietzsche.* Trans. By Walter Kaufmann, New York: Viking.

Norcross, J.C. & Goldfried, M.R. (Eds.). (1992). *Handbook of Psychotherapy Integration.* New York: Basic.

Pepper, R.S. (1991). The senior therapist's grandiosity: Clinical and ethical consequences of merging multiple roles. *Journal of Contemporary Psychotherapy, 21* (1), 63–70.

Pope, K.S. (1986). New trends in malpractice cases and changes in APA liability insurance. *Independent Practitioner, 6,* 23–26.

Pope, K.S. (1988). Dual relationships: A source of ethical, legal, and clinical problems. *Independent Practitioner, 8* (1), 17–25.

Pope, K.S. (1989). Therapist–patient sex syndrome: A guide to assessing damage. In G.O. Gabbard (Ed.), *Sexual Exploitation in Professional Relationships* (pp. 39–55). Washington, DC: American Psychiatric Press.

Pope, K.S. (1990). Therapist–patient sex as sex abuse: Six scientific, professional, and practical dilemmas in addressing victimization and rehabilitation. *Professional Psychology: Research and Practice, 21,* 227–239.

Pope, K.S. (1991). Dual roles and sexual intimacy in psychotherapy. *Ethics and Behavior, 1* (1), 21–34.

Pope, K.S. (1994). *Sexual Involvement with Therapists: Patient Assessment, Subsequent Therapy, Forensics.* Washington, DC: American Psychological Association.

Pope, K.S. & Bouhoutsos, J. (1988). Dual relationships in the practice of psychology. *Professional Psychology: Research and Practice, 19,* 123–135.

Pope, K.S. & Vasquez, M.J.T. (1998). *Ethics in Psychotherapy and Counseling: A Practical Guide for Psychologists.* San Francisco: Jossey-Bass.

Pope, K.S., Tabachnick, B.G., & Keith-Spiegel, K. (1987). Ethics of practice: The beliefs and behaviors of psychologists as therapists. *American Psychologist, 42* (1), 993–1006.

Ramsdell, P.S. & Ramsdell, E.M. (1993). Dual relationships: Client perceptions of the effect of client-counselor relationship on the therapeutic process. *Clinical Social Work Journal, 21* (2), 195–212.

Schank, J.A. (1998). Ethical issues in rural counseling practice. *Canadian Journal of Counseling, 32* (4), 270–283.

Schank, J.A. & Skovholt, T.M. (1997). Dual relationship dilemmas of rural and small-community psychologists. *Professional Psychology: Research and Practice, 28,* 44–49.

Sears, V.L. (1990). On being an "only" one. In H. Lerman & N. Porter (Eds.), *Feminist Ethics in Psychotherapy* (pp. 102–105). New York: Springer.

Sharkin, B.S. & Birky, I. (1992). Incidental encounters between therapists and their clients. *Professional Psychology: Research and Practice, 23* (4), 326–328.

Simon, R.I. (1989). Sexual exploitation of patients: How it begins before it happens. *Contemporary Psychiatry: Psychiatric Annals, 19* (2), 104–187.

Simon, R.I. (1991). Psychological injury caused by boundary violation precursors to therapist-patient sex. *Psychiatric Annals, 21,* 614–619.

Simon, R.I. (1992). Treatment boundary violations: Clinical, ethical, and legal considerations. *Bulletin of the American Academy of Psychiatry and Law, 20,* 269–287.

Simon, R.I. (1995). The natural history of therapist sexual misconduct: Identification and prevention. *Psychiatric Annals, 25,* 90–94.

Slack, C.M. & Wassenaar, D.R. (1999). Ethical dilemmas of South African clinical psychologists. *European Psychologist, 4*(3), 179–186.

Smith, A.J. (1990). Working within the lesbian community: The dilemma of overlapping relationships. In H. Lerman & N. Porter (Eds.), *Feminist Ethics in Psychotherapy* (pp. 92–96). New York: Springer.

Smith, D. (2003). Here are things every psychologist can do. *The APA Monitor, 34/1,* 5.

Smith, E.W.L., Clance, P.R., & Imes, S. (Eds.) 1998. *Touch in Psychotherapy: Theory Research and Practice.* New York: Guilford.

Sonne, J.L. (1994). Multiple relationships: Does the new ethics code answer the right questions? *Professional Psychology: Research and Practice, 25* (40), 336–343.

St. Germaine, J. (1996). Dual relationships and certified alcohol and drug counselors: A national study of ethical beliefs and behaviors. *Alcohol Treatment Quarterly, 14* (2), 29–45.

Staal, M.A. & King, R.E. (2000). Managing a multiple relationship environment: The ethics of military psychology. *Professional Psychology: Research and Practice, 31* (6), 698–705.

Stamm, B.H. (Ed.) (2003). *Rural Behavioral Health Care.* Washington, DC: APA Books.

Stockman, A.F. (1990). Dual relationships in rural mental health practice: An ethical dilemma. *Journal of Rural Community Psychology, 11* (2), 31–45.

Strasburger, L.H., Jorgenson, L., & Sutherland, P. (1992). The prevention of psychotherapist sexual misconduct: Avoiding the slippery slope. *American Journal of Psychotherapy, 46* (4), 544–555.

Thomas, J.L. (2002). On bartering. In A.A. Lazarus & O. Zur (Eds.) *Dual Relationships and Psychotherapy,* New York: Springer, pp. 394–408.

Tomm, K. (1993). The ethics of dual relationships. *The California Therapist,* January/February, 7–19.

Wassenaar, D.R. (1999). Ethical dilemmas of South African clinical psychologists: International comparisons. *European Psychologist. V. 4*(3) 179–186.

Williams, M.H. (1992). Exploitation and inference: Mapping the damage from therapist-patient sexual involvement. *American Psychologist, 47*, 412–421.

Williams, M.H. (1995). How useful are clinical reports concerning the consequences of therapist–patient sexual involvement? *American Journal of Psychotherapy, 49* (2), 237–243.

Williams, M.H. (1997). Boundary violations: Do some contended standards of care fail to encompass commonplace procedures of humanistic, behavioral and eclectic psycho-therapies? *Psychotherapy, 34,* 239–249.

Williams, M.H. (2000). Victimized by "victims": A taxonomy of antecedents of false complaints against psychotherapists. *Professional Psychology Research and Practice, 31* (1), 75–81.

Woody, R.H. (1998). *Fifty Ways to Avoid Malpractice.* Sarasota, FL: Professional Resource Exchange.

Yalom, I.D. (1980). *Existential Psychotherapy.* New York: Basic.

Yalom, I.D. (1997). *Lying on the Couch.* New York: Harper Perennial.

Younggren, J.N. & Skorka, D. (1992). The non-therapeutic psychotherapy relationship. *Law and Psychology Review, 16,* 13–28.

Zur, O. (2001). Out of office experience: When crossing office boundaries and engaging in dual relationships are clinically beneficial and ethically sound. *The Independent Practitioner, 21* (2), 96–100.

Zur, O. (2002). The truth about the Codes of Ethics: Dispelling the rumors that dual relationships are unethical. In A.A. Lazarus & O. Zur (Eds.) *Dual Relationships and Psychotherapy,* New York: Springer, pp. 55–64.

Zur, O. & Gonzalez, S. (2002). Multiple relationships in military psychology. In A.A. Lazarus & O. Zur (Eds.), *Dual Relationships and Psychotherapy,* New York: Springer, pp. 315–328.

Zur, O. & Lazarus, A. (2003). Letter to the Editor. *APA Monitor of Psychology, 34*(3), p. 5.

14

SOCIAL JUSTICE IN COMMUNITY PSYCHOLOGY

Jason Lillis, William T. O'Donohue, Michael Cucciare, and Elizabeth Lillis

Social justice plays a critical role in defining community psychology, yet this construct has evaded explication and critical analysis. This chapter examines the limitations of community psychology's liberal sociopolitical bias and presents an alternative conservative approach to social justice.

According to Wiley and Rappaport (2000), "Community psychology's aim is to foster a more just society" and is concerned with ".... social justice and progressive politics" (pp. 59–60). Prilleltensky (2001) noted that a central goal of community psychology is to eliminate oppression, discrimination, and violence and "To achieve that objective, we need to promote social justice and social action...." (p. 750). Prilleltensky and Nelson (1997) call for more social justice in the goals and interventions of community psychology. Dalton, Elias, and Wandersman (2001) identified social justice as a core value for the field, noting that ".... groups excluded from social justice in U.S. history have included women, persons of color, the poor, immigrants, workers, gay men and lesbians, and others" (p. 6).

The mainstream political left, amply represented in psychology, has influenced the definition of social justice in community psychology; however, political philosophers have explicated social justice in vastly different ways, rendering it multivocal. Critical analysis in community psychology has been absent with respect to defining social justice problems and methods of change, which has led to a dominant bias associated with a liberal worldview.

Moreover, social justice has taken on a powerful rhetorical function, implying the "goodness" of the motives and actions of the community psychologist. However, passive acceptance of the construct of social justice serves to limit critical evaluation of the goals and interventions of community psychology and ignore other, more conservative approaches to defining and achieving social justice. Specifically, the liberal worldview of community psychology has resulted in a complete lack of conservative ideas in the literature, depriving the field of potentially useful alternative conceptualizations of social justice problems, goals, methods of change, and interventions.

Ironically, community psychology advocates another important value—respect for diversity—yet does not practice this when it comes to sociopolitical ideas. Dalton et al. (2001) note that community psychology, "… recognizes and prizes the variety of communities and social identities, based on gender, ethnic or racial membership, sexual orientation, ability or disability, socioeconomic status, age. … It has become an important value in community psychology … a respect for diversity" (p. 18). Diversity of opinion is conspicuously omitted from that definition. Indeed, community psychology does not show any significant diversity of opinion in terms of defining social justice problems, goals, methods of change, and interventions.

It is has been argued that there is a liberal bias in the field of psychology as a whole. Redding (2001) noted that the field lacks sociopolitical diversity. Most psychologists are politically liberal, and research and advocacy efforts are guided by liberal sociopolitical views. One example of this is a study by Jost, Glaser, Kruglanski, and Sulloway (2003), which presents a theoretical perspective on the psychological motives underlying political conservatism. The authors use a variety of data, including speeches, interviews, and court verdicts, to support their theory that endorsement of politically conservative principles is fueled by two psychological factors: resistance to change and tolerance of inequality. This perpetually flawed study is another example of a political agenda under the guise of science.

The authors note that although there is a vast literature on conservatism, there is a dramatic absence of studies on liberalism. This, in and of itself, is evidence of a liberal bias. The message is clear: political conservatism is abnormal, and thus appropriate subject matter for psychology. One major flaw is that much of the data used in the meta-analyses was gathered using a number of scales that purport to measure conservatism. These scales were constructed to support the assumptions of the authors about what conservatism is (e.g., fearful, authoritarian, racist).

Jost et al. (2003) also use different definitions of conservatism interchangeably to support their conclusions. For example, they identify Stalin as a conservative because he wanted to preserve the status quo communist system in Russia. Furthermore, a variety of data (often anecdotal in nature) from different fields with varied epistemic and theoretical assumptions was integrated selectively, again to prove biased a priori assumptions. The authors of this chapter are currently writing a more comprehensive response to Jost et al. (2003) that will detail these shortcomings.

The state of community psychology is no different from the field as a whole. Thus, although the political right and left continue to debate what social justice is and how best to achieve it, this debate is absent in community psychology. The work of John Rawls (1971), which is the foundation of mainstream political liberalism in America, best characterizes the philosophy behind a liberal social justice. In order to elucidate this worldview, we summarize the work of John Rawls and show its influence in community psychology.

COMMUNITY PSYCHOLOGY AND JOHN RAWLS'S THEORY OF SOCIAL JUSTICE

A socially just society, according to Rawls (1971), redistributes resources to its least advantaged members. Rawls' theory is based on two concepts: the original position and the veil of ignorance. The "original position" is a hypothetical scenario in which a group of people, starting with no possessions, forms a society by establishing the basic rights and principles for dividing economic resources. Rawls assumes that in the original position people are self-interested, rational, and under a veil of ignorance. Behind the veil of ignorance, members of this group do not know what their social class, ethnicity, intelligence, and physical ability will be. However, individuals are aware that after society is designed, there will be a wide variety in the distribution of these characteristics. Each person purportedly then advocates for a system that would protect against potential disadvantages to him- or herself no matter what position is actually acquired, thus creating a socially just society that favors the least advantaged members.

Rawls advocates for a redistribution of economic resources when doing so benefits the least advantaged. Although he maintains that the hard working and talented may obtain a greater share of the economic resources, he claims that this is justified only if they share the additional wealth with the least advantaged. Rawls views a person's talents and abilities as undeserved, something for which society needs to correct. He envisions a government structure with four branches—Allocation, Stabilization, Transfer, and Distribution—that would (1) keep prices competitive, (2) guarantee full employment, (3) correct competitive pricing, and (4) correct the distribution of wealth.

Rawls's theory of social justice has been exceptionally influential and has formed the backbone of current liberal political ideology. Programs such as welfare and affirmative action can be attributed to his work.

Community Psychology's Worldview Bias

In community psychology, the influence of the political left (based on Rawls's theories) has led to a narrow definition of social justice problems and interventions characterized by the following.

- There are disadvantaged people who need help. These politically sanctioned minority groups include African-Americans, Hispanics, women, and homosexuals.
- These minority groups have and continue to experience disadvantages—for example, poverty, prejudice, exposure to violence, mental and physical health problems—that are the result of oppression.
- The disadvantaged are in need of assistance from the intellectual elite, who will design interventions to combat oppression.

The following examples illustrate this worldview bias in community psychology. In describing social justice, Dalton et al. (2001) write, "It is thus concerned with equality. … It also involves advocacy for policies that make resources for wellness available to all members of a community or society, especially its least privileged" (p. 16). According to the authors, these "least privileged" members of society are those who are currently being oppressed because of their race, ethnicity, gender, or sexual orientation. Oppression in America occurs primarily by White heterosexual males, who make up a "dominant group" granted "resources, power, and freedom … *not by their own efforts*" (p. 165; italics added). The disadvantaged groups are denied "access to power and resources" (p. 165). Prilleltensky (2003) notes that "It is only when the oppressed attain a certain degree of conscientization that mechanisms of resistance take place" and that "Oppression deprives individuals and collectives of these rights ..." (political and psychological well-being), "... whereas liberation promotes recovery (p. 195). Appropriate methods of change include: (1) resisting the dominant theory that economic growth is the main vehicle to well-being, (2) preventing exclusion and promoting liberation, (3) developing political activism, and (4) promoting acts of solidarity with other oppressed groups (Prilleltensky, 2003).

Community psychologists often posit that oppression, in its many forms, is to blame. Focusing on oppression as the key variable has led to a meta-framework by which many community psychologists operate.

- Find and define a disadvantaged group.
- Define problems of the group as the result of victimization, groups not having their fair share because of oppression.
- Define the process of helping as raising awareness, particularly political awareness, mobilizing community members to interact, obtaining political advocacy, working toward getting groups "what's owed" them.
- Define outcomes as consciousness-raising, political representation, "acts of solidarity," such as voting and holding community meetings.
- Through this political advocacy create government programs to redistribute opportunity and money.

This is a Rawlsian, liberal political solution: shift economic resources (programs) to disadvantaged populations that have been historically oppressed. The economic resources to fund these programs come from government actions such as taxes, which take resources from other members of society.

Problems with a Liberal Social Justice Based on Rawls

To examine the problems with a liberal social justice we must first discuss the limitations and inconsistencies of its intellectual basis.

Rawls Arrives at Illogical Conclusions about the Original Position

Scholars have questioned Rawls (e.g., Gauthier, 1974; Rasmussen, 1974), arguing that people in the original position would logically develop a much different society. Not all people are likely to view natural talents and abilities as undeserved, and it is questionable if they would agree to a society that punished rather then rewarded them, particularly as others indirectly experience the benefits of their talents and abilities. It is human nature to further one's self-interest, and each person is likely to want to keep what he or she creates. As such, under a Rawlsian system, resources must be taken forcefully (Rasmussen, 1974).

Rawls Fails to Give an Adequate Definition of "Least Advantaged"

Are certain people less advantaged than others, and on what dimensions? Who determines this? When is being disadvantaged no longer a matter of social justice? Choptiany (1973) notes that Rawls gives no specification of the "size of the inequality allowed in comparison with the amount of advantage provided" (p. 147). This means, simply, that there is no objective way to determine what "disadvantage" warrants intervention; furthermore, there is no way to determine how much intervention is enough.

The Rawlsian Government Violates Principles of Economics and Would Have Severe Negative Effects on the Economy

Economic resources would be required to fund the proposed four branches of the government, thus stunting economic growth. In addition, controlling prices thwarts the economy by arbitrarily assigning value to goods and services. Only the market itself can assign true value, which results from free exchanges by all individuals (Friedman & Friedman, 1980). Also, correcting the distribution of wealth leads to the desire for satisfaction and further extorts money that would stimulate economic growth. No government agency can decide what should be produced, who should produce it, what it should cost, and how people should be reimbursed. This would defeat the purpose of a free market.

Rawls's Theory Opens the Door to an Agenda of "Want Satisfaction" (Barry, 1973)

Life circumstances, viewed by Rawls as matters of social justice, could easily be perceived as simply wanting more than one has. So what are the limits to this satisfaction of want? How are claims of social injustice supported? Furthermore, how can we put a value or prioritization on different wants for different people? By treating wants as matters of social justice, we undertake the task of arbitrarily deciding the value of all aspects of living. There are many unintended negative consequences of this politics of victimization, including: infantalizing minorities, giving incentive for people to claim victim status, creating group polarization, and encouraging reverse discrimination. These consequences are explored in the next section.

The many problems with Rawls's theory of social justice hold true for community psychology's explication and operationalizing of social justice. Redistribution violates the principles of economics by arbitrarily assigning value and providing disincentives for economic achievement, leading to stunted economic growth and negatively affecting all members of society. Furthermore, there are no objectively correct answers in deciding what people ought to receive as their just due. Trying to solve this problem will lead to "want satisfaction" in the form of a politics of victimization.

The Politics of Victimization Creating a politics of victimization, whereby groups of people are encouraged to claim victim status to obtain what is owed to them, has a number of unintended adverse consequences.

1. It provides incentive for people to be victims. If victims deserve advocacy efforts in order to combat oppressive circumstances and claim their rightful stake, then there is less need for them to take personal responsibility and work hard to change their current circumstances. Victims are dependent on their advocates, who fight for what is "deserved." The mindset is "How do I get what is owed?" instead of "How do I make the most of my life, fighting barriers that exist and maximizing my potential?"
2. Labeling people as victims can lead to attribution effects. They may see themselves as unable to advance in life by their own efforts. They may come to attribute their successes to luck or others, while seeing their failures as characteristic of their oppressed nature.
3. Currently, women, African Americans, Hispanics, Native Americans, Asian Americans, and homosexuals, to name a few, are viewed as historically oppressed according to community psychology. These groups combined constitute more than two-thirds of the U.S. population. With all these victims, where is the oppression coming from? More important, how will we adjudicate claims of victimhood? How many more groups should be added to the list: the elderly, who are fighting ageism; the overweight, who are fighting the oppressive forces of fast food and the media? Which groups deserve economic reparations and

what are our priorities? How do we identify and stop individual oppressors?

4. Labeling people into oppressed and nonoppressed groups can create prejudice and deepen a cycle of hatred. Social psychologists have documented many phenomena that fuel prejudice and racism, including:

Scapegoating: This is the tendency for people to find a target for their anger, someone to blame. Identifying people as oppressed would seem to feed the idea of scapegoating the oppressors, thus fueling prejudice and racism (Gilbert, Fiske, & Lindzey, 1998).

Ingroup and Outgroup: This is the tendency for people to favor those in their socially identified groups. Rather than letting people decide on their own what groups they want to identify with (e.g., college students, suburbanites, music lovers, etc.), community psychologists proscribe group membership based on historical oppression, thus fueling an ingroup bias against all others. This serves to create increased and arbitrary polarization between the so-called haves and have-nots (Gilbert et al., 1998).

Categorization: By putting people into categories instead of letting them define themselves, community psychologists create a categorization bias. We group all Hispanics into the "oppressed Hispanic" group, and all White people into the "nonoppressed, dominant, white" group. This supports stereotypes and fuels prejudice and racism (Gilbert et al.,1998).

5. Identifying people as oppressed often gives them the right to hate. For example, feminists can call all men "rapists" (McKinnon, 1987). This hinders male–female relations and is an example of reverse discrimination. In addition, men are not accorded the same rights as women in many cases because women's categorization as oppressed allows them more leeway to speak and act without penalty. This kind of double standard can only serve to fuel hatred by sending the message that it is okay to hate as long as you're part of an oppressed group.

The many problems with Rawls's analysis hold true for community psychology, which focuses on problematic mechanisms of change: eradicating alleged oppression through community and government action. This liberal social justice promotes the adverse consequences we have described and serves to perpetuate current circumstances in disadvantaged groups. More important, there is no efficacy data to support this approach. For example, there are no data showing that the socioeconomic status of minorities rises after a community psychology intervention or that prejudice causes socioeconomic discrepancies that advocacy changes. Community psychology simply has not hit any homeruns in this area that would warrant the de facto dismissal of alternative views.

The Economics of Social Justice

Examined more closely, the core issue of social justice is economics and economic disparities. Historically, a "disadvantaged" group is no longer seen as oppressed if they are doing well economically, for example, Jews, one of the most historically persecuted groups in history, and Asian Americans, who had to face higher admission standards than Whites in original affirmative action programs (Sowell, 1983). Community psychologists, however, would have us believe that certain racial groups, for example, African Americans, are poorer than average mostly due to oppression and political underrepresentation.

Sowell points out that the success of a given group can be attributed to the group's culture, which rewards some behaviors over others, determining skills, orientation toward work, and economic performance. Thus, in Sowell's view, the primary social justice intervention is to target cultural practices that support good economic behavior. The market rewards certain behaviors and penalizes others without regard for race or culture. Sowell cites the following as evidence.

- Experiences denied to black slaves in America, for example, incentives to exercise initiative (entrepreneurial activities), owning and managing economic resources, buying and selling goods or services—were also denied to West Indies Blacks, who have subsequently risen much faster economically in America despite suffering the same discrimination.
- Remarkable examples of politically subordinate and oppressed peoples that have prospered far beyond the level of political majority and socially powerful. Examples include the Jews in Europe, the Chinese in Southeast Asian countries such as Indo-China, Thailand, Vietnam, and the Italians in Argentina. These groups faced harsh extreme discrimination, and oppression, yet rose economically, and later socially.
- Historically, the relationship between political success and economic success has been more inverse than direct. People without entrepreneurial skills tend to flock to politics, civil service,

and military jobs. Furthermore, attempts to advance groups economically through political means has often had paradoxical effects, because such attempts are often met with counterchauvinism. The true mechanisms of economic advancement have still not been addressed.

Economic performance differences among groups are quite real and quite large. Liberals blame discrimination for the so-called "underrepresentation" of different racial and ethnic groups in various occupations, institutions, activities, and income levels, as if there are no substantial cultural differences among the various groups. This assumption is nowhere demonstrated historically but rather falsified many times over (Sowell, 1983). According to Sowell, the key variables are ability to work hard and long, the ability to save money, and entrepreneurial skills and sensibilities.

In addition, antecedent political biases obscure the correct identification of social problems. Political approaches must be emotionally acceptable to the people addressed, and must offer an actual solution within the political domain (Sowell, 1983). Thus, no matter what variables actually play a role in change, political leaders emphasize factors that can be addressed by law—usually moral condemnation of other groups—while ignoring factors such as group differences, skill levels, and cultural values/practices.

These political misconceptions, however, can serve the political leadership despite being counterproductive (Sowell, 1983). For example, redistributing resources to an "oppressed group" can negatively affect the economy as a whole by increasing the national deficit and inflation. In addition, other groups may react harshly to this arbitrary decision to take their money, straining race relations. These consequences would seem to outweigh the benefits. However, it is still in the leadership's best interest to pursue these benefits. If the oppressed group rises as society as a whole rises, the leaders suffer because they serve no function. This is the same for the intellectual elite. By promoting "social justice causes" for oppressed groups, they gain favor, publication, and promotions, whether or not their ideas or interventions help the groups they champion. This has come to be known as the poverty industry.

Sowell's analysis describes the many problems with attributing socioeconomic outcomes to oppression and political underrepresentation. Community psychology has spent too long on this narrow leftist definition of social justice, resulting in the unfair dismissal of alternative (e.g., conservative) viewpoints that would be valuable in defining social justice problems, interventions, and methods of change.

CONSERVATIVE DEFINITIONS OF SOCIAL JUSTICE: PROVIDING AN ALTERNATIVE

Hayek's Theory

The intellectual basis for a conservative social justice can be traced to Frederick A. Hayek (Hayek, 1944; Butler, 1983). According to Hayek, the construct of social justice has no meaning (Butler, 1983). We, as a society, simply cannot decide what people ought to have in any reliable, scientific, or metaphysical way. To do so, a society would first need to centralize power in an institution that would strive for social justice by distributing resources according to some clear, accurate, and absolute "moral standard."

To accomplish this task, such an institution—which would be susceptible to extreme abuses of its absolute power—would have to decide the "correct" moral standard motivating this distribution of resources. Contributions could be overestimated and resources would be assigned to areas that are seen by some elite as "worthy." This will result in decreased incentives for efficiency and innovation, while fewer resources are allocated to areas that promote broad economic growth. There would be many competing claims for resource allocation and no conceivable way of adjudicating these claims. Because we do not have the capacity to process the mass amounts of information necessary to make these decisions, nor an effective way to implement them, Hayek maintains that any attempt to achieve social justice will inevitably fail, crippling the economy (Feser, 1997).

Hayek endorses a fair and just market system in which no person or institution is responsible for distributing wealth. The market is driven by supply and demand, and each person gets to vote with his or her resources.

- People are free to buy and sell goods and services.
- Each exchange is voluntary and reflects independent appraisals of value for a given good or service.
- Individuals must be attuned to how others allocate value in order to produce goods or services in demand at a fair price.
- Social justice is achieved by creating more freedom and liberty, while giving people economic literacy tools that will help them be better producers and consumers.

There is nothing more just than a free economic transaction, which increases value for everyone involved. In any given exchange, each person walks away happier, because by definition he or she has made a voluntary choice. For example, when Bill pays $5.00 for John's book, Bill values the book more than he values the $5.00, and John values the $5.00 more than the book. The market offers incentive for people to be efficient, solve problems, and produce something in demand by society. The price mechanism guides people into different areas of work, which allows the economy as a whole to grow and creates more resources for all members of society, while keeping them free from coercion and tyranny.

Throughout history, these economic principles have been the engine of socioeconomic change (Sowell, 1983). Groups across the world have experienced a rise in living standards as a result of hard work, sound economic management, and entrepreneurial skills, often in the face of extreme prejudice and discrimination. Government redistribution has never resulted in a rise in living standards for disadvantaged groups. In fact, government redistribution has resulted in many catastrophic failures for entire societies (communist Russia, East Germany, China, and others in which tens of millions died in the twentieth century).

Hayek's theory of social justice is internally consistent, calling for the repudiation of the construct. In all situations, the market decides who gets what, and everyone has a chance to put his or her efforts into an area that offers better rewards. There are a number of problems Hayek's theory avoids, including defining the least advantaged, deciding what people ought to have, and creating a centralized institution that could thwart economic growth.

An approach like Hayek's that promotes liberty and the market has the following advantages.

- The market produces more resources on the whole, minimizing poverty in general. The Federal Reserve Board reported that the net worth of Americans in the lowest income quintile (lowest twenty percent) rose twenty-five percent between 1998 and 2001 (Kemp, 2003). America also has a significantly reduced homeless population as a result of a market economy.
- The market promotes economic mobility. In America, eighty-six percent of tax filers in the bottom income quintile had exited this quintile by the end of a decade. In addition, an individual in the bottom quintile had a better chance of rising to the top quintile than remaining at the bottom (Kemp, 2003).

- The market fosters progressive societal values. People are given the incentive to solve problems better, cheaper, and faster, providing a natural mechanism for combating societal problems and leading to better living conditions for all.
- The market combats prejudice and discrimination, which are detrimental to efficient economic arrangement. It allows for the successful Black investor and the lesbian CEO. Everyone is allowed to market his or her skills and rise to the top regardless of race, sex, religion, or sexual orientation.

Examples of Conservative Approaches

Throughout history, the engine of socioeconomic improvement has never been "victim helping." It is difficult to understand why community psychology has not attempted to combat social problems by promoting improved economic behavior. This section outlines such an approach, based on models of Hayek (1944) and Sowell (1983). A conservative approach to social change would:

- Focus on individuals, not groups, identifying specific needs and deficits rather than assuming them based on ethnic or racial origin. There are numerous successful African Americans, Hispanics, and women, as well as numerous unsuccessful White men.
- Study individuals who have succeeded in raising their own living standards, analyze what has worked for groups and individuals in the past, and disseminate this information to others.
- Teach relevant financial skills such as financial management, ownership, investing, entrepreneurism, orienting to long-term goals, and building positive work orientation.
- Provide incentives for "smart" economic choices by individuals, while giving businesses incentives to create opportunities.

The following are examples of conservative principles in action.

Creating Opportunities through Ownership: Mali's Makeshift Cuisinarts

In a village in the African country of Mali, a miraculous change in living standards has occurred. Producing peanut butter, a primary local industry, once took all the time and energy of the women and children in Mali. Now, a peanut-processing machine reduces the time it takes to grind fifteen pounds of peanuts from ten hours to ten minutes, while improving the quality of the peanut butter produced. This is the result of a United Nations-sponsored program to aid poverty, which provided the $8,000 machine to the village for $4,000 (once a village raises half, the rest is sponsored).

The women of the village pay twenty-five cents to use the machine, and some are paid to manage it. The surplus funds generated by the machine (total revenue after management salaries and maintenance) have been used to rig up a lighting system for the village, leading to safer streets and clinics, as well as for nighttime educational opportunities. With dramatically increased free time, women are branching out into other businesses such as dyeing clothes, making soap, and cultivating rice. Children are now free to learn to read and write. The machine continues to generate money, which is used to improve the village.

This program is an example of achieving social justice goals by promoting sound economic principles. The machine promotes pride of ownership—the villagers own, operate, maintain, and pay to use the machine—while creating opportunities for entrepreneurial activities. The villagers take care of the machine because they have an ownership stake in it. They have learned to use their newfound free time to market other talents and abilities. The villagers have gained valuable knowledge about managing both financial resources and human resources.

Thus, the agenda for community psychology could be to create similar opportunities for disadvantaged people in this country by working with either the government or a private financer. Community psychologists can develop programs to provide equipment vital to some industry through loans with little or no interest rate, promoting ownership while creating financial opportunities.

Tax Incentives: Jack Kemp's Free Enterprise Zones One novel idea is to use entrepreneurial capitalism creatively to combat poverty and social problems. Free enterprise zones provide incentives, such as tax and regulatory relief, for businesses to locate in rural or inner-city areas suffering from high unemployment. This practice creates jobs, increases local tax revenue, and rejuvenates neighborhoods. It has been particularly successful when coupled with state assistance through business seminars, industrial site information, community profiles, and financial assistance for small business startups. Besides increased revenue and jobs, neighborhoods often become safer as people take pride in their work and have a stake in the businesses that operate there.

In other words, creating the context to reinforce better economic behavior (teaching skills, promoting ownership, giving people a stake) helps combat a host of other social problems in the process. Thus, the job of the community psychologist could be to lobby for tax incentives that would give businesses incentives to locate in poor neighborhoods, bringing jobs, teaching work skills, and making the neighborhood safer.

Small Business Loans: The SBA The Small Business Administration (SBA) provides loans to small businesses across the country. In the 1990s, the SBA helped approximately 435,000 small businesses obtain about $95 billion in loans. Small businesses account for approximately seventy-five percent of the new jobs added to the economy. The SBA provides special funding opportunities for women and minorities, including the minority small business program, microloans, and the publication of Spanish-language informational materials. In 1964, the SBA began to attack poverty through the Equal Opportunity Loan (EOL) Program. The EOL Program relaxed the credit and collateral requirements for applicants living below the poverty level in an effort to encourage new businesses that had been unable to attract financial backing but were, nevertheless, sound commercial initiatives.

The SBA has had a huge impact on minorities in business. A recent report (Minorities in Business, 2001) claims that minorities now own fifteen percent of American businesses and that ninety-nine percent of those are small businesses. These businesses totaled approximately $600 billion in revenue, paying out almost $100 billion in payroll. Thus, the agenda for community psychology could be to educate minorities about small business loan opportunities. Community psychologists could also be a source for referrals to all kinds of support resources necessary to start a business.

Philanthropy: Microsoft Philanthropy has long been ignored by community psychologists. This is strange, given the many corporations and individuals that have the money and want it used in a morally conscious way. Following are examples of how Microsoft has combined business and community initiatives to help people.

- *ClubTech* Funded by a $100 million donation from Microsoft, Club Tech will support the technology outreach efforts of Boys and Girls Clubs of America. The program will be extended to more than 3.3 million children and teens through every Boys and Girls Club in the nation by 2010. Technology centers and curricula will be established, accompanied by program management and computer training for staff members. Microsoft will work with the Boys and Girls Clubs to integrate all aspects of the technology, from overall club management to specific programs covering topics such as educational enhancement, character and leadership development, the arts, and sports and fitness.

- *College Assistance.* Microsoft has worked with the United Negro College Fund (UNCF) and the Hispanic Association of College Universities (HACU) to provide major cash donations, free software, scholarships, and annual training symposia for computer science and information technology personnel.

Thus, community psychologists could attempt to lobby for and organize philanthropic donations. They could spend time meeting with wealthy individuals and organizations to discuss the important moral aspects of giving back to society, while noting the many worthy causes that fall under the community psychology agenda.

Mentoring: State of Florida Mentoring is an approach to community assistance largely ignored by community psychology. The state of Florida has initiated a program that pairs minority- and woman-owned companies with established corporations making more than $1 million per year (Lauer, 2002). Its goal is to help minority businesses expand while giving them a way to participate in state contracts by being linked with big businesses. The program enables smaller, minority-owned companies to get vital support: seminars, formal meetings, and frank evaluations with recommendations for improvement. The mentor relationship also helps the sponsoring corporation, which gains access to new subcontractors and opens up new relationships with future clients.

The program seems to be working. In fiscal year 1998–1999, the governor's agencies spent $151 million with minority businesses, a number that increased 160 percent to $392 million by 2000–2001. As predicted by the governor's office, the figure increased by another twenty percent by the end of fiscal year 2002. Thus, the agenda for community psychology could be to organize and provide resources to help out minority-owned businesses.

Education: School Vouchers One of the biggest obstacles to economic success that urban minority (and nonminority) children face is poor schooling. Children graduate from high school without the ability to effectively read, write, and perform simple mathematics. This puts them at a huge disadvantage in the job market. Instead of teaching children to blame others, proponents of school vouchers say we should simply teach more effectively. School vouchers give parents the opportunity to send their children to a school that will teach them the fundamentals they need to go on to college or compete in the job market.

Wolf, Peterson, and West (2001) presented data on a pilot school voucher program in Washington, DC. One thousand randomly selected children were given vouchers to attend the private school of their choice. A control sample of more than 5000 children who applied for but did not receive school vouchers was used as a comparison. The authors reported the following results.

- African-American students who used the voucher averaged ten national percentage rank points higher in math and eight national percentage rank points higher in reading relative to those in the control group (both statistically significant results).
- In the private school where vouchers were used, the classes were significantly smaller, more homework was assigned, and eighty-one percent of parents reported satisfaction with the quality of their child's education as opposed to less than sixty percent in the control group.
- It is interesting that students who switched to private schools were more likely, after only two years, to provide tolerant responses to questions about civil liberties. For example, approximately one-half of private school students polled said they would permit a member of a group they disliked to live in their neighborhood, compared with less than one-quarter of public school controls.

Thus, community psychologists could organize support in favor of school choice and higher academic standards. Community psychologists could also conduct research to elucidate the relationship between early education and socioeconomic outcomes later in life.

Teaching Financial Skills: The MBDA The Minority Business Development Agency (MBDA), part of the U.S. Department of Commerce, is specifically designed to foster the creation, growth, and expansion of minority-owned businesses in the United States. It provides free financial information, and educational and consulting services. Specifically, the agency provides access to public and private debt and equity financing, directs minorities to market opportunities, helps coordinate and leverage public and private resources, and helps businesses form strategic alliances. The following are specific examples.

- Citizens Trust Bank, a minority-owned bank in Atlanta, will leverage the resources of the MBDA to help expand opportunities for minority-owned business by providing access to capital across the United States. The primary goal of this endeavor is to offer minority business owners an opportunity to move beyond theory-based workshops and seminars to the actual closing of financial lending transactions.
- On April 17, 2003, minority business entrepreneurs in San Francisco learned how to get on the "Fast Track to Business Opportunities and Access to Capital." This intense four-hour seminar/showcase was sponsored by the San Francisco regional office of MBDA, Wells Fargo, and the Asian Business Association, Inc. Attendees learned about buyers' budget forecasts for 2003–2004 and beyond, and a panel of high-profile agencies and business and community leaders explained their needs and the people and assistance available to get one's company in the process and expand a business (www.mbda.gov).
- The MBDA provides free resources online, including courses in acquisitions, basic loan criteria, business taxes, e-commerce, management, evaluating a business idea, startup businesses, manufacturing, and customer relations.

Thus, the community psychology agenda could include teaching financial skills to those in need, both for the small business entrepreneur and the average person aspiring to reach middle-class status. This could encompass education not only for business loans but for buying a home, opening a retirement account, managing bills, spending within budget limits, and avoiding credit card debt.

These seven examples merely scratch the surface. There are many others that illustrate conservative principles of change in action. With so many examples to build on, it is a wonder that community psychology continues to ignore the possibility that there are alternatives to the narrow view of social justice it takes.

RECOMMENDATIONS FOR CHANGE IN COMMUNITY PSYCHOLOGY

1. Abandon the rhetoric of social justice. Instead, explicate the purpose of using the construct by stating the matter of social concern, hold up a model of social change, and allow for critical debate of this claim. Problems described as matters of social

justice, and programs to ameliorate them, should be open to debate by the scientific community.

2. Clearly define change goals. Abandon the victim-helping approach for an economically driven, skills-based approach.
3. Use existing programs, such as the ones mentioned in this chapter, to generate novel ideas about how to use economic principles to benefit the disadvantaged.
4. Implement programs on a small scale at first. Use outcome measures that matter, such as better academic performance scores, higher income levels, and decreases in crime. An empirical approach should track both intended and unintended effects of the program. If preliminary results on a small scale are promising, the program might warrant expansion. Let the data determine the usefulness of the approach.

REFERENCES

Barry, B. (1973). Liberalism and want-satisfaction: A critique of John Rawls. *Political Theory, 1* (2), 134–154.

Beers, D. (1989). *Social Consciousness and Individual Freedom.* New York: Freeman.

Butler, E. (1983) *Hayek, His Contribution to the Political and Economic Thought of Our Time.* London: Temple Smith.

Choptiany, L. (1973). A critique of John Rawls's principles of justice. *Ethics, 83* (2), 146–150.

Dalton, J.H., Elias, M.J., & Wandersman, A. (2001). *Community Psychology: Linking Individuals to Communities.* Belmont, CA: Thomson Learning.

Feser, E. (1997). Hayek on social justice: Reply to Lukes and Johnston. *Critical Review, 11* (4), 581– 606.

Friedman, M. & Friedman, R. (1980). *Free to Choose.* New York: Harcourt.

Gauthier, D. (1974). Justice and natural endowment: Toward a critique of Rawls' ideological framework. *Social Theory and Practice, 3,* 3–26.

Gilbert, D.T., Fiske, S.T., & Lindzey, G. (1998). *The Handbook of Social Psychology.* Boston: McGraw-Hill, Oxford University Press.

Hayek, F.A. (1944). *The Road to Serfdom.* Chicago: University of Chicago Press.

Hobhouse, L.T. (1922). *The Elements of Social Justice.* New York: Henry Holt.

Jost, J., Glaser, J., Kruglanski, A., & Sullowat, F. (2003). Political conservatism as motivated social cognition. *Psychological Bulletin, 129* (3), 339–375.

Kemp, J. (2003). The rich are getting richer, and so are the poor. *Empower America on-line* Retrieved 7/1/2003 from http://www.empoweramerica.org/stories/storyReader.

Lauer, N.C. (2002). Mentoring goes corporate: State launches minority initiative. *Tallahassee Democrat,* May 16.

McKinnon, C.A. (1987). *Feminism unmodified: Discourses on life and law.* Cambridge, MA: Harvard University Press.

Prilleltensky, I. (2001). Value-based praxis in community psychology: Moving toward social justice and social action. *American Journal of Community Psychology, 29*(5), 747–778.

Prilleltensky, I. (2003). Understanding, resisting, and overcoming oppression: Toward psychopolitical validity. *American Journal of Community Psychology, 31*(1), 195–201.

Prilleltensky, I. & Nelson, G. (1997). Community psychology: Reclaiming social justice. In D. Fox & I. Prilleltensky (Eds.), *Critical Psychology: An Introduction,* pp. 166–184.

Rasmussen, D.B. (1974). A critique of Rawls' theory of justice. *Personalist, 55*, 303–318.

Rawls, J. (1971). *A Theory of Justice.* Cambridge, MA: Belknap Press of Harvard University Press.

Redding, R.E. (2001). Sociopolitical diversity in psychology: The case for pluralism. *American Psychologist, 56*(3), 205–215.

Sowell, T. (1983). *The Economics and Politics of Race.* New York: Morrow.

Small Business Administration (2001). *Minorities in business.* Washington, DC: Author.

Wiley, A. & Rappaport, J. (2000). Empowerment, wellness, and the politics of development. In D. Cicchetti & J. Rappaport (Eds.), *The Promotion of Wellness in Children and Adolescents,* pp. 59–99. Boston: McGraw-Hill.

Wolf, P.J., Peterson, P.E., & West, M.R. (2001). Results of a school voucher experiment: The case of Washington, D.C. after two years. Paper presented at the annual meeting of the *American Political Science Association,* San Francisco.

15

SOCIOPOLITICAL DIVERSITY IN PSYCHOLOGY: THE CASE FOR PLURALISM

Richard. E. Redding

There is a struggle about what is sayable within our discipline, and about what need not be said, about what can be assumed and what requires explanation, about what questions can be asked and what constitutes legitimate answers (Kitzinger, 1991, p. 49). Although psychology celebrates diversity, which has become one of the profession's core values (see American Psychological Association, 1992; Fowers & Richardson, 1996) and strives to be inclusive by recognizing the value and legitimacy of diverse beliefs, the profession lacks sociopolitical diversity. Most psychologists are politically liberal, and conservatives are vastly underrepresented in the profession.

APA's ethical principles urge psychologists to be sensitive to cultural differences. Moreover, "We have a central responsibility to examine our biases and the ways in which these biases contribute to perpetuating a particular political point of view" (Silverstein, 1993, p. 305). Despite these ideals, the lack of sociopolitical diversity continues. Sociopolitical views that guide the research, advocacy, or professional practice of psychologists most often are liberal.

This lack of political diversity has unintended negative consequences and is detrimental to psychology in ways that conflict with the profession's core values and ethical principles. It biases research on social policy issues, damages psychology's credibility with policymakers and the public, impedes serving conservative clients, results in de facto discrimination against conservative students and scholars, and has a chilling effect on liberal education. This chapter discusses these problems and presents four strategies for increasing sociopolitical pluralism in psychology.

THE CONSERVATIVE ABSENCE

Social policy issues are often at the forefront of the "culture wars" (Hunter, 1991). Conservative and liberal worldviews on such issues represent "two distinct conceptions of moral authority—two different ways of apprehending reality, of ordering experience, of making moral judgments" (Hunter, 1991, p. 128). This may be due to individual differences in views on human nature and the effective remedies for social problems (Hunt, 1999; Hunter, 1991; Tomkins, 1963) and views on the extent to which individuals are responsible for their life circumstances (Weiner, 1995; Williams, 1984). In addition, conservative and liberal worldviews may hinge on intrinsic (e.g., reliance on individually defined moral truths) versus extrinsic (e.g., reliance on natural law or God) orientations to the sources of moral authority (e.g., Hunter, 1991, 2000), on tough-mindedness versus tender-mindedness (Eysenck, 1954; Stone & Schaffner, 1988), and on an orientation toward authoritarian–paternalistic versus egalitarian–nurturing family models (Lakoff, 1996; Milburn & Conrad, 1996).

If one accepts the common distinction between political liberalism and conservatism—with the former representing progressive values, an emphasis on communitarianism, and support for government-sponsored social welfare programs and the latter representing traditional values, an emphasis on self-reliance, and opposition to government welfare programs—it is safe to say that conservatives are vastly underrepresented in psychology. It is well documented that, like social scientists in general, both academic and practicing psychologists are much more liberal than the general population and most other professionals (see Lipset & Ladd, 1970; McClintock, Spaulding, & Turner, 1965; Tetlock & Mitchell, 1993). Psychology departments rank fifth in the percentage of professors who are politically liberal, according to a national survey of twenty-seven academic disciplines (Roper Center, 1991).

To obtain data about party affiliation, eighty-five psychology faculty and graduate students at the University of Virginia were surveyed. Of these seventy-four percent were Democrats (half were liberal Democrats), but only five percent were Republicans. Participants also were asked to rate their political orientation on a one (very liberal) to eight (very conservative) scale. With a mean of 3.1, the resulting distribution was highly skewed toward liberalism. A similar survey of psychology faculty at Stanford University found no Republicans (Sacks & Thiel, 1995).

The absence of the conservative voice is also demonstrated in the liberal social policies often proposed by psychological science (Fox, 1993; Lakoff, 1996; Prilleltensky, 1994; see also Denner, 1992; Tetlock & Mitchell, 1993). For instance, a past APA president urged psychologists to advocate "radical" leftist positions and "explicitly blend our data and values in order to make strong arguments for the kinds of [radical] change we think is necessary" (Fox, 1991, p. 165). Indeed, social policy articles in psychology journals typically espouse liberal sociopolitical views (see Prilleltensky, 1994, for lengthy citation lists).

To obtain a sampling of the relative proportion of conservative (right of center) and liberal (left of center) views represented, this author performed a content analysis of articles appearing in the *American Psychologist* between 1990 and 1999. As the flagship journal of the largest professional organization for psychologists in the world, the *American Psychologist* is widely cited and often carries articles on social policy issues.

Three coders (one politically conservative, one liberal, and one centrist) independently classified articles containing political views on social issues as either liberal or conservative. Coders were asked to judge whether the articles recognized traditional/status quo versus progressive/change-oriented themes or positions on social issues; advanced conservative versus liberal themes or positions on "culture wars" issues (e.g., abortion, affirmative action, welfare policy, crime control, rights of gay individuals); advanced either anti- or pro-government involvement in and spending on welfare and social programs; were elitist/meritocracy-oriented versus egalitarian/social justice-oriented in their values; or favored capitalist/self-reliance versus socialist/communitarian values.

With an interrater reliability of ninety-three percent, the raters judged that ninety-seven percent of the articles advanced liberal themes or policies; only one of the thirty-one articles reflected more conservative views. The same analysis of articles appearing in the *Journal of Social Issues*—the banner publication of APA Division 9, the Society for the Psychological Study of Social Issues—showed that ninety-six percent of the articles expressing political views were liberal. For example, the death penalty issue included numerous articles opposing the death penalty but no articles supporting it; the grassroots organizing issue included numerous articles about liberal group organizing but no articles about conservative group organizing; and the affirmative action issue included many articles supporting affirmative action but no articles opposing it. Yet these are hotly debated social issues in the larger society.

THE PROBLEMATIC CONSEQUENCES OF LIBERAL HEGEMONY

Biases in Policy Research

Psychologists who research social issues often have values invested in those issues (Maracek, Fine, & Kidder, 1997), and psychology's liberal Zeitgeist influences research on social problems. As clearly illustrated by Ryan (1971) and Seidman (1983), how one defines a problem goes a long way in determining the proposed solution. "What one finds in psychological research often hinges on what one is looking for and how hard one looks" (Tetlock & Mitchell, 1993, pp. 249–250). If liberal questions are asked, one is likely to get liberal answers. One is unlikely to get conservative answers, however, if one fails to characterize problems from a conservative perspective. Science frequently is interpreted in a manner consistent with the values and beliefs of the scientists doing the research (see MacCoun, 1998; Suedfeld & Tetlock, 1992; Unger, 1983, for reviews).

As studies have shown, sociopolitical biases influence the questions asked, the research methods selected, the interpretation of research results, the peer review process, judgments about research quality, and decisions about whether to use research in policy advocacy (see Abramowitz, Gomes, & Abramowitz, 1975; Lord, Ross, & Lepper, 1979; Mahoney, 1977; Miller & Pollack, 1994; Wilson, DePaulo, Mook, & Klaaren, 1993).

Consider Adorno, Frenkel-Brunswick, Levinson, and Sanford's (1950) *The Authoritarian Personality*, which characterized right-wing conservatives as having an authoritarian personality, and Altmeyer's (1988) subsequent work on right-wing authoritarianism. Research using Adorno et al.'s F scale, a commonly used measure of authoritarianism, has consistently found that right-wing radicals score much higher in authoritarianism than left-wing radicals (see McClosky & Chong, 1985).

But as Ray (1989) showed in his analysis of eight studies on authoritarianism, the studies are biased to favor the theory that conservatives are more likely than liberals to be authoritarian (see Suedfeld, 2004). Items on the F scale are strongly oriented toward identifying right-wing, not left-wing, authoritarians. McClosky and Chong's study using left-wing as well as right-wing authoritarianism scales found authoritarianism in both ideological camps. For other examples of how construct definition and measurement are influenced by researchers' liberal views, see Gilbert's (1993) discussion of advocacy research on date and acquaintance rape and discussions of the liberal bias pervading much of political psychology and justice research (Tetlock, 1994; Tetlock & Mitchell, 1993; Suedfeld, 2004).

The following examples illustrate how psychologists' liberal sociopolitical values influence social policy research.

Adolescent Competence As an example of liberal bias affecting problem definition and the questions researchers choose to address, consider research on adolescents' legal competence. Psychologists have suggested two liberal but somewhat contradictory positions on whether adolescents are "competent." The first position is that adolescents should be allowed to make medical treatment decisions (e.g., abortion decisions) because they are "cognitively competent" to do so (Interdivisional Committee on Adolescent Abortion, 1987; Melton, 1983; Melton & Russo, 1987; Redding, 1993). The second position is that adolescents should not be tried or punished as adults because they are "immature" and thus not fully culpable for their crimes (Grisso, 1997; Redding, 1997b; see also Scott, Reppucci, & Woolard, 1995).

By focusing on cognitive competence rather than the psychosocial maturity variables differentiating adult from adolescent judgment, the researchers' position that adolescents should be afforded greater decision-making autonomy (Melton, 1983) enabled them to favor the liberal conclusion that adolescents should be allowed to make certain medical treatment decisions without parental consent (Redding, 1998; Scott et al., 1995). Yet focusing on psychosocial immaturity in the context of juveniles' criminal culpability enabled psychologists to argue against conservative get-tough-on-crime policies of adjudicating juveniles as adults (e.g., Grisso, 1997; Redding 1997b; see also Morse, 1997).

Symbolic Racism An example of liberal bias affecting research methodology is research on symbolic racism (e.g., McConahay, 1986; Sears, 1988), which operationally defines and measures racism partly as a function of political attitudes toward policies such as affirmative action, welfare, school busing, and "traditional American values, particularly individualism" (Kinder, 1986, p. 156). The research equates racism with political conservatism and traditional values (Tetlock, 1994). "Racists, according to this approach, are by definition conservatives; and conservatives, again by definition, are racists" (Sniderman & Tetlock, 1986, p. 181). Sniderman and Tetlock invite us to consider "how the social science community would react to conservative researchers who operationalized their concept of symbolic Marxism with items that focused on support for the civil liberties of American communists or on opposition to aid to right-wing governments" (p. 182).

Gay and Lesbian Parenting An example of liberal bias affecting research interpretation and its use in advocacy is researchers who advocate that parental sexual orientation should be irrelevant in child custody decisions (Conger, 1977; Green & Bozett, 1991; Patterson & Redding, 1996). Much of the extant research that finds no negative effects of gay parenting on children has serious limitations, for example, small sample sizes, nonrepresentative and self-selected samples, reliance on self-reporting subject to social desirability biases, and lack of longitudinal data. These limitations are often downplayed by advocates, who also frequently fail to consider fully the potential importance of having both male and female nurturance and role models for children (see Belacastro et al., 1993; Booth & Crouter, 1998; Rohner, 1998; Wardle, 1997).

The liberal bias also is evident in the interpretation of results (Wardle, 1997), with researchers sometimes "disregard[ing] their own results" (Belacastro et al., 1993, p. 117) suggesting negative effects of gay parenting on children's development. To be sure, psychologists' advocacy in this area is a response to status quo legal policies lacking empirical evidence for the assumptions that underlie them (Ball & Pea, 1998). However, as Baumrind (1995) pointed out, "It would be useful for … hypotheses positing deficits to be formulated by conservative, as well as liberal, scientists" (p. 135).

The Bell Curve An example of how conservatively oriented research may be held to a higher standard than research supporting liberal positions (Tetlock & Mitchell, 1993) is provided by the controversy surrounding *The Bell Curve* (Herrnstein & Murray, 1996). Because it espouses conservative sociopolitical views, *The Bell Curve* has been judged by many as "socially irresponsible" science whose "pro-fascist" authors and funders lack personal and professional integrity (Kincheloe, Steinberg, & Gresson, 1996, pp. 41, 408–409).

Holding research having significant implications for public policy, or implications with which the researcher disagrees, to higher or different standards of scientific proof poses dangers for the integrity of scientific research (Tetlock, 1994). "If when a study yields an unpopular conclusion it is subjected to greater scrutiny, and more effort is expended toward its refutation, an obvious bias to 'find what the community is looking for will have been introduced'" (Loury, 1994, p. 142). This is illustrated by the statement of one scholar who, with respect to research on gender differences in cognitive abilities, said, "I impose the highest standards of *proof* … on claims about biological inequality" (Fausto-Sterling, 1992, p. 11).

Hereditarian views of intelligence have long been contentious because they tend to undercut egalitarian social policies. Those espousing such views have been subjected to withering personal attacks from colleagues, driving some to abandon intelligence research altogether (Gottfredson, 1999; Scarr, 1999). (For a disturbing account of the censorship of politically unpopular research by scientific journals, see Halpern, Gilbert, & Coren 1996.)

Consequences of Research Bias

The aforementioned cases provide just a few examples of how psychologists' liberal values "organize facts" (Rein, 1976, p. 250; see also Kunda, 1990). As several researchers have acknowledged, "Our reading of the scientific literature supports our political agenda" (Silverstein & Auerbach, 1999, p. 399). It is possible, of course, that psychology's tenets may be overwhelmingly liberal yet accurate. In other words, the liberal worldview may be the correct one.

To date, however, psychological research has been strongly biased toward validating the "flattering" psychological portrait of liberalism and the "unflattering" portrait of conservatism. Psychologists have not devoted the same attention to proposing, developing, and testing conservative perspectives on social issues as they have to liberal perspectives (Tetlock & Mitchell, 1993). A variety of mechanisms serves to reward conformity to dominant sociopolitical paradigms, including graduate training, peer review, grant/award systems, professional awards and recognitions, and ingroup influences among the informal networks to which professionals belong (Sternberg, 1998).

The failure to consider, develop, and test conservative ideas has invidious effects on intellectual honesty, creativity, and progress in scientific research (see Azar, 1997; Scarr, 1997). It also decreases the ecological validity of psychologists' research. A culture's common wisdom is a useful source for evaluating the ecological validity of psychological research, particularly social policy research (Redding, 1998). Because the sociopolitical wisdom of psychologists is skewed heavily toward the liberal perspective, we may not fully consider the common wisdom and concerns of the larger, more conservative society when we define social problems or conduct and evaluate research. Lacking political diversity, we maintain a dominant liberal discourse that may result in the biased evaluation or exclusion of conservative ideas and undue confidence in the validity of liberal paradigms, thus undermining the accuracy of our scientific theories and findings.

PSYCHOLOGY'S CREDIBILITY IN QUESTION

Organized psychology's advocacy efforts have historically supported liberal political agendas (Suedfeld & Tetlock, 1992). The profession has become increasingly politicized as the APA's advocacy efforts have expanded. A perusal of the *APA Monitor* since 1990 regarding political stances taken by the APA Council of Representatives reflects only liberal views on contentious social issues in the so-called culture wars (see Hunter, 1991). Many of these policies lack sufficient scientific foundation (Suedfeld & Tetlock, 1992), which may provide an example of why psychology's efforts to influence law and policy have not been as successful as many had hoped (see Redding, 1998).

Psychology's manifestly liberal stance undermines its credibility. Scientific findings are rendered suspect. For example, Senator Hatch—quoting Bayer (1981)—questioned whether "psychologists want to move into a position where 'the findings of their research are now almost perfectly predictable from their political views'" (Hatch, 1982, p. 1036). As shown in the results of a national survey of trial judges' attitudes about social science research evidence (Redding & Reppucci, 1999), "judges may believe that the results of empirical research are unreliable, because they have been distorted by the scientists' liberal values" (Tanford, 1990. p. 153). One federal judge complained that psychologists' opinions in a school-testing discrimination case were "more the result of a doctrinaire commitment to a preconceived idea than they are the result of scientific inquiry" (*Pase v. Hannon,* 1980, p. 836).

Whom Do We Serve?

The lack of sociopolitical diversity in psychology may impede our ability to serve conservative clients. The value-laden nature of psychotherapy and social interventions has been well documented, with therapists' sociopolitical values influencing clinical diagnosis, intervention, and treatment (see Bayer, 1981; Cushman, 1995; Prilleltenskv, 1990; Woolfolk, 1998). Studies have shown that a mismatch in therapist–client sociopolitical values may bias clinical judgment even more than differences in race, gender, or socioeconomic status (see Abramowitz & Dokecki, 1977; Mazer, 1979).

Gartner et al. (1990) presented case histories differing only in the client's political–religious orientation to 363 clinical psychologists, who provided information on their own political orientation and rated their degree of empathy for the client. The ideological match between therapist and client affected therapists' empathy for the clients, with politically liberal therapists having less empathy for conservative clients (and vice versa). In addition, because a shifting process often occurs in therapy, whereby the client's values gravitate toward those of the therapist (Bergin, Payne, & Richards, 1996), there is the ethical concern that therapists may impose their liberal values on conservative clients (see Flanagan & Sommers, 1986). Cushman (1995), for example, has advocated that psychotherapy should include discourses aimed at helping clients understand how the moral status quo (e.g., consumerism or competitiveness) may be psychologically unhealthy.

Furthermore, treatment outcome research underscores the importance of understanding, appreciating, and empathizing with clients' values, with a rough congruence in therapist–client values being key to therapeutic success (Bergin et al., 1996; Sue, 1998). The therapeutic bond, which is one of the most important determinants of treatment outcomes, is adversely affected when the worldviews of therapists and clients differ too greatly (Sue, 1998). In effect, psychology's pervasive liberal Zeitgeist may adversely affect treatment or program effectiveness with politically conservative clients and communities.

De Facto Discrimination in the Educational Process

The lack of political diversity may result in discrimination against conservative students and scholars. One of the most robust findings in social psychology is that people tend to have affinity for those sharing their attitudes and values and often dislike those whose values differ too much from their own (Byrne et al., 1975; Rosenbaum, 1986).

An important dimension along which we judge others is the degree to which their sociopolitical values match ours (Rokeach, 1960, 1973).

In his cognitive modeling of conservative and liberal worldviews, Lakoff (1996) illustrated the strong negative stereotypes that each group often holds of the other, as did Hunter (1991) in his sociological analysis of the culture wars. Indeed, some studies have suggested that sociopolitical bias may be as strong as, or stronger than, racial or ethnic bias (see Haidt, Rosenberg, & Horn, 2000; Hyland, 1974; Rokeach & Mezei, 1966: Rokeach, Smith, & Evans, 1960). "Belief in a common vision of reality, or rather a shared, social construction of reality, may be a far more potent social glue than the color of one's skin, cultural heritage, or gender" (Shafranske & Malone, 1996, p. 564).

Gartner's (1986) empirical study suggests discrimination in graduate school admissions. Professors in APA-approved clinical psychology departments were sent graduate student applications (including grade point average, Graduate Record Examination scores, and a personal statement) that differed only in whether the applicant volunteered that he was a conservative Christian. Professors rated the nonconservative applicant significantly higher in all areas. Professors had fewer doubts about the abilities of nonconservatives, felt more positively about their ability to be good psychologists, and rated them as more likely to be admitted to their graduate program. Because the mock applicants had identical academic qualifications, the findings suggest an admissions bias against religious conservatives, which violates the APA's ethical principles and antidiscrimination laws (Gartner, 1986).

There is a probable selection effect among those entering graduate school, as well as de facto discrimination in faculty hiring (Cheney, 1995; Nisbet, 1997). Professions and organizations tend to select those who share their values (Cable & Judge, 1997). An academic department "will decide whose conversations it finds interesting, helpful, or illuminating" (Levinson, 1988, p. 178). With social science disciplines demanding "at least a rough allegiance to a leftist perspective as qualification for membership in the faculty" (Gross & Levitt, 1994, p. 34), "a certain politics [is] simply assumed" (Dickstein, 1994, p. 43). People often opt out of careers that they later discover to be inconsistent with, or unsupportive of, their values. Perhaps this is why there are so few conservatives in psychology, the prevailing liberalism being a strong disincentive for prospective graduate students and professors who are conservative (Gross & Levitt, 1994).

Conservatives have few role models in the profession, and few like-minded colleagues with whom to collaborate on researching social issues. In addition, conservatives may feel, rightly or wrongly, that their professional success is dependent on staying in the political closet. Particularly in applied disciplines of psychology (e.g., clinical, community, and applied social), in which sociopolitical issues often are the subject of inquiry, the discrepancy between conservative values and those of the liberal sociopolitical majority are salient for conservatives. This may decrease their likelihood of educational success and job satisfaction (see Meglino, Ravlin, & Adkins, 1989; Shih, Pittinsky, & Ambady, 1999). Minority status produces feelings of psychological distinctiveness that may negatively affect job satisfaction (Milliken & Martins, 1996; Niemann & Dovidio, 1998).

The lack of political diversity also has a chilling effect on liberal education. Conservative sociopolitical views are not nearly represented in the psychology curriculum to the same extent as liberal views, which often are expressly incorporated into curricular materials (Bergin, 1983). One community psychology text (Duffy & Wong; 1996), for example, explicitly criticizes Reagan–Bush social policies while praising Clinton policies. Another leading text (Levine & Perkins, 1997) concludes with a liberal critique of the Republican "Contract With America." The liberal bias in curricular materials makes it difficult for students to distinguish between science and politics and deprives students of a true liberal arts education, which should expose them to differing political perspectives on social issues. Although conservative views may be readily accessible to students outside of the academy, the issue is whether conservative perspectives are given voice in the classroom, particularly by professors.

Furthermore, political self-censorship operates to limit academic freedom and stifle classroom debate, particularly when negative attributions are assigned to those espousing unpopular views (see Halpern et al., 1996; Loury, 1994). Rokeach (1960) observed that closed-mindedness exists among liberal academics who espouse tolerance but do not practice it with regard to conservative views and those who hold them (Fish, 1999). To succeed in academia, conservatives feel they must accommodate the liberal views of their professors or colleagues and often find the academic climate hostile to their politics (Cheney, 1995; D'Souza, 1991; Kimball, 1990; Rauch, 1993; Sacks & Thiel, 1995). This may make them hesitant to express their views (Loury, 1994).

Strategies for Increasing Sociopolitical Diversity

The pervasive liberal Zeitgeist in psychology affects our roles and contributions as researchers, policy advocates, clinicians, and educators. Do we want a professional environment in which our liberal worldview prevents us from considering valuable strengths of conservative approaches to social problems; where the public and policymakers dismiss our research and advocacy because it is seen as too intertwined with our political beliefs; where psychologists fail to appreciate the phenomenology and values of conservative clients and communities; or where conservatives are reluctant to enter the profession, and we tacitly discriminate against them if they do so? Psychology's core values and ethical principles would answer these questions in the negative.

Four Strategies for Increasing Political Diversity in Psychology

Explore Conservative Alternatives Both liberal and conservative paradigms have important and unique contributions to offer. A psychology that merely echoes the received wisdom of the liberal wing of the Democratic Party (or any other orthodoxy) will not succeed by the standards of scientific endeavor because we claim—in our journals, in our classrooms, in our conversations with those who wield power—to represent a self-correcting scientific community (Tetlock 1994, pp. 515, 528).

We must question the liberal wisdom of our profession, challenge its assumptions, and explore conservative alternatives, not because the liberal wisdom is necessarily incorrect, but because it is incomplete. In so doing, we also help protect against politically biased research. Lord, Lepper, and Preston (1984) found a debiasing effect when psychology students considered whether their evaluation of research would have been the same had it produced the opposite result. Brenner, Koehler, and Tversky (1996) came to the same conclusion when students evaluated the strength of opposing arguments. (For a systematic application of this approach, see Tetlock, 1994.)

Tribe (1972) suggested that alternative views be identified and fleshed out at each iteration of research design and policy analysis. Toward this end, Tetlock and Mitchell (1993) put together a taxonomy of the sociopolitical assumptions inherent in social policy research. They proposed "as a corrective to [the] ideological tunnel vision" (Tetlock & Mitchell, 1993, p. 235) inherent in psychology's liberal bias that researchers systematically test hypotheses derived from each of the sociopolitical models. They outlined this approach in their 2 (conservative vs. liberal) × 2 (flattering vs. unflattering psychological portraits of each political perspective) × 2 (cognitive vs. motivational aspects of the portraits) taxonomy. Researchers can use the taxonomy as a guide for formulating and testing hypotheses, including those flowing from the "flattering" portrait of conservatism and the "unflattering" portrait of liberalism.

Some may argue, however, that psychology's task is to challenge traditional assumptions. This would make it unnecessary to explore or develop conservative views, which represent a societal status quo that already is reified in psychology (Fox, 1993; Prilleltensky, 1994; Sampson, 1993). Many conservatives, however, view the status quo as too liberal. Those arguing that psychology is not liberal or radical enough find little comfort in the fact that psychology is far more liberal than the American polity and ignore that worthwhile change comes from the right as well as the left. Rather than setting out to challenge or affirm traditional versus nontraditional assumptions, psychologists should test all assumptions against data and relevant theory.

Expand the Domain of Diversity In my view, we should consider sociopolitical values to be a key component of cultural diversity (Bergin et al., 1996). Sociopolitical beliefs reflect people's deeply held core values and moral beliefs (Hunter, 1991; Kerlinger, 1984; Lakoff, 1996; Tomkins, 1963), and the APA's (1992) ethical principles urge psychologists to be sensitive to cultural differences. A definition of cultural diversity that incorporates sociopolitical values, however, necessitates the empowerment of conservatives in the profession. Because "empowerment is not a scarce resource which gets used up" (Rappaport 1987, p. 142), empowering conservatives does not mean we disempower others. Insofar as sociopolitical values are concerned, conservatives are a vastly underrepresented and marginalized minority in psychology. This is incompatible with our respect for diversity and a host of other ethical principles. We should emphasize the strengths of the "other" (conservative) and critically evaluate how we may unwittingly contribute to their oppression, even when that oppression is unintended, subtle, or tacit.

To increase diversity in psychological research and practice, the profession should take steps to overcome the disincentives and de facto discrimination that may prevent conservatives from entering the profession. A critical mass of conservative psychologists is necessary to provide a supportive environment, comfortably allowing for the exploration and development of conservative views (Niemann & Dovidio, 1998). We should reach out to conservatives in graduate student recruiting and faculty hiring—ironically, sort of affirmative action in reverse—for the sake of sociopolitical and intellectual diversity (see Cox & Blake, 1991; Nemeth, 1986, 1994).

As Justice Powell pointed out, diversity brings "experiences, outlooks, and ideas that enrich the training of [students] and better equip … graduates to render with understanding their vital service to humanity"

(*Regents of the University of California v. Bakke,* 1978, p. 320). Minority influences stimulate creativity, novel and divergent thinking, consideration of alternatives, and deep as opposed to shallow cognitive processing (Cox & Blake, 1991; Nemeth, 1986, 1994), as well as behavioral variation that stimulates adaptation and change (Colarelli, 1998). It is also possible that, under the appropriate circumstances, negative stereotypes of conservatives may be ameliorated through direct and continuous interaction with conservatives and their viewpoints (see Nemeth, 1986; Pettigrew, 1997).

Enrich the Curriculum With the persuasive power that professors have over their students and the ethical duty to be pedagogically objective and even-handed (APA, 1992; Friedlich & Douglass, 1998), comes the obligation to foster students' engagement with liberal as well as conservative (or status quo) political views. Engagement with multiple perspectives fosters critical thinking, produces more complex reasoning styles and attitudes (Kitchener & King, 1994), and facilitates values clarification, moral development, and social responsibility (Grube, Mayton, & Ball-Rokeach, 1994). When students seek to integrate opposing views, it enhances perspective taking and information seeking, improves understanding and decision-making quality, and creates attitude change (Johnson et al., 1985).

In the classroom, we need a true dialectic that examines and challenges liberal and conservative perspectives on social issues. (For an excellent example in psychology, see Suedfeld & Tetlock, 1992). When studying social problem definition, for example, students might consider Ryan's (1971) *Blaming the Victim,* alongside Sykes's (1992) *A Nation of Victims: The Decay of the American Character,* which critiques the social policy implications of Ryan's view. Given the lack of politically conservative readings in psychology, instructors may need to seek sources from relevant social science disciplines such as political science, economics, public policy, or law.

Separate Science from Advocacy Psychologists should engage in advocacy only when there is strong empirical evidence bearing on the social policy issue in question (Redding, 1998). For example, to the extent that child custody laws are grounded in empirically false assumptions about the negative effects of gay parenting, psychologists have an important role to play in bringing relevant research to lawmakers' attention (see Patterson & Redding, 1996). However, when these laws are based on moral views about homosexuality, psychologists have no role to play because psychology can neither validate nor invalidate moral beliefs.

A case in point is advocacy for the Equal Rights Amendment (ERA). Research showing the harmful effects of discrimination, along with psychology's collective value of respecting human dignity, leads many psychologists to the conclusion that the APA should oppose discrimination. But just as the APA Council of Representatives acknowledged when it passed a resolution supporting it, "[the ERA] is a matter of human rights rather than of scientific fact" (APA, 1988, p. 59). In endorsing particular social policies, we may exploit our professional status by creating the impression that psychological science has identified the most appropriate means for achieving desired social ends; otherwise, we would not undertake advocacy as psychologists (Suedfeld & Tetlock, 1992).

We also commit what philosophers call the naturalistic fallacy—deriving a moral "ought" from an empirical "is" by conflating values with "scientific facts" (Kendler, 1993). Melton (1990) committed the naturalistic fallacy in arguing that "psychological jurisprudence" dictates certain moral–political positions such as opposition to Judge Bork's nomination to the Supreme Court, as did Lakoff (1996) in arguing that empirical developmental psychology supports liberal social policies (Redding, 1997a). Although the naturalistic fallacy principle is not accepted by all (see Plaud & Volgeltanz, 1994), "abiding by the implications of the naturalistic fallacy enables psychology to gain its freedom from those who use it for their own political goals" (Kendler, 1996, p. 28).

In general, policymakers need "information and analyses which cover the waterfront and which are as objective and value-neutral as humanly possible" (Streib, 1988, p. 257). As an ideal, this is never wholly attainable, given the inseparability of science and values. However, we can and should make an effort to distinguish between scientific knowledge and our political views. We have an ethical obligation not to go beyond our expertise, particularly in view of psychology's increasing impact on society (Prilleltensky, 1994). Judge Bazelon, recognized as probably one of the more liberal judges ever to sit on the federal bench, urged psychologists to disclose their biases and "acknowledge the existence of alternative hypotheses and explanations" (Bazelon, 1982, p. 119, quoting APA ethical guidelines). In the same way, deciding whether research is sufficiently reliable for dissemination to policymakers is a judgment call that should not be driven by the political agenda of researchers.

CONCLUSION

Sociopolitical values should be included under the rubric of cultural diversity. We should encourage conservatives to join our ranks and foster a true sociopolitical dialogue in our research, practice, and teaching. It is in our self-interest to do so. Otherwise, "We pay a terrible price that is a consequence of partisan narrow-mindedness" (Sarason, 1986, p. 905). Political narrowness and insularity limit and deaden a discipline.

Increasing political diversity will require second-order change in the profession. We must examine our political biases and their effects on our work. Do we implicitly or explicitly dismiss, marginalize, or stereotype conservative views and those who hold them? No area of human inquiry is free of implicit assumptions and ideology, however, there is a difference between politics writ large and politics writ small. We cannot escape the latter because ideology is inescapable. It is a question of giving equal time to opposing views and of openness to true diversity in sociopolitical thought. Conservative views must be sayable, seriously considered, and seen as respectable alternative perspectives. An abundance of diverse views is the ideal for invigorating education and scholarship, clinical practice, and professional integrity.

REFERENCES

Abramowitz, C.V. & Dokecki, P.R. (1977). The politics of clinical judgment: Early empirical returns. *Psychological Bulletin, 84,* 460–476.

Abramowitz, S.L., Gomes, B., & Abramowitz, C.V. (1975). Publish or politic: Referee bias in manuscript review. *Journal of Applied Social Psychology, 5,* 187–200.

Adomo, T.W., Frenkel-Brunswik, E., Levinson, D.J., & Sanford, R.N. (1950). *The Authoritarian Personality.* New York: Harper.

Altmeyer, B. (1988). *Enemies of Freedom: Understanding Right-Wing Authoritarianism.* San Francisco: Jossey-Bass.

American Psychological Association. (1988). *APA Council Policy: Reference Book.* Washington, DC: Author.

American Psychological Association. (1992). Ethical principles of psychologists and code of conduct. *American Psychologist, 47,* 1597–1611.

Azar, B. (1997, August). When research is swept under the rug. *APA Monitor,* 18.

Ball, C.A. & Pea, J.F. (1998). Warring with Wardle: Morality, social science and gay and lesbian parents. *University of Illinois Law Review, 1998,* 253–339.

Baumrind, D. (1995). Commentary on sexual orientation: Research and policy implications. *Developmental Psychology, 31,* 130–136.

Bayer, R. (1981). *Homosexuality and American Psychiatry: The Politics of Diagnosis.* New York: Basic.

Bazelon, D.L. (1982). Veils, values, and social responsibility. *American Psychologist, 37,* 115–121.

Belacastro, P.A., Gramlich, T., Nicholson, T., Price, J., & Wilson, P. (1993). A review of data-based studies addressing the effects of homosexual parenting on children's sexual and social functioning. *Journal of Divorce and Remarriage, 20,* 105–122.

Bergin, A.E. (1983). On Garfield, Hatch, and psychology's values. *American Psychologist, 38,* 958–959.

Bergin, A.E., Payne, I.E., & Richards, P.S. (1996). Values in psychotherapy. In E.P. Shafranske (Ed.), *Religion and the Clinical Practice of Psychology* (pp. 297–321). Washington, DC: American Psychological Association.

Booth, A. & Crouter, A.C. (1998). *Men in Families: When Do They Get Involved and What Difference Does It Make?* Mahwah, NJ: Erlbaum.

Brenner., L.A., Koehler, D.J., & Tversky, A. (1996). On the evaluation of one-sided evidence. *Journal of Behavioral Decision Making, 9,* 59–70.

Byrne, D., Gouaux, C., Griffitt, W., Lamberth, J., Murakawa, N., Prasad, M., Prasad, A., & Ramirez, M. (1975). The ubiquitous relationship: Attitude similarity and attraction. *Human Relations, 24,* 201–207.

Cable, D.M. & Judge, T.A. (1997). Interviewers' perceptions of person–organization fit and organizational selection decisions. *Journal of Applied Psychology, 52,* 546-561.

Cheney, L.V. (1995). *Telling the Truth: Why Our Culture and Our Country Have Stopped Making Sense and What We Can Do About It.* New York: Simon & Schuster.

Colarelli, S.M. (1998). Psychological interventions in organizations: An evolutionary perspective. *American Psychologist, 53,* 1044–1056.

Conger, J.J. (1977). Proceedings of the American Psychological Association, Incorporated, for the year 1976: Minutes of the annual meeting of the Council of Representatives. *American Psychologist, 32,* 408–438.

Cox, T. & Blake, S. (1991). Managing cultural diversity: Implications for organizational competitiveness. *Academy of Management Executives, 5,* 45–56.

Cushman, P. (1995). *Constructing the Self, Constructing America: A Cultural History of Psychotherapy.* Reading, MA: Addison-Wesley.

Denner, B. (1992). Research as moral crusade. *American Psychologist, 47,* 81–82.

Dickstein, M. (1994). Correcting PC. In E. Kurzweil & W. Phillips (Eds.), *Our Country, Our Culture: The Politics of Political Correctness* (pp. 42–49). New York: Partisan Review Press.

D'Souza, D. (1991). *Illiberal Education: The Politics of Race and Sex on Campus.* New York: Free Press.

Duffy, K.G. & Wong, F.Y. (1996). *Community Psychology.* Boston: Allyn & Bacon.

Eysenck, H.J. (1954). *The Psychology of Politics.* London: Routledge & Kegan Paul.

Fausto-Sterling, A. (1992). *Myths of Gender.* New York: Basic.

Fish, S. (1999). *The Trouble with Principle.* Cambridge, MA: Harvard University Press.

Flanagan, R. & Sommers, J. (1986). Ethical considerations for the peace activist psychologist. *American Psychologist, 41,* 723–724.

Powers, B.J. & Richardson, F.C. (1996). Why is multiculturalism good? *American Psychologist, 51,* 609–621.

Fox, D.R. (1991). Social science's limited role in resolving psycholegal social problems. *Journal of Offender Rehabilitation, 17,* 159–166.

Fox, D.R. (1993). Psychological jurisprudence and radical social change. *American Psychologist, 48,* 234–241.

Friedlich, J. & Douglass, D. (1998). Ethics and the persuasive enterprise of teaching psychology. *American Psychologist, 53,* 549–562.

Gartner, J., Hannatz, M., Hohmann, A., Larson, D., & Gartner, A.F. (1990). The effect of patient and clinician ideology on clinical judgment: A study of ideological counter-transference. *Psychotherapy, 27,* 98–106.

Gartner, J.D. (1986). Antireligious prejudice in admissions to doctoral programs in clinical psychology. *Professional Psychology: Research and Practice, 17*, 473–475.

Gilbert, N. (1993). Examining the facts: Advocacy research overstates the incidence of date and acquaintance rape. In R.J. Gelles & D.R. Loseke (Eds.), *Current Controversies on Family Violence* (pp. 120–132). Newbury Park, CA: Sage.

Gottfredson, L.S. (1999). Jensen, Jensenism, and the sociology of intelligence. *Intelligence, 26*, 291–300.

Green, G.D. & Bozett, F.W. (1991). Lesbian mothers and gay fathers. In J.C. Gonsiorek & J.D. Weinrich (Eds.), *Homosexuality: Research Implications for Public Policy* (pp. 197–214). Beverly Hills, CA: Sage.

Grisso, T. (1997). Society's retributive response to juvenile violence. *Law and Human Behavior, 20*, 229–247.

Gross, P. & Levitt, N. (1994). *Higher Superstition: The Academic Left and Its Quarrels with Science.* Baltimore: Johns Hopkins University Press.

Grube, J.W., Mayton, D.M., & Ball-Rokeach, S.J. (1994). Inducing change in values, attitudes, and behaviors: Belief system theory and the method of value self-confrontation. *Journal of Social Issues, 50*, 153–174.

Haidt, J., Rosenberg, E., & Horn, H. (2000). *Diversity Is Like Cholesterol: Some (Demographic) Is Good, Some (Moral) Is Bad.* Unpublished manuscript, University of Virginia.

Halpern, D.F., Gilbert, R., & Coren, S. (1996). PC or not PC? Contemporary challenges to unpopular research findings. *Journal of Social Distress and the Homeless, 5*, 251–271.

Hatch, O.G. (1982). Psychology, society, and politics. *American Psychologist, 37*, 1031–1037.

Herrnstein, R.J. & Murray, C. (1996). *The Bell Curve: Intelligence and Class Structure in American Life* (rev. ed.). New York: Free Press.

Hunt, M. (1999). *The New Know-Nothings: The Political Foes of the Scientific Study of Human Nature.* New Brunswick, NJ: Transaction.

Hunter, J.D. (1991). *Culture Wars: The Struggle to Define America.* New York: Basic.

Hunter, J.D. (2000). *The Death of Character.* New York: Basic.

Hyland, M. (1974). The anticipated belief theory of prejudice: Analyses and evaluation. *European Journal of Social Psychology, 4*, 179–200.

Interdivisional Committee on Adolescent Abortion. (1987). Adolescent abortion: Psychological and legal issues. *American Psychologist, 42*, 73–78.

Johnson, R., Brooker, C., Stutzman, J., Hultman, D., & Johnson, D.W. (1985). The effects of controversy, concurrence seeking, and individualistic learning on achievement and attitude change. *Journal of Research in Science Teaching, 22*, 197–205.

Kendler, H.H. (1993). Psychology and the ethics of social policy. *American Psychologist, 48*, 1046–1053.

Kendler, H.H. (1996). The politics of the APA—self-inflicted wounds: A response to O'Donohue and Dyslin. *New Ideas in Psychology, 14*, 27–29.

Kerlinger, F.N. (1984). *Liberalism and Conservatism: The Nature and Structure of Social Attitudes.* Hillsdale, NJ: Erlbaum.

Kimball, R. (1990). *Tenured Radicals: How Politics Has Corrupted Our Higher Education.* New York: Harper & Row.

Kincheloe, J.L., Steinberg, S.R., & Gresson, A.D. (Eds.) (1996). *Measured Lies:* The Bell Curve *Examined.* New York: St Martin's.

Kinder, D.R. (1986). The continuing American dilemma: White resistance to radical change 40 years after Myrdal. *Journal of Social Issues, 42*, 151–171.

Kitchener, S. & King, P. (1994). *Developing Reflective Judgment: Understanding and Promoting Intellectual Growth and Critical Thinking in Adolescents and Adults.* San Francisco: Jossey-Bass.

Kitzinger, C. (1991). Politicizing psychology. *Feminism and Psychology, 1*, 49–54.

Kunda, Z. (1990). The case for motivated reasoning. *Psychological Bulletin, 108,* 480–498.

Lakoff, G. (1996). *Moral Politics: What Conservatives Know That Liberals Don't.* Chicago: University of Chicago Press.

Levine, M. & Perkins, D.V. (1997). *Principles of Community Psychology: Perspectives and Applications* (2d ed.). New York: Oxford University Press.

Levinson, S. (1988). *Constitutional Faith.* Princeton, NJ: Princeton University Press.

Lipset, S.M. & Ladd, H.C. (1970, November). And what the professors think. *Psychology Today, 106,* 49–51.

Lord, C.G., Lepper, M.R., & Preston, E. (1984). Consider the opposite: A corrective strategy for social judgment. *Journal of Personality and Social Psychology, 47,* 1231–1243.

Lord, C.G., Ross, L., & Lepper, M.R. (1979). Biased assimilation and attitude polarization: The effects of prior theories on subsequently considered evidence. *Journal of Personality and Social Psychology, 37,* 2098–2109.

Loury, G.C. (1994). Self-censorship. In E. Kurzweil & W. Phillips (Eds.), *Our Country, Our Culture: The Politics of Political correctness* (pp. 132–144). New York: Partisan Review Press.

MacCoun, R.J. (1998). Biases in the interpretation and use of research results. *Annual Review of Psychology, 49,* 259–287.

Mahoney, M.J. (1977). Publication prejudices: An experimental study of confirmatory bias in the peer review system. *Cognitive Therapy and Research, 1,* 161–175.

Maracek, J., Fine, M., & Kidder, L. (1997). Working between worlds: Qualitative methods and social psychology. *Journal of Social Issues, 53,* 631–644.

Mazer, D.B. (1979). Toward a social psychology of diagnosis: Similarity, attraction, and clinical evaluation. *Journal of Counseling and Clinical Psychology, 47,* 586–588.

McClintock, C.G., Spaulding, C.B., & Turner, H.A. (1965). Political orientations of academically affiliated psychologists. *American Psychologist, 20,* 211–221.

McClosky, H. & Chong, D. (1985). Similarities and differences between left-wing and right-wing radicals. *British Journal of Political Science, 15,* 329–363.

McConahay, J.B. (1986). Modem racism, ambivalence, and the modem racism scale. In J.F. Dovido & S.L. Gaertner (Eds.), *Prejudice, Discrimination, and Racism* (pp. 91–125). Orlando, FL: Academic.

Meglino, B.M., Ravlin, E.C., & Adkins, C.L. (1989). A work values approach to corporate culture: A field test of the value congruence process and its relationship to individual outcomes. *Journal of Applied Psychology, 74,* 427–432.

Melton, G.B. (1983). Toward "personhood" for adolescents: Autonomy and privacy as values in public policy. *American Psychologist, 38,* 99–103.

Melton, G.B. (1990). Law, science, and humanity: The normative foundation of social science in law. *Law and Human Behavior, 24,* 315–332.

Melton, G.B. & Russo, N.F. (1987). Adolescent abortion: Psychological perspectives on public policy. *American Psychologist, 42,* 69–72.

Milburn, M.A. & Conrad, S.D. (1996). *The Politics of Denial.* Cambridge, MA: MIT Press.

Miller, N. & Pollack, V.E. (1994). Meta-analysis and some science-compromising problems of social psychology. In W.R. Shadish & S. Fuller (Eds.), *The Social Psychology of Science* (pp. 230–261). New York: Guilford.

Milliken, F.J. & Martins, L.L. (1996). Searching for common threads: Understanding the multiple effects of diversity in organizational groups. *Academy of Management Review, 21,* 402–433.

Morse, S.J. (1997). Immaturity and responsibility. *Journal of Criminal Law and Criminology, 88,* 15–67.

Nemeth, C.J. (1986). Differential contributions of majority and minority influence. *Psychological Review, 93,* 23–32.

Nemeth, C.J. (1994). The value of minority dissent. In S. Moscovici, A. Mucchi-Faina, & A. Maass (Eds.), *Minority Influence* (pp. 3–15). Chicago: Nelson-Hall.

Niemann, Y.F. & Dovidio, J.F. (1998). Relationship of solo status, academic rank, and perceived distinctiveness to job satisfaction of racial/ethnic minorities. *Journal of Applied Psychology, 83*, 55–71.

Nisbet, R.A. (1997). *The Degradation of the Academic Dogma*. New Brunswick, NJ: Transaction.

Pase v. Hannon. (1980). 506 F. Supp. 83.

Patterson, C.J. & Redding, R.E. (1996). Lesbian and gay families with children: Implications of social science research for policy. *Journal of Social Issues, 52*, 29–50.

Pettigrew, T.F. (1997). Generalized intergroup contact effects on prejudice. *Personality and Social Psychology Bulletin, 23*, 173–185.

Plaud, J.J. & Volgeltanz, N. (1994). Psychology and the naturalistic ethics of social policy. *American Psychologist, 49*, 967–968.

Prilleltensky, I. (1990). The politics of abnormal psychology: Past, present, and future. *Political Psychology, 11*, 767–785.

Prilleltensky, I. (1994). *The Morals and Politics of Psychology: Psychological Discourse and the Status Quo*. Albany, NY: State University of New York Press.

Rappaport, J. (1987). Terms of empowerment/exemplars of prevention: Toward a theory for community psychology. *American Journal of Community Psychology, 15*, 121–147.

Rauch, J. (1993). *Kindly Inquisitors: The New Attacks on Free Thought*. Chicago: University of Chicago Press.

Ray, J.J. (1989). The scientific study of ideology is too often more ideological than scientific. *Personality and Individual Differences, 10*, 331—336.

Redding, R.E. (1993). Children's competence to provide informed consent to mental health treatment. *Washington and Lee Law Review, 50*, 695–753.

Redding, R.E. (1997a). Empirical psychology meets the politics of family values. *Contemporary Psychology, 42*, 1092–1093.

Redding, R.E. (1997b). Juveniles transferred to criminal court: Legal reform proposals based on social science research. *Utah Law Review, 1997*, 709–763.

Redding, R.E. (1998). How common-sense psychology can inform law and psycholegal research. *University of Chicago Law School Roundtable, 5*, 107–142.

Redding, R.E. & Reppucci, N.D. (1999). Relationships between lawyers' sociopolitical attitudes and their judgments of social science in legal decision making. *Law and Human Behavior, 23*, 317–54.

Regents of the University of California v. Bakke. (1978) 438 U.S. 265.

Rein, M. (1976). *Social Science and Public Policy*. New York: Penguin.

Rohner, R.P. (1998). Father love and child development: History and current evidence. *Current Directions in Psychological Science, 7*, 157–161.

Rokeach, M. (Ed.) (1960). *The Open and Closed Mind*. New York: Basic.

Rokeach, M. (1973). *The Nature of Human Values*. New York: Free Press.

Rokeach, M. & Mezei, L. (1966, January 14). Race and shared belief as factors in social choice. *Science, 151*, 167–172.

Rokeach, M., Smith, P.W., & Evans, R.I. (1960). Two kinds of prejudice or one? In M. Rokeach (Ed.), *The Open and Closed Mind* (pp. 132–168). New York: Basic.

Roper Center. (1991, July/August). Politics of the professoriate. *Public Perspective, 2*, 86–87.

Rosenbaum, M.E. (1986). The repulsion hypothesis: On the nondevelopment of relationships. *Journal of Personality and Social Psychology, 51*, 1156–1166.

Ryan, W. (1971). *Blaming the victim*. New York: Pantheon.

Sacks, D.O. & Thiel, P.A. (1995). *The Diversity Myth: "Multiculturalism" and the Politics of Intolerance at Stanford*. Oakland, CA: Independent Institute.

Sampson, E.E. (1993). Identity politics: Challenges to psychology's understanding. *American Psychologist, 48*, 1219–1230.

Sarason, S.B. (1986). And what is the public interest? *American Psychologist, 41,* 899–905.

Scarr, S. (1997, May/June). Toward a free market in research ideas. *APS Observer, 10,* 33–34.

Scarr, S. (1999). On Jensen's integrity. *Intelligence, 26,* 227–232.

Scott, E.S., Reppucci, N.D., & Woolard, J.L. (1995). Evaluating adolescent decision making in legal contexts. *Law and Human Behavior, 19,* 221–244.

Sears, D.O. (1988). Symbolic racism. In P.A. Katz & D.A. Taylor (Eds.), *Eliminating Racism: Profiles in Controversy* (pp. 53–84). New York: Plenum.

Seidman, E. (1983). Unexamined premises of social problem solving. In E. Seidman (Ed.), *Handbook of Social Intervention* (pp. 48–67). Beverly Hills, CA: Sage.

Shafranske, E.P. & Maloney, H.N. (1996). Religion and the clinical practice of psychology. In E.P. Shafranske (Ed.), *Religion and the Clinical Practice of Psychology* (pp. 561–586). Washington, DC: American Psychological Association.

Shih, M., Pittinsky, T.L., & Ambady, N. (1999). Stereotype susceptibility: Identity salience and shifts in quantitative performance. *Psychological Science, 10,* 80–83.

Silverstcin, L.B. (1993). Reply to commentaries. *Journal of Family Psychology, 7,* 305–306.

Silverstcin, L.B. & Auerbach, C.F. (1999). Deconstructing the essential father. *American Psychologist, 54,* 397–407.

Sniderman, P.M. & Tetlock, P.E. (1986). Reflections on American racism. *Journal of Social Issues, 42,* 173–187.

Sternberg, R.J. (1998). Costs and benefits of defying the crowd in science. *Intelligence, 26,* 209–216.

Stone, W.F. & Schaffner, P. E. (1988). *The Psychology of Politics* (2d ed.). New York: Free Press.

Streib, V.L. (1988). Academic research and advocacy research. *Cleveland State Law Review, 36,* 253–259.

Sue, S. (1998). In search of cultural competence in psychotherapy and counseling. *American Psychologist, 53,* 440–480.

Suedfeld, P. (2004). Post-modernism, identity politics, and other political influences in political psychology. In K. Monroe (Ed.), *Political Psychology.* New York: Erlbaum.

Suedfeld, P. & Tetlock, P. (Eds.) (1992). *Psychology and Social Policy.* New York: Hemisphere.

Sykes, C.J. (1992). *A Nation of Victims: The Decay of the American Character.* New York: St. Martin's.

Tanford, J.A. (1990). The limits of a scientific jurisprudence: The Supreme Court and psychology. *Indiana Law Journal, 66,* 137–173.

Tetlock, P.E. (1994). Political psychology or politicized psychology: Is the road to scientific hell paved with good intentions? *Political Psychology, 15,* 509–529.

Tetlock, P.E. & Mitchell, G. (1993). Liberal and conservative approaches to justice: Conflicting psychological portraits. In B.A. Mellers & J. Baron (Eds.), *Psychological Perspectives on Justice: Theory and Applications* (pp. 234–258). New York: Cambridge University Press.

Tomkins, S.S. (1963). Left and right: A basic dimension of ideology and personality. In R.W. White (Ed.), *The Study of Lives* (pp. 388–411). New York: Atherton.

Tribe, L.H. (1972). Policy science: Analysis or ideology? *Philosophy and Public Affairs, 2,* 66–110.

Unger, R.K. (1983). Through the looking glass: No wonderland yet! (The reciprocal relationship between methodology and models of reality). *Psychology of Women Quarterly, 8,* 9–32.

Wardle, L.D. (1997). The potential impact of homosexual parenting on children. *University of Illinois Law Review, 1997,* 833–920.

Weiner, B. (1995). *Judgments of Responsibility: A Foundation for a Theory of Social Conduct.* New York: Guilford.

Williams, S. (1984). Left–right ideological differences in blaming victims. *Political Psychology, 5,* 573–581.

Wilson, T.D., DePaulo, B.M., Mook, D.G., & Klaaren, K.J. (1993). Scientists' evaluations of research: The biasing effects of the importance of the topic. *Psychological Science, 4,* 322–325.

Woolfolk, R.L. (1998). *The Cure of Souls: Science, Values, and Psychotherapy.* San Francisco: Jossey-Bass.

The Editors

Rogers H. Wright, Ph.D. After receiving his doctorate from Northwestern University, Dr. Wright joined the Department of Psychiatry at the University of California at Los Angeles. In 1957 he began his independent practice of psychology in Long Beach, California, and continued in that city, and later in San Diego as well, for the next forty years. This was the era before licensure, insurance reimbursement, or societal recognition of psychology in private practice, and he spent the next thirty-five years indefatigably fighting to establish psychology as an autonomous profession.

Predicting that most Americans would soon have some form of health insurance, he reasoned that if psychology were not recognized statutorily as a health profession eligible for third-party payment, then clinical psychologists—who during and after World War II became increasingly important contributors to mental health service delivery—would essentially be eliminated from the marketplace. Consequently, he joined other local psychologists in lobbying for and passing a local ordinance regulating the practice of psychology. In 1959 his efforts to procure California licensure resulted in the first mandatory regulation of the practice of psychology by a major state.

Finding the then academically oriented American Psychological Association (APA) impervious to his entreaties, Wright pulled together a group of fourteen activists determined to change both the APA's disinterest in professional practice and the insurance industry's denial of third-party reimbursement to psychologists. Tactically persuasive and cajoling as required, this strident, frequently shrill, and sometimes combative group earned the affectionate appellation of "The Dirty Dozen" from grateful professional colleagues. The surviving members of the Dirty Dozen were feted in a series of award ceremonies at the 1999 APA convention for their sustained activities, which changed the APA forever and established psychology as an autonomous profession.

Although remaining controversial, Dr. Wright exerted his influence through important APA positions and offices. He served three different terms on the APA Council of Representatives and was the second independent practitioner elected to the APA Board of Directors. He also served on the Board of Professional Affairs, as well as a host of committees, task forces, and advisory panels. He was elected president of Division 12 and founding president of Division 31. Failing to enlist the APA in advocacy, he co-founded and was founding president of the Council for the Advancement of the Psychological Professions and Sciences (CAPPS), which in its first year made more presentations on Capitol Hill than the APA had done in its entire previous history. So effective was CAPPS that within three years of its founding the APA sponsored its own advocacy organization, the Association for the Advancement of Psychology (AAP), which in later years recruited Dr. Wright for a seven-year term as its chief executive officer. He served two terms as president of the California Psychological Association (CPA), and was instrumental in making CPA an imago to be emulated by the emerging state psychological associations.

Wright earned his B.A., M.A., and Ph.D., all with distinction, from Northwestern University and, like many early clinical psychologists, interned with the Veterans Administration. He is a fellow of the APA, a diplomate in Clinical Psychology of ABPP, the recipient of an honorary doctorate, and a distinguished practitioner of the National Academies of Practice. Among his numerous awards are the APA's Award for Distinguished Contributions to Applied Psychology as a Professional Practice and the American Psychological Foundation's Gold Medal for a Lifetime of Contributions to Practice. He is currently retired from practice and lives in Spring Valley, California, with his wife, Charlotte.

Nicholas A. Cummings, Ph.D., Sc.D. As stated in the citation that awarded him the 2003 APF Gold Medal for Lifetime Achievement in Practice, Dr. Cummings "not only consistently predicted the future of professional psychology for the past half century, he helped create it." Always the visionary, he joined Rogers Wright and the other fearless members of the legendary "Dirty Dozen" at the forefront of battles for licensure, third-party reimbursement, and psychological advocacy.

In the late 1950s, he wrote and implemented the first comprehensive prepaid psychotherapy benefit while at Kaiser Permanente in San Francisco. In addition, he conducted research demonstrating that the medical costs saved by psychological services more than offset the cost of the behavioral interventions. It was this research that persuaded insurers to recognize psychotherapy as an important benefit in health insurance. Within the first two years of becoming the first chair of the APA's Committee on Health Insurance, he wrote and implemented legislation in six states mandating reimbursement for psychological services if psychiatric services are covered.

In the drive to involve psychology in advocacy, Cummings cofounded with Rogers Wright and Ernest Lawrence the Council for the Psychological Professions and Sciences (CAPPS, not to be confused with CAPP, which came much later). In its first year, CAPPS testified more often on Capitol Hill than the APA had done in its entire prior history. The success of CAPPS led to the formation of the Association for the Advancement of Psychology, which subsequently superseded CAPPS and flourishes to this day.

As APA president, Cummings continued his commitment to civil rights by appointing the first Committee on Ethnic Minority affairs and the first Task Force on Lesbian and Gay Issues. Even before assuming the office of President-Elect, he noted that beginning with his presidency the next three APA conventions were to be held in states that did not support the Equal Rights Amendment (ERA). Women psychologists had asked that these conventions be canceled, but the Council of Representatives balked on the grounds that the APA would be sued for breach of contract. After much soul-searching, Cummings declared that if these contracts were not rescinded, he would resign as president and lead a counterconvention. The Council was thrown into chaos, but eventually acceded, and the APA became the first national organization to cancel existing contracts in support of the ERA. Gloria Steinem readily accepted Cummings' invitation to be the convention speaker.

Anticipating the industrialization of healthcare—particularly behavioral healthcare—Cummings' founded American Biodyne as a model of ownership of managed care. He promised to limit American Biodyne to 500,000 covered lives, but when two years passed and psychology continued to ignore his warnings, he took his foot off the brake and American Biodyne grew in the next five years to 14.5 million covered lives in thirty-nine states. To this day it remains the only behavioral managed care company that uses effective interventions to achieve efficiency instead of session limits, precertification, case management, and other bean-counter cost-cutting techniques. In 1992, approaching 70 years of age and despairing that psychology had missed a great opportunity, he sold American Biodyne, which quickly changed when it came under the ownership of business interests.

Unable to convince the APA's Education and Training Board to permit practicing clinicians to hold faculty rank, in 1969 he founded the California School of Professional Psychology (CSPP) and its subsequent four campuses, a move that launched the professional school movement. Before leaving CSPP in 1976, he founded the National Council of Schools of Professional Psychology (NCSPP), which continues to thrive. Other organizations that Cummings founded include the National Academies of Practice (limited to 150 distinguished practitioners each in the fields of dentistry, medicine, nursing, optometry, osteopathic medicine, pharmacy, psychology, social work, and veterinary medicine), and the American Managed Behavioral Healthcare Association. He is also a co-founder of the California Psychological Association, the San Francisco Bay Area Psychological Association, and the San Joaquin County Psychological Association. In addition to serving as APA president in 1979, he has been president of APA Division 12 (Clinical Psychology) and Division 29 (Psychotherapy) and the California Psychological Association. He is a Fellow of APA Divisions 1, 12, 13, 29, 31, and 42.

Cummings has served the government in a pro bono capacity, and has testified before Congress eighteen times. He was a consultant to President Kennedy's Mental Health Task Force and a member of President Carter's Mental Health Commission. For a number of years he served as consultant to the Health Economics Branch of the then Department of Health, Education, and Welfare (now Department of Health and Human Services), the U.S. Subcommittee on Health, and the U.S. Finance Committee.

Cummings has always prided himself in being a practicing psychologist in the trenches. Throughout his professional career, he has seen no fewer than forty to fifty patients a week despite all his other activities. He maintains a profound involvement in research and is the author or editor of twenty-eight books (five coauthored with his psychologist daughter, Janet) and more than four hundred journal articles and book chapters. He is the recipient of numerous awards, not only from psychology, but also medicine, nursing, and the Greek classics, and has received five honorary doctorates. Currently, he serves as distinguished professor at the University of Nevada, Reno, and president of the Cummings Foundation for Behavioral Health. He chairs the boards of both The Nicholas & Dorothy Cummings Foundation and the University Alliance for Behavioral Care.

Contributors

Christine E. Caselles, Ph.D. received her doctorate from the University of Northern Illinois. She is currently director of the Early Intensive Intervention Program at Community Services for Autistic Adults and Children (CSAAC) in Rockford, Maryland. Dr. Caselles is also involved in all aspects of planning a large-scale, multisite research project on the outcome of intensive early intervention.

Michael Cucciare, M.A. is an advanced graduate student in the doctoral psychology program at the University of Nevada, Reno. His research interests include medical psychology, psychosocial assessment, and the development of psychosocial interventions for high utilizers of healthcare services.

Christopher Dyslin, Ph.D. received his doctorate in clinical psychology from Northern Illinois University. His interests include the influence of politics on psychology. He is the author of three other books, and has published more than twenty journal articles and book chapters.

Katherine A. Fowler, B.S. is an advanced graduate student in the clinical psychology doctoral program at Emory University. Her principal interests include the assessment of psychopathic personality and the problem of pseudoscience in contemporary clinical psychology. She works with Dr. Scott Lilienfeld.

William Glasser, M.D. is one of the few psychiatrists who focuses on mental health as totally separate from mental illness. He is president of the William Glasser Institute, whose many instructors teach choice theory and reality therapy all over the world as the way to mental health. Glasser was board certified in psychiatry in 1961. He has written more than twenty books to support his ideas.

Linda S. Gottfredson, Ph.D. received her doctorate in social psychology from Johns Hopkins University and is a professor in the School of Education, University of Delaware. Her interests include industrial/organizational psychology and the evaluation of intellectual abilities.

Scott O. Lilienfeld, Ph.D. is associate professor of psychology at Emory University. He is the editor of *The Scientific Review of Mental Health Practice* and a past president of the Society for a Science of Clinical Psychology. He serves on the editorial boards of numerous journals, including the *Journal of Abnormal Psychology* and *Psychological Assessment,* and is the recipient of the 1998 David Shakow Award for Early Career Contributions to Clinical Psychology from APA Division 12. His primary interests include the assessment and causes of personality disorders and the problem of pseudoscience in contemporary clinical psychology.

Elizabeth Lillis, B.A. is pursuing a Ph.D. in clinical psychology at the University of Nevada, Reno. Her research interests include couples communication, individual psychotherapy in the context of relationships, and dialectical behavior therapy.

Jason Lillis, M.A. is a doctoral candidate in the clinical psychology program at the University of Nevada, Reno. His research interests include sexual victimization, substance abuse, and the link between politics and psychology.

Jeffrey M. Lohr, Ph.D. is a professor of psychology at the University of Arkansas–Fayetteville. He is the former chief financial officer of Clinical Psychology, Ltd., Fayetteville, Arkansas. He is on the boards of the Council for Scientific Medicine and Mental Health, the Association for Applied and Preventive Psychology, and the editorial board of *The Scientific Review of Mental Health Practice.* He is a member of the Association for the Advancement of Behavior Therapy and the American Psychological Society.

Steven Jay Lynn, Ph.D. is a professor of psychology at the State University of New York at Binghamton. He is a diplomate of both clinical and forensic psychology (ABPP), and a former president of the APA's Division of Psychological Hypnosis. He serves on eleven editorial boards, including the *Journal of Abnormal Psychology.* Dr. Lynn has published more than two hundred articles and book chapters, and has written or edited thirteen books, several of which have received awards from professional organizations. His research program is funded by the National Institute of Mental Health.

William T. O'Donohue, Ph.D. is the Nicholas Cummings Professor of Organized Behavioral Healthcare Delivery in the department of psychology at the University of Nevada, Reno. He received his doctorate in psychology from the State University of New York, Stony Brook, and a masters degree in philosophy from Indiana University. He holds adjunct appointments in the departments of philosophy and psychiatry at the University of Nevada, and the department of psychology at the University of Hawaii, Manoa. He is the author or editor of more than twenty-five books.

Richard E. Redding, J.D., Ph.D. is associate professor of law at Villanova University, associate professor of psychology at Drexel University, and director of the J.D./Ph.D. program in law and psychology at Villanova and Drexel Universities. Previously, he was assistant professor and associate director of the Institute of Law, Psychiatry and Public Policy at the University of Virginia. Professor Redding received his doctoral degree from the University of Virginia and his law degree from Washington and Lee University. He has published more than seventy-five book chapters and articles in leading scientific and legal journals, serves on the editorial boards of several peer-reviewed journals, and is the associate editor of the *Journal of Forensic Psychology Practice.* He serves as consultant to the U.S. Department of Justice, Office of Juvenile Justice and Delinquency Prevention.

John K. Rosemond, M.S. is a psychological associate in North Carolina. He is a nationally syndicated columnist in parenting and family issues, and the author of ten books on parenting and family issues. He is a sought-after speaker by many organizations in the United States and abroad. He serves as director of The Center for Affirmative Parenting in Gastonia, Georgia. He proudly refers to himself as a husband of thirty-five years, the father of two, the grandfather of six, and what he calls a "certified psychological heretic."

Ofer Zur, Ph.D. is a licensed psychologist, forensic consultant, and pioneer of the managed-care–free private practice movement. His teachings and writings focus on independent practice, ethics, critical thinking, boundaries, and dual relationships. For many years he taught at graduate schools such as the California School of Professional Psychology in Alameda, California, and CIIS in San Francisco. He is the co-editor with A.A. Lazarus, Ph.D., of *Dual Relationships and Psychotherapy* (Springer, 2002). Dr. Zur's interest in dual relationships arises from his outrage at the harm inflicted on clients by the practice of distant, dogmatic, inflexible, and ideologically based, rather than patient-based, therapies. His focus includes exposing how therapists have developed self-serving beliefs and practices at the expense of patient care.

Index

Rogers H. Wright, Ph.D., is a past president of Division 12 and founding president of Division 31 of the American Psychological Association, and co-founded and was founding president of the Council for the Advancement of the Psychological Professions and Sciences (CAPPS). Wright is a fellow of the APA, a diplomate in Clinical Psychology of ABPP, the recipient of an honorary doctorate, and a distinguished practitioner of the National Academies of Practice.

Nicholas A. Cummings, Ph.D., Sc.D., is currently distinguished professor, University of Nevada, Reno, and president of the Cummings Foundation for Behavioral Health. He chairs the boards of both The Nicholas & Dorothy Cummings Foundation and CareIntegra. He is past president of the APA as well as its Divisions 12 (Clinical) and 29 (Psychotherapy), is the recipient of five honorary doctorates for contributions to psychology, education, and the Greek Classics, and was awarded psychology's Gold Medal for a "lifetime of contributions to practice."

Printed and bound by CPI Group (UK) Ltd, Croydon, CR0 4YY

22/10/2024

01777620-0013